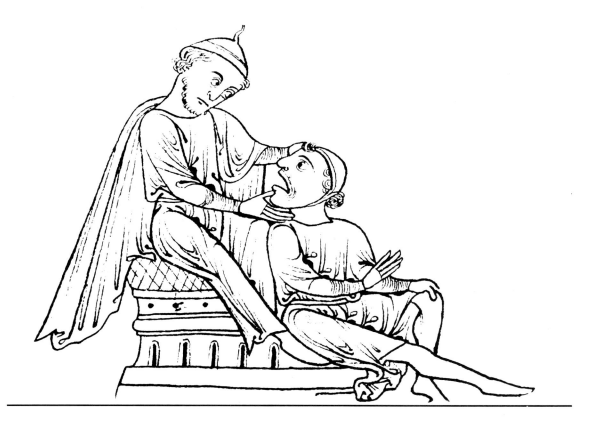

DENTISTRY

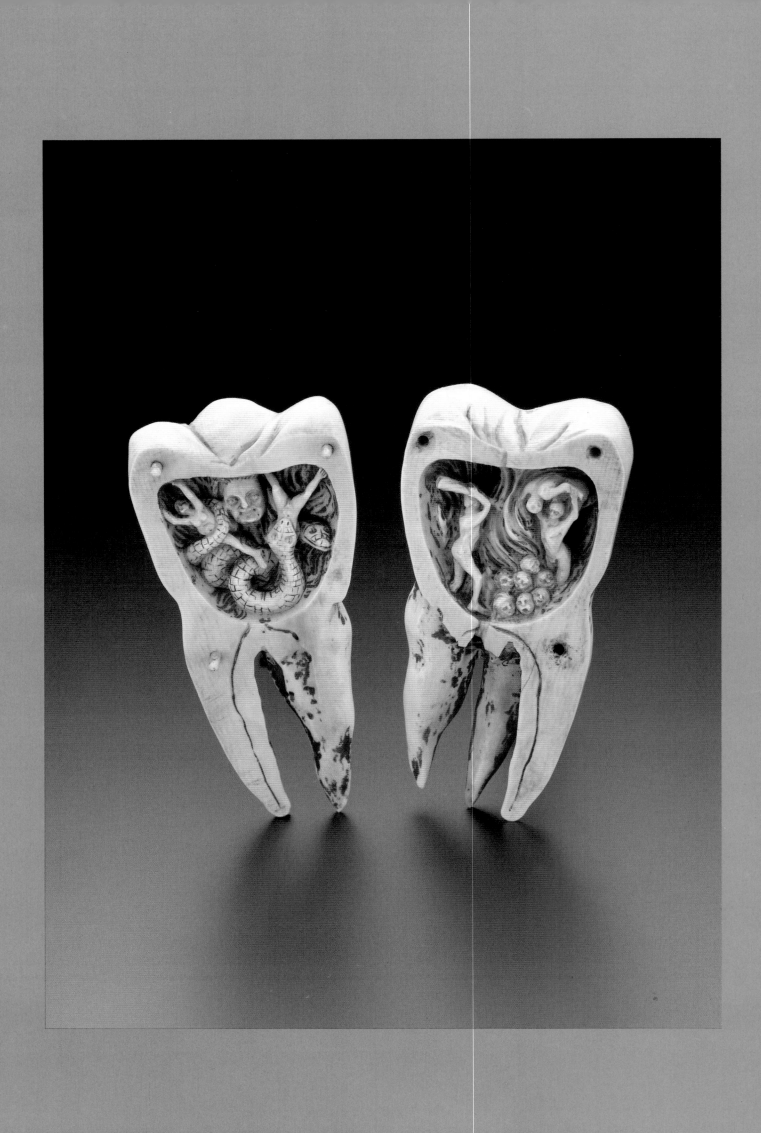

DENTISTRY

·

AN ILLUSTRATED HISTORY

MALVIN E. RING, D.D.S., M.L.S., F.A.C.D.

ABRADALE PRESS
HARRY N. ABRAMS, INC., PUBLISHERS

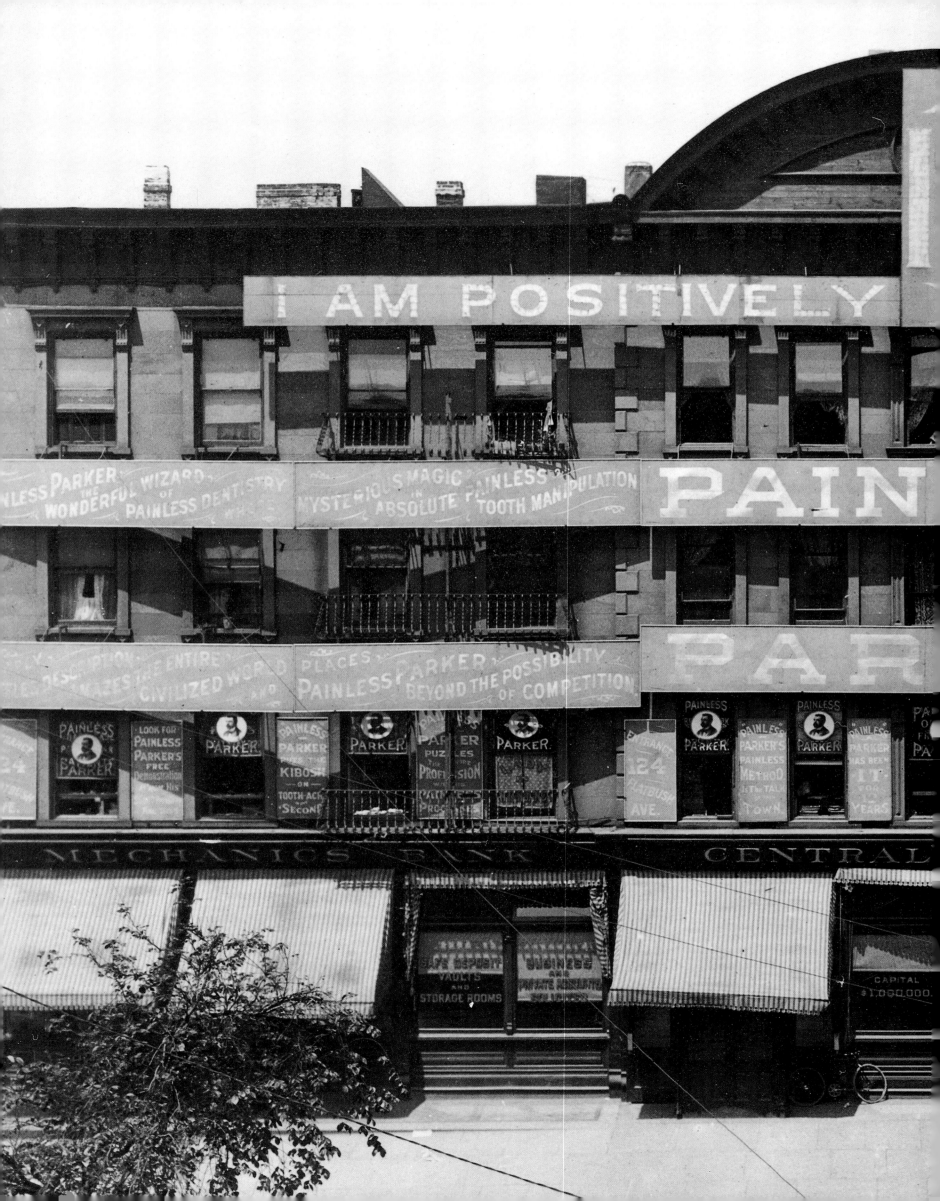

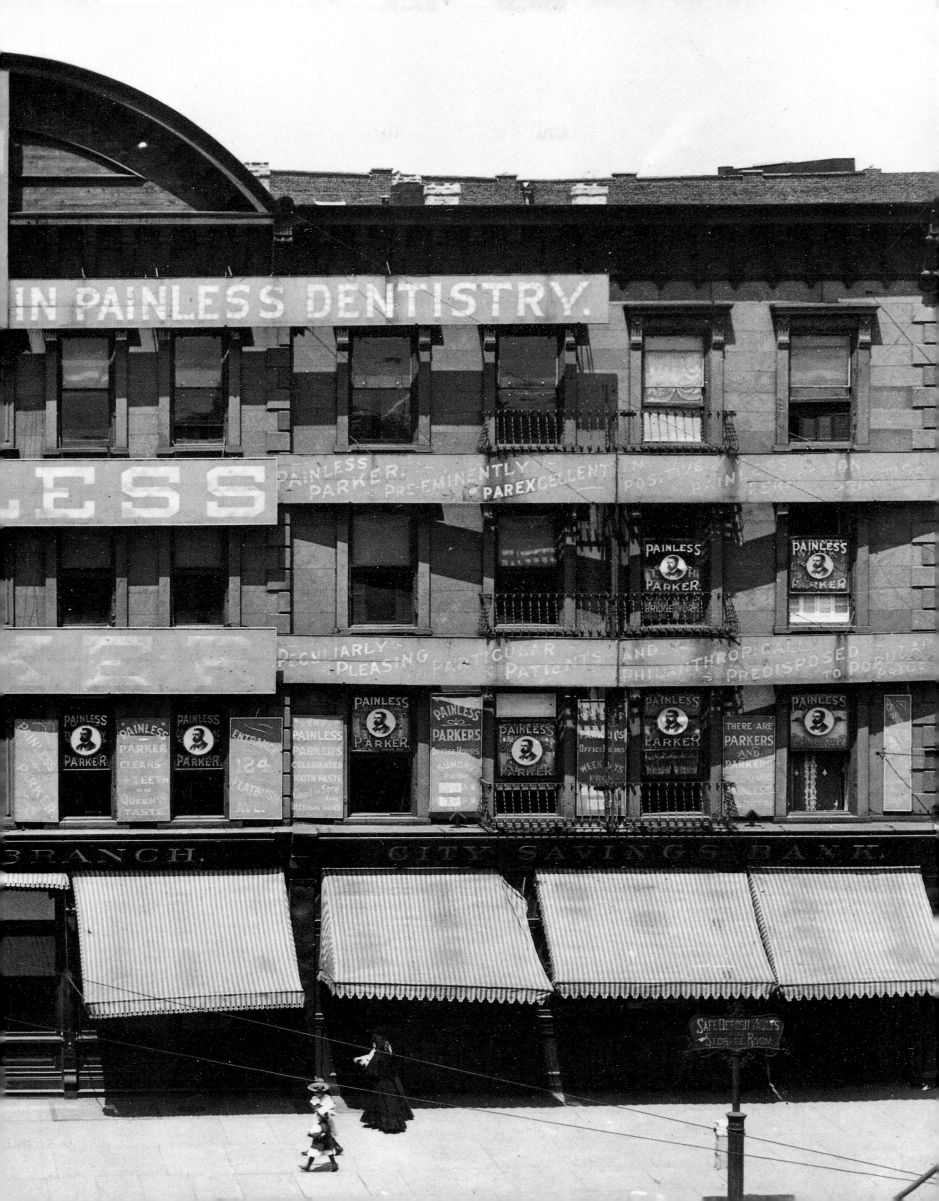

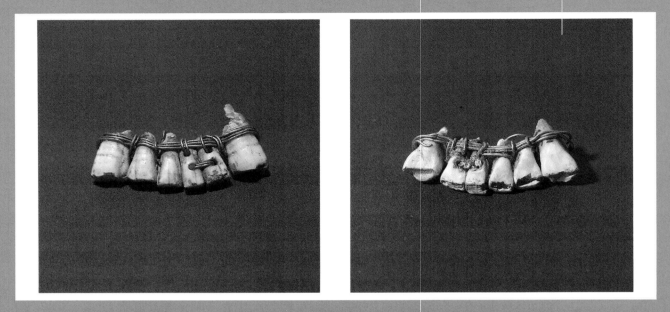

CONTENTS

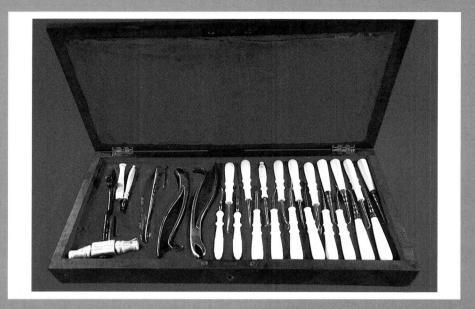

PREFACE AND ACKNOWLEDGMENTS

From the very earliest times, humans have been plagued by dental problems and have sought a variety of means to alleviate them. The first dental healers were physicians, but by the Middle Ages the barber-surgeons of Europe had specialized in the care of the teeth. These practitioners learned by trial and error but also by observation, and by the fifteenth century they had made more progress in their new-fledged field than had the doctors in the long-established practice of medicine. The pace of achievement redoubled in the eighteenth century, when the immortal Pierre Fauchard through his great treatise *Le chirurgien dentiste* solidly established dentistry as a true profession. No longer mired in superstition and ignorance, the field was based at last on sound rational and scientific principles.

Today the profession of dentistry is looked upon by the public with respect and admiration. Yet some dental specialists and many laymen know nothing about the struggles that took place to advance the profession or the great contributions that have been made by dentistry to human welfare—the most significant of which has been surgical anesthesia.

Dentists and dental researchers employed by government agencies and individual practitioners struggling to meet professional demands would do well to examine the history of dentistry and use that knowledge as a directional. The *only* guide to what lies ahead is the study of the past. The great Roman orator Cicero was well aware of this when he said, "Not to know what has been transacted in former times is to continue always as a child. If no use is made of the labors of past ages, the world must remain in the infancy of knowledge." How much more important it is to be aware of our historical antecedents today, when changes are occurring so rapidly that only by keeping our eyes steadily on what went before can we progress with intelligence and confidence. In the words of one of the most illustrious dentists this country has produced, the late Dr. J. Ben Robinson, founder of the American Academy of the History of Dentistry, "The dental profession will continue to flounder, to perpetuate its handicaps, and to fail its true purpose as long as it lacks an intelligent understanding of its historical background."

Thus, the study of dental history is in every way worthwhile. It is also fascinating, illuminating, and entertaining. In a word, it is fun! So, in bringing knowledge to his readers, the author hopes he is also bringing them enjoyment.

The publication of *Dentistry: An Illustrated History* marks the culmination of many years of writing and research both in this country and abroad. I wish to express my deepest thanks to all those who aided me, whether with advice, or by helping me to locate documentary material, or by providing one or more of the excellent photographs that adorn this book.

Many of my colleagues in the dental profession deserve special recognition here: Milton B. Asbell, Cherry Hill, New Jersey; Amadeo Bobbio, São Paulo, Brazil; François Brunner, Lyons, France; R. A. Cohen, Leamington Spa, England; Gordon E. Dammann, Lena, Illinois; F.E.R. DeMaar, The Hague; J. A. Donaldson, East Molesey, England; Clifton O. Dummett, Los Angeles; Are C. Edwards, Paris; the late Samuel Fastlicht, Mexico City; Rafi Fisher, Ramat Gan, Israel; Focion Febres-Cordero, Caracas; Jacques Fouré, Paris; Otto Francke, Stockholm; Erich Geiser, Adliswil, Switzerland; Richard A. Glenner, Chicago; James E. Harris, Ann Arbor; Walter Hoffmann-Axthelm, Freiburg, Germany; Kuninori Homma, Niigata, Japan; Yasuo Ishii, Fukui, Japan; Gary D. Lemen, Sacramento; Ake B. Löfgren, Göteborg, Sweden; H. Berton McCauley, Baltimore; Louis B. Marry, Villeneuve-lès-Avignon, France; Leif Marvitz, Copenhagen; Noringa Moriyama, Tokyo; Bernard S. Moskow, Ridgewood, New Jersey; Sataro Motoyama, Tokyo; Lawrence L. Mulcahy, Jr., Batavia, New York; Frank J. Orland, Chicago, Illinois; Jean-Jacques Quenouille, Orchamps, France; Peter Schulz, Cologne; Ben Z. Swanson, Jr., London; Ralph S. Voorhees, Montgomery, Texas; and Mitsuo Yatsu, Matsudo, Japan.

I am indebted as well to many persons in fields other than dentistry for the success of my efforts: Janet Brady Berk, History of Medicine Librarian, School of Medicine and Dentistry, University of Rochester; Isabel Caballero, History of Medicine Librarian, School of Medicine, University of Miami; Allan D. Charles, Professor of History, University of South Carolina, Union; Gardner P. H. Foley, Professor Emeritus, Baltimore College of Dental Surgery, Dental School, University of Maryland, Baltimore; David L. Gunner, Professor, Department of Anatomy, Harvard Medical School, Cambridge, Mass.; the late Everett Jackson, Museum Specialist, Smithsonian Institution, Washington, D.C.; Brett A. Kirkpatrick, Director of the Library, New York Academy of Medicine, New York; Patricia C. Knudson, Deputy Director, Health Sciences Library, University of Maryland, Baltimore; Samuel Kottek, Professor of the History of Medicine, Hebrew University–Hadassah Medical School, Jerusalem; Aletha Kowitz, Director, Bureau of Library Services, American Dental Association, Chicago; Felicity Nowell-Smith, Curator, Museum of the History of Medicine, Academy of Medicine, Toronto; Minnie Orfanos, Librarian, Dental Library, Northwestern University, Chicago; Egon Peters, Director of Public Relations, Bundesverband der Deutschen Zahnärzte, Cologne; Dr. Samuel X. Radbill, Philadelphia; Philip Szczepanski, photographer, University of Maryland, Baltimore; Menachem Schmelzer, Librarian, Jewish Theological Seminary of America, New York; Lilli Sentz, History of Medicine Librarian, Health Sciences Library, State University of New York at Buffalo; James Ulrich, photographer, Educational Communications Center, State University of New York at Buffalo; Philip Weimerskirch, Director, Burndy Library, Norwalk; Richard J. Wolfe, Curator, Rare Books and Manuscripts, Francis A. Countway Library of Medicine, Boston; David Wilk, Librarian, Israel Institute for the History of Medicine, Jerusalem; the late Yigael Yadin, Professor of Archaeology, Hebrew University, Jerusalem; Helena Zinkham, Curator of Prints, New-York Historical Society, New York.

To the staffs of the publishing houses responsible for the production of this book go my heartfelt thanks: to Darlene Barela Warfel, who conceived the idea for the book and saw it through to completion, and Myrna Oppenheim, who was always there when she was needed—both of the C. V. Mosby Company; and to the fine and competent workers, both past and present, of Harry N. Abrams, Inc., who changed this book from dream to reality: Barbara Lyons, whose guidance and judgment were invaluable; Ellyn Allison, whose editing unified the book and brought it to its finished state; Cindy Deubel, who gathered many pictures from the far reaches of the earth; and Carol Robson, who was responsible for the handsome design. There have been many other persons involved in the production of this book, and I wish to acknowledge my gratitude to them for helping to make it a pleasure to hold and to read!

Malvin E. Ring, D.D.S., M.L.S., F.A.C.D.
January 1985

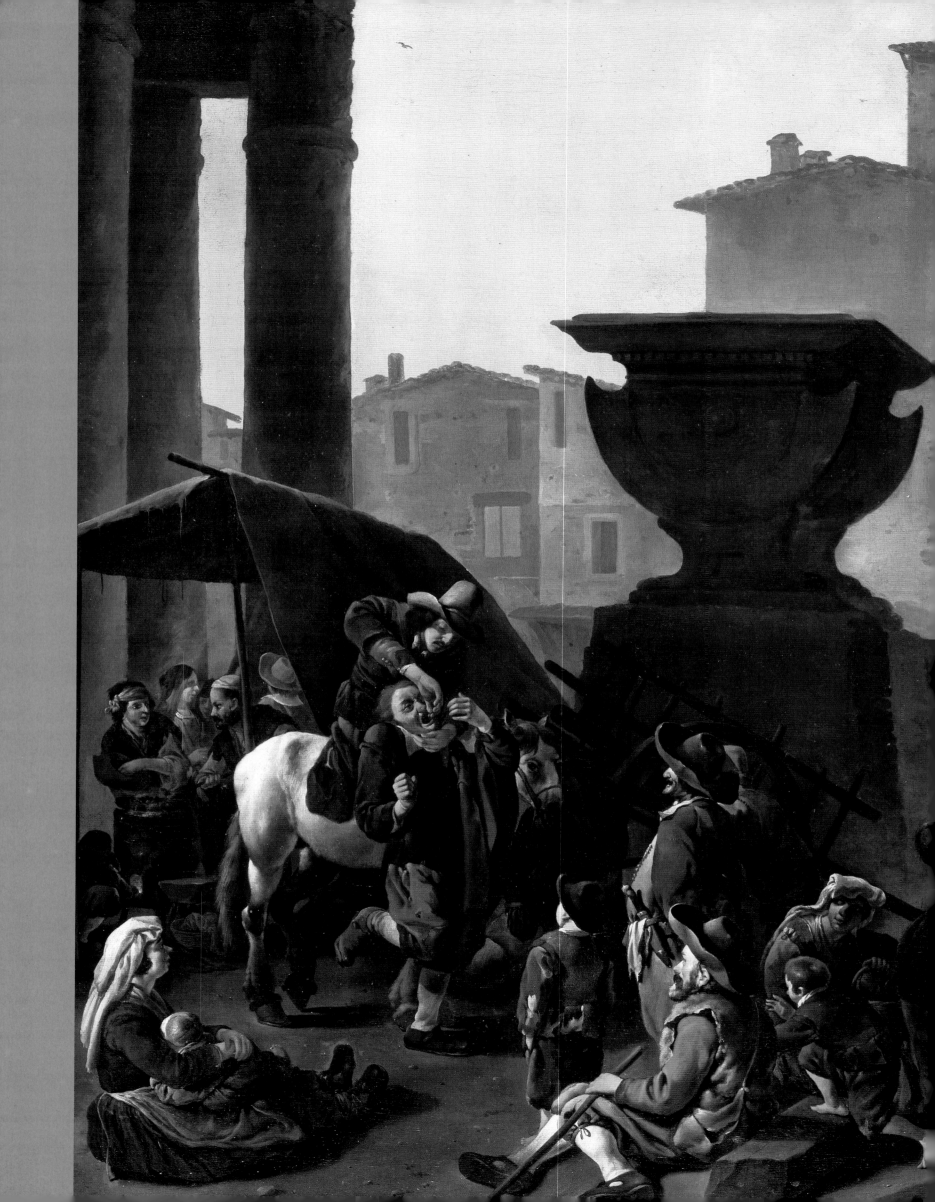

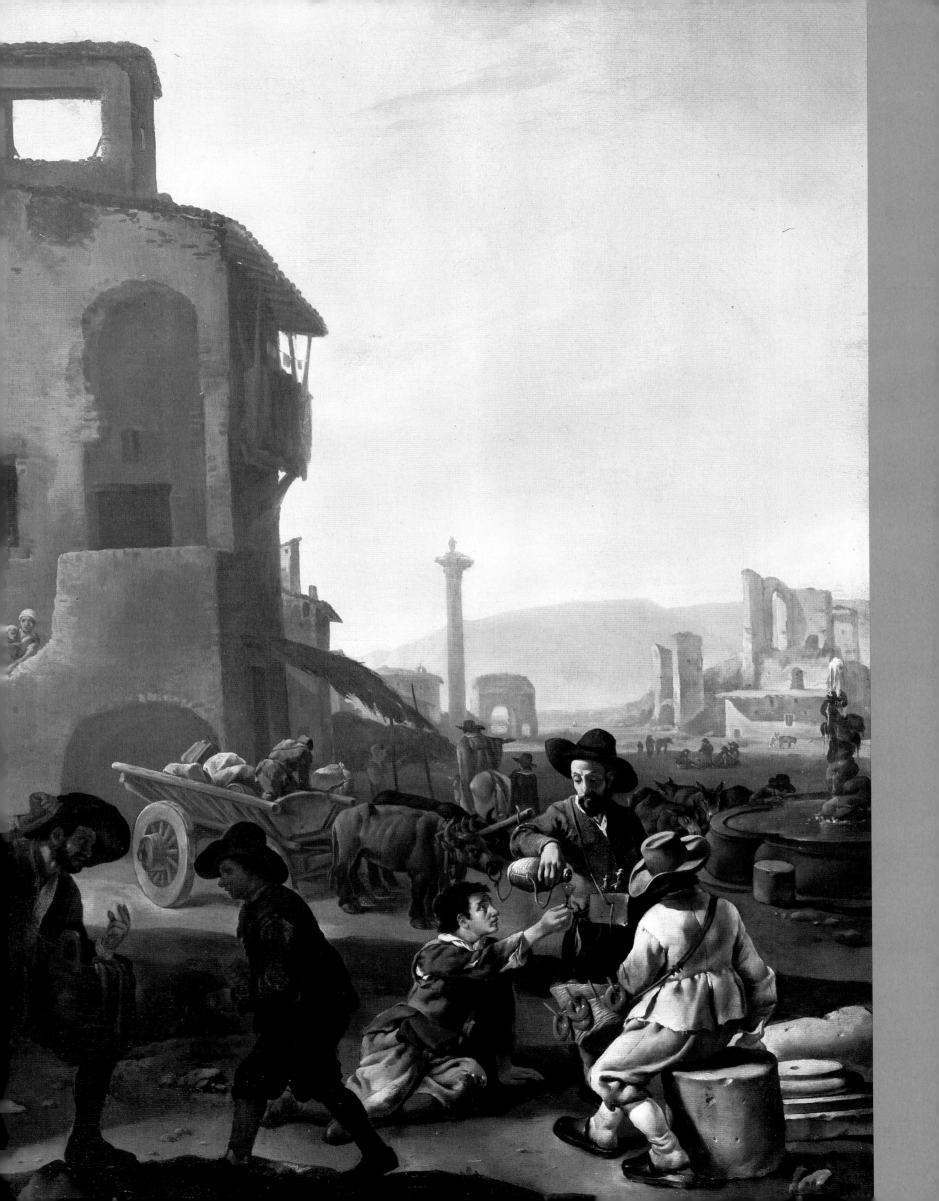

For my beloved wife, Hilda, without whose unswerving support and devotion and unstinting assistance this book could never have been written.

And for Darlene Barela Warfel, of the C. V. Mosby Company, who conceived the idea of the book and whose encouragement and valued guidance brought an idea to fruition.

Page 1

Figure 89, see description on page 109.

Page 2

Figure 17, see description on page 28.

Pages 4–5

The Painless Parker dental parlors flourished in New York City, especially during the late 1920s and 1930s. The chain's flamboyant advertising became a byword. The sign on this building on Flatbush Avenue in Brooklyn extends nearly a full city block, and the word "it" is two stories high. Museum of the City of New York. The Byron Collection.

Page 6

Figure 19, see description on page 29.

Page 7

Dr. Holton Ganson of Batavia, New York, owned this dental instrument chest about 1840. Dr. Ganson was a physician who devoted part of his practice to dental treatment. Holland Land Office Museum, Batavia, New York.

Pages 10–11

The focus of interest in this lively street scene in an imaginary town is a dentist on horseback extracting a tooth. The Dutch genre artist Johannes Lingelbach painted it in 1651. Rijksmuseum, Amsterdam.

DENTISTRY

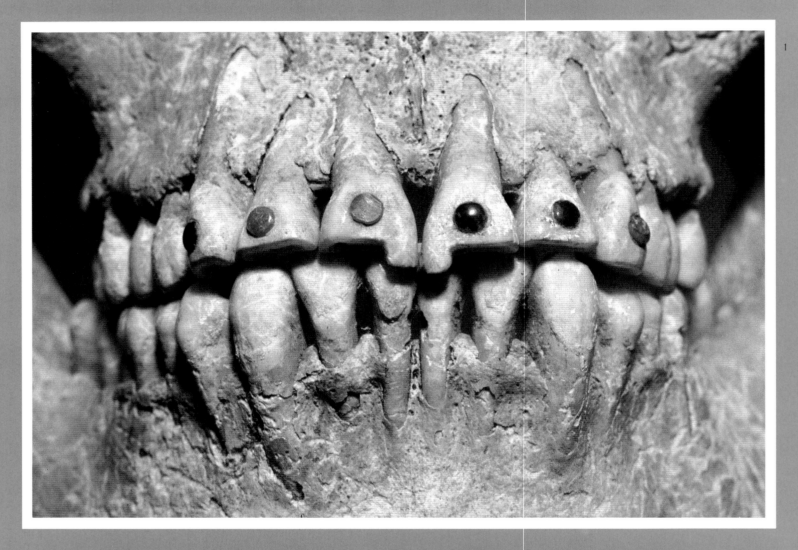

1

The teeth of this Mayan skull of the ninth century A.D. have numerous inlays of jade and turquoise. Museo Nacional de Antropología, Mexico City.

2

Dr. Pedro Beltranena shows how the Mayas may have prepared cavities for inlays using a bow drill.

3

Dr. Samuel Fastlich has suggested that the Mayas used tube drills and bow drills of this sort in preparing cavities for dental inlays.

I
THE PRIMITIVE WORLD

Pre-Columbian America

The Mayas

It is believed that the Indians of the Western Hemisphere arrived there approximately 15,000 years ago, having crossed over from Asia on a then-existing land bridge across the Bering Strait. They migrated east into the woodlands of North America, and south into Mesoamerica and South America, where a number of nations developed, all with certain basic similarities of culture. Principal among these were the Aztecs, a fierce, warlike people who resided in the area of what is now central Mexico; the Mayas, a more peaceful people with a highly developed culture who inhabited the Yucatán Peninsula, as well as present-day Guatemala and Honduras; and the Incas, also a highly advanced people, who lived in the Andes Mountains of today's Peru.

When the Spanish conquistadors subdued the great Mayan nation, they were determined to destroy its culture, root and branch. The Mayas had developed a written language, and central to their culture was a huge collection of parchments with hieroglyphic writings chronicling their history and traditions. One spiritual leader of the Spaniards in Yucatán, the fanatical Bishop Diego de Landa, ordered that since these were pagan writings, and thus words of the devil, they were to be destroyed. And so a great bonfire was built in the public square of the town of Maní and these priceless manuscripts were consigned to the flames. A Spanish chronicler who recorded the scene for the edification of Spaniards across the sea naively wrote that as the manuscripts were cast into the fire the people "made a great cry of woe." This was not to be wondered at, said Edward Thompson, an archaeologist who did much pioneering work in the area, for the people saw "not only the sacred things calcining in the fervent heat, but also the written lore, the accumulated knowledge of their race, going up in smoke and cinders."

The destruction of the written records of these industrious people robbed future scholars of an irreplaceable treasure. Despite many exploratory missions, rigorous excavations, and exhaustive research through the years, we still know less about the Mayan civilization than we know of the more ancient cultures of Egypt and Mesopotamia. Though separated from us in time by only a few centuries, the Mayas are more remote than the people of ancient Babylon! We do know, however, that they carried on extensive agriculture and were successful in selectively breeding better crops. Their highly advanced architecture included great pyramids surmounted by magnificent temples, numerous public buildings, and imposing palaces. These they decorated with elaborately carved friezes and low-relief sculpture as well as wall paintings.

The nation's history began about 2500 B.C., but the culture achieved its greatest heights from about A.D. 300 to about A.D. 900. After that, for some inexplicable reason (possibly exhaustion of the soil as a result of intensive farming) it went into a slow but steady decline, so that when the Toltecs, who preceded the Aztecs in the Valley of Mexico, subdued the Mayas about 1000, their glory was only a shadow of its former self.

The Mayas had a well-developed system of mathematics. In addition to their skill in architecture, they had an excellent understanding of time and fashioned a successful calendar. Essentially a Stone Age people, for their tools were of flint and their weapons of wood edged with sharpened obsidian, they nevertheless were accomplished smelters and forgers of gold, silver, and, to a lesser extent, bronze. Their lapidaries were very skillful, turning out beautifully carved jewelry of jadeite, hematite, onyx, turquoise, and other semiprecious stones.

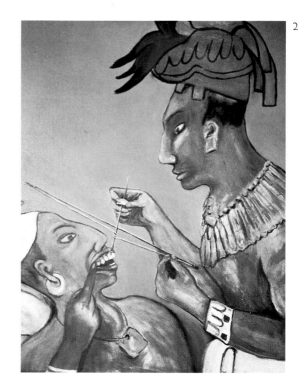

2

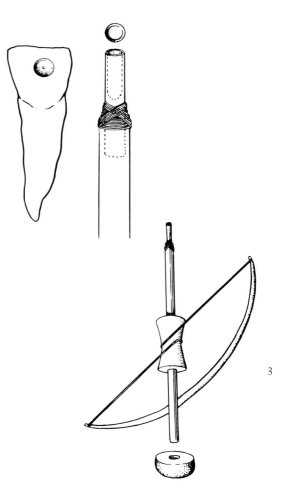

3

The teeth of this terra-cotta head from Veracruz, Mexico, of A.D. 200–500, have been painted with a coal-black resin that stands out sharply against the light brown clay. Many native populations of the Americas stain their teeth for cosmetic purposes. Albright-Knox Art Gallery, Buffalo. Gift of Thomas Robins, Jr.

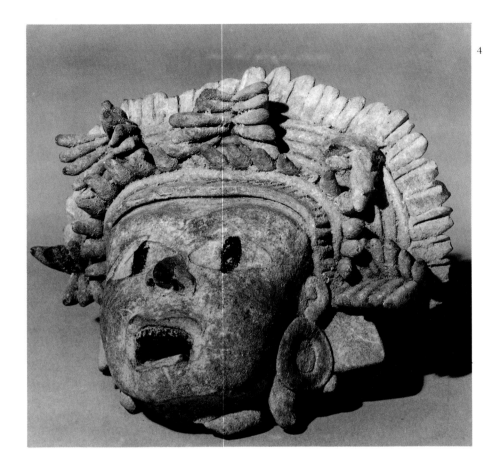

4

Yet although they excelled in working stone and metal, no true restorative or corrective dentistry was performed by these people for the maintenance or improvement of oral health. They developed their skills in working on the teeth strictly for ritual or religious purposes. Some investigators claim personal adornment was a principal incentive. We know, however, that the Mayas had elaborate religious ceremonies in which blackening of the teeth and scarification of the face or torso played a part. Thus, it is reasonable to assume that tooth mutilation and ornamentation served a cultic purpose.

The Mayas were skilled in placing beautifully carved stone inlays in carefully prepared cavities in the upper and lower anterior teeth, and occasionally in the bicuspid teeth. These inlays were made of a variety of minerals, including jadeite (a silicate related and similar in appearance to Oriental jade); iron pyrites; hematite (which they called "bloodstone"); turquoise; quartz; serpentine (which when in combination with dolomite, magnesite, or calcite has an appearance similar to jade); and cinnabar, the ore from which mercury is extracted.

There is no doubt that the cavities were prepared in living teeth. A round, hard tube similar in shape to a drinking straw, made in early times of jade and later of copper, was spun between the hands or in a rope drill, with a slurry of powdered quartz in water as the abrasive, cutting a perfectly round hole through the enamel and into the dentin. X rays have shown that if the pulp was inadvertently penetrated, the inlay was nevertheless put in place; then the pulp died and a periapical abscess resulted.

The stone inlay was ground to fit the cavity so exactly that many have remained in situ for a thousand years. In order to supplement frictional retention, the space between the inlay and the cavity wall was sealed with cements. Modern spectrographic examination of the remnants of these cements show that they were made of a variety of minerals, principally calcium phosphate. Also found in the cement residues were particles of silicon, but we do not know whether the silicon was mixed in the cement to form a stronger adhesive or if it was part of the abrasive used to cut the cavity.

The Mayas also filed their teeth in a variety of ways. It is probable that each design had a particular tribal or religious significance, since more than fifty different patterns have been identified. The incisal edges of some teeth were filed with a single cut; some had double cuts; some had the distal portions of the edges removed, leaving the mesial portions intact; and some were filed to points.

Diego de Landa kept extensive notes on the culture of the people, and we ironically have him to thank for our knowledge of some of their practices, including tooth filing. Of the Yucatán Mayas he said, "They had the habit of allowing their teeth to be filed like those of a saw. It was done for reasons of vanity. The skill was practiced by elderly women using certain stones and water."

An interesting controversy has arisen over a skull fragment found far to the south of the Mayan area in Esmeraldas, Ecuador (now in the collection of the Museum of the American Indian in New York City). First described by Marshall H. Saville in 1913, it is a part of a maxilla with all of the posterior teeth present except for the third molars. The two incisors contain round gold inlays on their labial surfaces. It is quite apparent that these two incisors were jammed into the tooth sockets, fracturing the alveolar process. One of the incisors was filed on the mesial surface of the crown to make it fit into the available space. Many specialists, especially Bernhard Weinberger, one of America's great dental historians, are of the opinion that this was an early instance of tooth transplantation from one individual to another. However, Samuel Fastlicht of Mexico City, without a doubt the world's leading authority on Pre-Columbian dentistry, disputes this for an obvious reason: there is no bone regeneration in the lines of fracture. Thus, the implantation was obviously done postmortem, possibly in preparing the body for burial according to religious beliefs similar to those held by the ancient Egyptians.

There is strong evidence, on the other hand, that the Mayas practiced the implantation of alloplastic (nonorganic) material in living persons. While excavating at the Playa de los Muertos in the Ulúa Valley of Honduras in 1931, Wilson Popenoe and his wife found a mandible fragment of Mayan origin, dating from about A.D. 600 (fig. 5). This fragment, now in the Peabody Museum of Archaeology and Ethnology at Harvard University, has been studied by Amadeo Bobbio of São Paulo, Brazil, a world-acknowledged authority on implants. He observed that three tooth-shaped pieces of shell had been placed in the sockets of three missing lower incisor teeth. Contrary to an earlier opinion that they, too, had been inserted after death, Bobbio's X rays, taken in 1970, showed compact bone formation around two of the implants, bone radiographically similar to that which would surround a blade implant of today. Consequently, these are the earliest endosseous (within bone) alloplastic implants yet discovered.

This mandible found by Dr. and Mrs. Wilson Popenoe in Honduras in 1931 has three pieces of shell in place of the natural lower incisors. Dating from about A.D. 600, the fragment is our earliest example of a presumably successful endosseous alloplastic implant operation on a living person. Peabody Museum of Archaeology and Ethnology, Harvard University, Cambridge, Massachusetts.

5

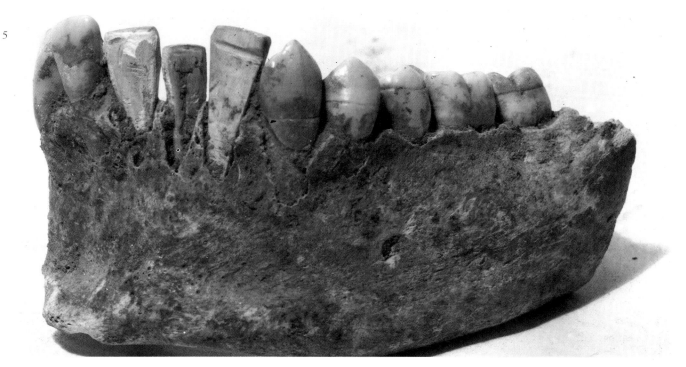

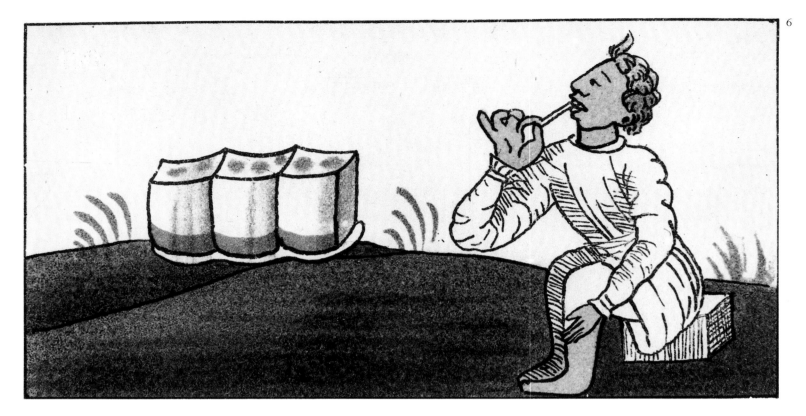

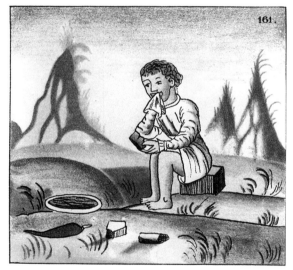

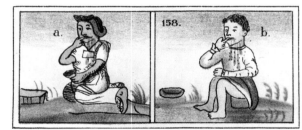

These drawings from Fray Bernardino de Sahagún's sixteenth-century treatise *Historia general de las cosas de Nueva España* probably illustrate how the Aztecs of Mexico treated certain oral diseases. Ibero-Amerikanisches Institut, Preussischer Kulturbesitz, Berlin.

The Valley of Mexico

In the ancient palace of Tepantitla, at the ceremonial center of Teotihuacán, which lies in central Mexico, is to be found one of the best-preserved Pre-Columbian frescoes. It depicts scenes of the paradise of Tlaloc, the rain god. The early native chroniclers described this paradise where happiness and delight reigned, where life consisted of games, pleasure, song, and dance. Among the figures who are singing, catching butterflies, and otherwise enjoying themselves is a man filing the teeth of another, using for the purpose a narrow, sharpened flint (fig. 7). It is thus possible that the early Mexicans filed the teeth hoping to achieve a state of bliss in the "earthly paradise."

Some 350 years after Teotihuacán was abandoned, the barbarian Aztecs settled in the Mexican highlands in the vicinity of what is today Mexico City. They conquered neighboring tribes and, like the Romans of classical times, adopted customs of those they conquered.

They, too, practiced tooth mutilation, filing their teeth as well as inlaying them with stone. One of the most important sources for our knowledge of early dental practices among the Aztecs is the writing of a Spanish monk who arrived in the New World just after the conquest. Fray Bernardino de Sahagún was a young man when he undertook his mission. He had an insatiable desire to chronicle the customs of the conquered Indians, and he learned their language and wrote a large part of his great work *Historia general de las cosas de Nueva España* in the Nahuatl tongue.

Sahagún spent his adult life examining and recording every aspect of the culture of the newly conquered land. Among other things, he studied diseases of the mouth and how they were treated with herbs and botanicals. He translated the names of the teeth into Nahuatl and mentioned fractured and loose teeth, calculus formation, and caries (which the Aztecs believed were caused by a worm and which they relieved by chewing on a hot chili). He reported the native belief that only those children born during a full moon would have a harelip (probably because our Man in the Moon for the Mexicans was a rabbit!). He reported that cavities in teeth were filled with a powder of snail shells, sea salt, and the herb *tlalcacaoatl*, but archaeological evidence of such fillings is lacking.

Sahagún makes the only reference to tooth extraction we have found in all Aztec lore. He says that when a patient suffered from toothache, the practice was to grind up a worm, mix it with turpentine, and paint it on the cheek. At the same time a grain of salt was placed in the cavity and the tooth covered with heated pepper. An incision was then made in the gum and the herb *tlalcacaoatl* was placed in it. And then, if the toothache and infection still remained, the tooth was extracted.

Since the Aztecs were warlike, they suffered many wounds and apparently became quite adept at suturing, using strands of hair. Sahagún mentions suturing wounds of the lips and cheeks.

Sahagún began writing his great work about 1547 and completed it sometime before 1577. Although under orders to turn over all copies of his work to the Crown (ostensibly for the royal archives, but more probably to be destroyed), Sahagún managed to rewrite his work from notes he had hidden away. Not until 1829 was it published, and for a century and a half it has proved a priceless source of information.

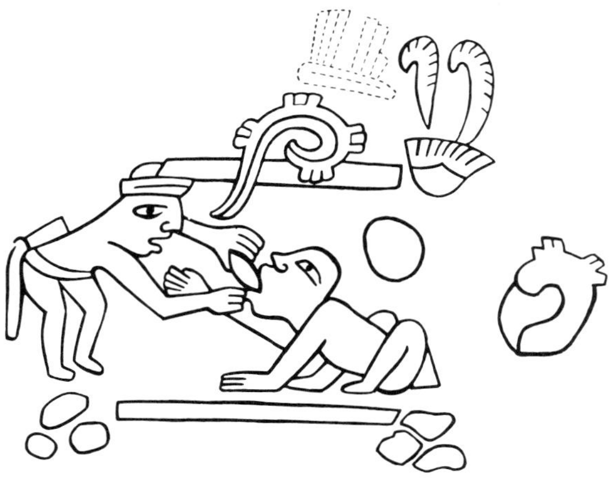

7

Miguel Covarrubias's modern copy of a fresco in the Temple of Tepantitla at Teotihuacán, a ceremonial center near Mexico City, shows an Indian of some fifteen hundred years ago filing the teeth of a companion, presumably for ritual purposes. Museo Nacional de Antropología, Mexico City.

The Incas

Also a highly developed people, the Incas dominated the Peruvian highlands and spread out along the coast in the early 1400s. They conquered other peoples and, like the Aztecs, absorbed the lore and adopted the practices of those they dominated. They themselves were brutally conquered by Francisco Pizarro in 1533, and much of their culture was destroyed.

Their treatment of disease was closely linked to their religious beliefs, and magic was intermingled with their attempts at rational therapeutics. Thus, though illness was looked upon as a sin that could be expiated only upon confession to specified priests, numerous herbal remedies were resorted to.

As with the Mayas, much of what we know of Inca civilization derives from the writings of a chronicler. Sebastián Garcilaso de le Vega, who was himself descended from the Incas, wrote extensively of his forebears. He recounted the treatment of dental and oral problems, describing the excision of carious material from a tooth with a burning stick. Balsam of Peru, a resin from the tree *Myroxylon pereirae*, was used to treat gingival diseases, and in severe cases, cautery was resorted to. He wrote that the root of a plant was heated until it glowed and then was partially split down the middle. After that, "when it was very hot they pressed it on the teeth, putting one part on one side of the gums, and the other on the other side, and left it there until it was cool." The inflamed and hyperplastic gingival tissue was undoubtedly burned away to permit the development of new and healthy granulation tissue. Apparently leaves of the coca bush were chewed during the operation to provide relief from pain. Teeth in need of extraction seem first to have been loosened by working a caustic resin around and under the detached gingiva. Then the loosened tooth was presumably knocked out with a sharp blow from a stick.

The Incas did not ornament their teeth, but skulls found in Ecuador, the northernmost area they penetrated, show mutilation by filing, inlaying of gold, and what appears to be the insertion of hammered gold into previously prepared cavities in the gingivo-labial surfaces of the incisor teeth.

North America

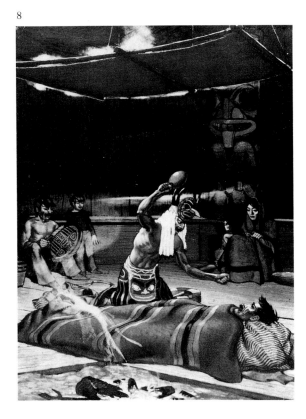

While his apprentice beats a drum, a shaman of the West Coast Tlingit tribe of North America exorcises evil spirits from a sick man in this contemporary painting by W. Langdon Kihn. © 1945 National Geographic Society.

When Columbus landed on the shore of the North American continent, the Indians he found there had an essentially Stone Age culture. They had learned to cope with their environment through a complex system of magical beliefs and superstitions, and they relied on magic to treat both sickness and disease.

Though the tribes were many and distinct, their medical practices were very similar. Central to their system was the shaman, or medicine man. He was either the chief or second in command and importance after the chief. His fellow tribesmen believed that his powers were divinely conferred upon him, and so they felt that he could not only cure diseases but also enlist the help of the gods in furthering an individual's endeavors or those of the tribe as a whole. In addition, not only could he coax out an afflicting spirit from the body of a sick patient but he could also send "disease spirits" to infect whomever he chose. Consequently, the shaman was greatly feared, and he exercised profound influence. His techniques were clearly described by Frederick W. Hodge (*Handbook of American Indians North of Mexico*, 1907): "He inquired into the symptoms, dreams and transgressions of the taboos by the patient, whom he examined, and then pronounced his opinion as to the nature . . . of the ailment. He then prayed, exhorted or sang, the last, perhaps to the accompaniment of a rattle; made passes with his hand, sometimes moistened with saliva, over the part affected; and finally placed his mouth over the most painful spot and sucked hard to extract the . . . illness."

Today among the Navajos there is a female healer called a "hand trembler" whose profession may reflect the ancient shamanistic practices. She can only diagnose, however, not cure. She begins her ministrations by going into a trance, and her hand moves without apparent control of her conscious mind. Thus she obtains intuitive clues about the patient's illness. Although skeptical about her abilities at first, the white doctors on the reservation have come to accept her because her method apparently works well. When patients should be treated at a medical clinic, she is quick to refer them there, and practically all dental patients find their way to the reservation's dental clinic.

The Reverend William Leach, writing in 1855 in Omaha, Nebraska, described a Pawnee medicine man's treatment of toothache caused by an inflamed third molar. He "danced around the patient in a semicircle, rattling a gourd . . . [then] he took a small stone knife and cut an 'x' on Running Wolf's cheek, directly over the throbbing tooth. He sucked at the cut lightly . . . [and] pretended to draw out the fang . . . then dashed it into the fire. 'The Evil Spirits cannot use it again,' he said triumphantly!" This patient was fooled into believing his tooth had been removed, but in fact extraction was frequently resorted to, the offending tooth generally being knocked out rather than drawn. A vivid description of such an operation was given by a traveler to North Carolina in the early years of the nineteenth century: "They have several Remedies for the toothache, which often drive away the pain. But if they fail, they have recourse to punching out the Tooth with a small Cane set against the same on a Bit of Leather. Then they strike the Reed and so drive out the tooth; and howsoever it may seem to the Europeans, I prefer it before the common way of drawing teeth by those Instruments that endanger the Jaw, and a flux of blood often follows which this Method of a Punch never is attended withal. Neither is it half the pain."

Another method of extraction involved the use of a buckskin thong, which was tied at one end to the offending tooth and at the other to some firm object from which the sufferer suddenly jerked away. The patient might also lie on his back, with one end of a thong tied to the aching tooth and the other to a strong stick, which was pulled sharply to make the tooth come out.

The Indians' dental health was much better before the advent of the white man. In 1935 an investigator of the Hopi in Arizona was told by a chief that his people's need for gold crowns on their teeth was, "alas, a result of their having taken to hot coffee and other luxuries of the white man," and there seems to be ample evidence to support his belief. The famous French traveler Michel de Montaigne, who wrote of his visit to this country in the late 1700s, declared: "As my testimonies have told me, it is verie rare to see a sicke body amongst them; and they have further assured me they never saw any man there ... toothless." The celebrated Colonial physician Dr. Benjamin Rush also noted that the eastern tribes "appear to be strangers to diseases and pains of the teeth." In those areas where contact with European civilization was minimal, dental disease remained infrequent until well into the twentieth century. In the 1930s, Weston Price examined the teeth of 87 Indians living in remote parts of the Yukon Territory, and only 4 teeth out of 2,464 (0.16 percent) had caries, whereas among those living closer to white settlements, percentages ranged from 25 to 40.

Though their diet probably protected from dental caries those Indians living without contact with the white man, it nevertheless also caused certain dental problems. One of the principal causes of toothache was severe attrition of the biting surfaces of the teeth, resulting ultimately in pulp exposure, due to the coarse and gritty nature of Indian food. The mortars and pestles that they used to grind their maize were of stone, and inevitably grit was incorporated into their foodstuffs.

In addition to tooth destruction by wear, periodontal disease was a frequent problem, even among the younger people. Skulls unearthed from Indian burial mounds bear evidence of severe alveolar bone resorption and loss of teeth. Although we have no evidence that any type of physical cleaning or scaling of the teeth was done by the Indians, we do know that they held a clean mouth in high regard and had a variety of concoctions with which they attempted to cleanse the teeth.

Tobacco, an Indian discovery, they valued not only for the pleasurable effects of smoking, but also because they attributed a clean mouth to its use. Unfortunately, those who chewed tobacco abraded their teeth very rapidly because they mixed ground mussel shells and lime with the tobacco leaves to give the wad the proper consistency.

More popular were gums, resins, and plant roots, chewed not only to prevent toothache or gum diseases but to clean the mouth. A Quaker botanist, William Bartram, who in 1788 toured the Cherokee country in the South, described a species of *Silphium* whose gum the Indians collected. This was dried into hard semipellucid drops of a pale amber color with a very agreeable fragrance and slightly bitter taste, and the Indians chewed them to cleanse their teeth and sweeten their breath.

When preventive treatment had failed and disease had invaded a tooth, several methods of cure might be tried before extraction was resorted to. In some tribes a leather-working awl heated red hot was poked into carious lesions, and almost everywhere herbs, roots, and grasses were applied in hopes of easing the pain and curing dental affliction. One almost universal remedy for dental ills among the Indians, later adopted by white settlers, was the bark of the prickly ash tree (*Zanthoxylum americanum*), called by the Europeans the "toothache tree." The early Pennsylvania Germans learned from the local Indians to decoct the bark of the root of the white poplar tree and apply this hot to an aching tooth.

Equally popular though less efficacious were magical and superstitious practices of many kinds. Some Indians "cured" toothache by cutting out a piece of sod before sunrise, breathing upon it three times, and restoring it to the same place from which it was taken. In certain tribes it was customary never to throw into the fire the remains of anything one had chewed (a quid of tobacco or the skin of an apple into which one had bitten) lest the fire chew one's teeth! And it was important upon seeing a shooting star to spit immediately lest one lose a tooth. To insure that his teeth would stay sound for the rest of his life a member of the Cherokee tribe need only catch a green snake, hold it horizontally by neck and tail, move it seven times back and forth between his two rows of teeth, and then turn it loose. No food prepared with salt was eaten for four days after this operation.

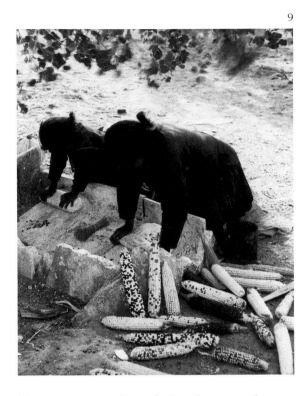

Navajo women grind corn for bread in a stone bin. Grit in the food eventually wears down even the healthiest teeth. National Archives, Washington, D.C.

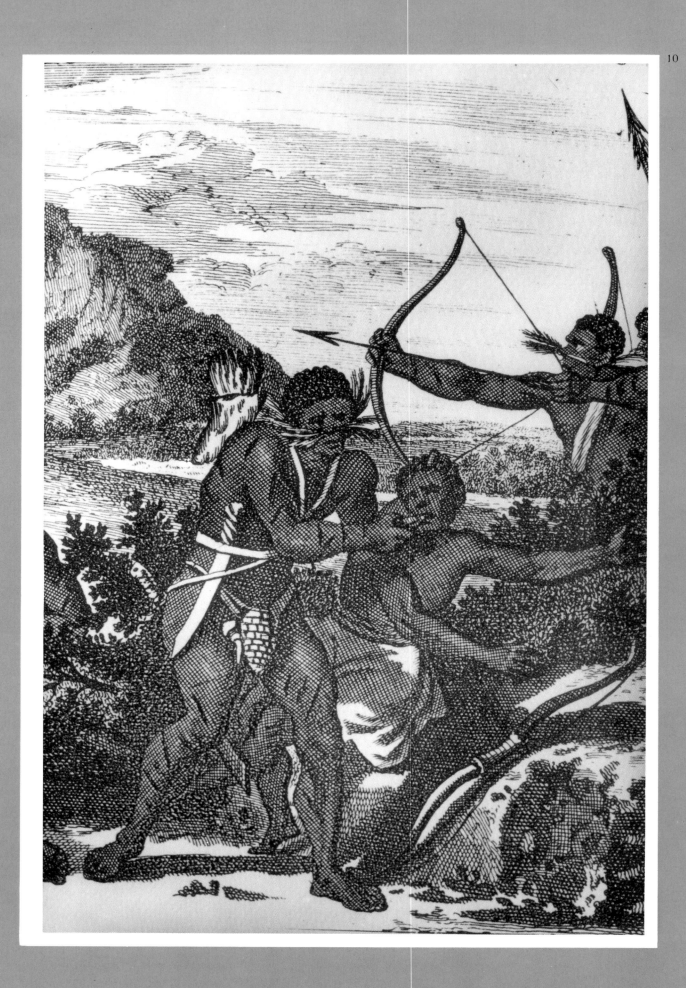

Contemporary Nonindustrialized Societies

Few primitive societies of modern times have developed systems for care of even the most minor dental ailments. As among pre-Conquest American Indians, relief from dental ills is generally sought from a shaman or witch doctor or someone else in the tribe designated to offer "medical" treatment.

Although, like us, they almost universally prize healthy teeth, primitive people frequently mutilate or destroy one or more of theirs, either as a means of tribal identification or for religious reasons. Some file their anterior teeth to points to increase the ferocity of their appearance (certain South American Indians of the Amazon Valley do this to imitate the dreaded piranha fish). A coarse diet, too, contributes to the dental problems of primitive peoples, as do certain specific practices. For example, the Eskimo women of northern Greenland chew sealskin to make it pliable for boot soles, and because of the toughness of the leather their teeth in time become worn down to the gum line.

Add to all this the fact that no satisfactory dental care exists for them and it becomes obvious why most primitive people lose their teeth earlier than their contemporaries in advanced societies. It is indeed remarkable that there are occasional individuals with exceptionally strong, healthy teeth. The author Joy Adamson, who visited the bush country of Kenya in the early 1960s, described a healing ritual in which a truly remarkable set of teeth played an important part. "The medicine man held a very large wood mortar—weighing thirty-four pounds and over two feet long, and made of a tree trunk—balanced by his teeth. He held it between his pointed teeth. How could he hold such a heavy weight? He told me this was thanks to a medicine he had put on his tongue." With the heavy trunk high over his head, he leaned backward and, balancing the mortar, walked several times around a patient who lay stretched flat on the ground. (The shaman told Adamson he also specialized in snakebites and in charms for protection against lions.)

It is to a medicine man such as this one that most African tribesmen go in order to alleviate toothache, and elsewhere in the world primitive peoples consult similar experts. Early in the Christian Era, the Han people of China forcibly dispossessed the inhabitants of the southwestern part of the land. The latter moved into wild mountainous areas and are today known as the hill peoples of Yunnan. They have stubbornly clung to their ancient ways in spite of the efforts of the Chinese Communist regime to bring them into the twentieth century. They, too, have a medicine man, or *mawpa*, who is believed to possess occult powers that enable him to disarm the spirits of illness. Because of his powers of sorcery he is able to exorcise demons, and the demons of toothache are among those driven out of a sufferer's body by his ministrations.

One of the most pervasive practices among primitive peoples is the mutilation of the dentition by removal of one or more of the teeth. Travelers to Africa in the 1600s reported this practice among the natives, and it is still widely carried on there today.

The Mbotgote, who inhabit the forests of the island of Malekula in the Coral Sea, about a thousand miles northeast of Australia, have preserved an ancient way of life. For most of the year they are cut off by the swollen rivers from contact with the civilizing influences of the modern world, which are confined to the coastal regions. Only about 150 of these people remain today, living in three villages. They cling to their belief in the power of ancestral spirits, and this colors almost every action in their daily lives. Ritual is a most important part of their culture. As part of the initiation rite into a special society for Nimangi women, each candidate must submit to having her upper right central incisor tooth knocked out. Having spent ten days without working and having limited her diet to soft, mushy foods so that her gums have become inflamed, she lies flat on her back with a short piece of wood clenched between her teeth. She is pinned to the ground hand and foot by relatives, and a kinsman straddles her and places a short stick on the tooth to be removed. This he hits with a stone and after a number of

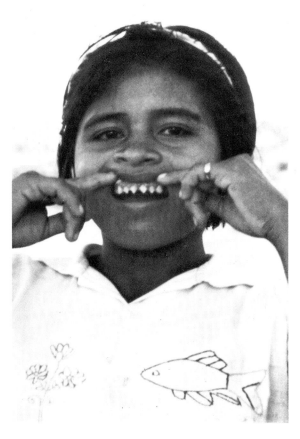

This girl of the Ticuana tribe of Brazil proudly displays her teeth, filed as a mark of beauty when she was nine years old.

10

In 1670 Oliver Dapper published an account of his travels in the African kingdom of Monoemugi, in the present-day Congo. This illustration from his book shows one native knocking out the upper central incisors of another, a custom of the people.

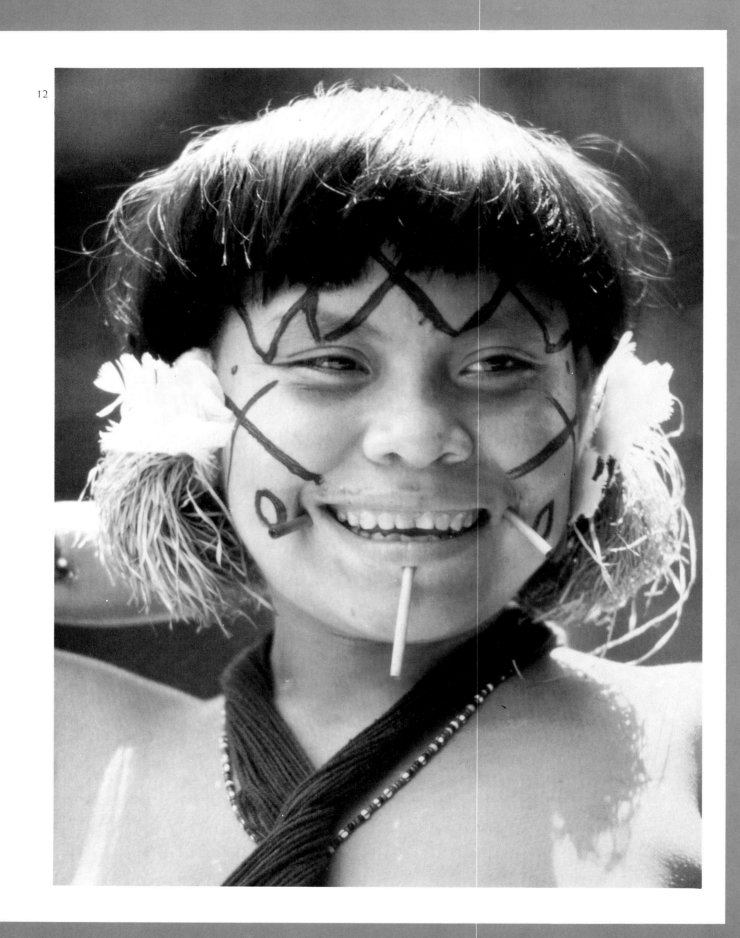

12

Beginning in early childhood, girls of the Yano-
mami tribe, who inhabit the far reaches of the Ori-
noco River in Venezuela, insert sharpened slivers
of hardwood and bamboo into their lips and
cheeks as a beauty enhancer.

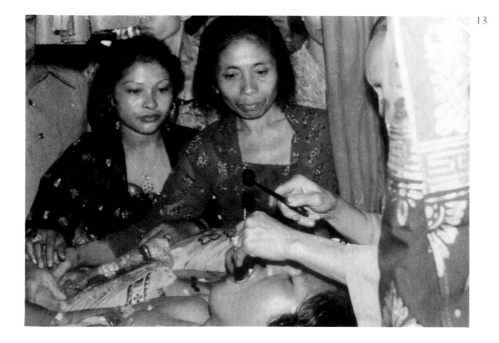

13

After reaching puberty, the young people of Bali have the incisal edges of their six upper front teeth chipped away—symbolic protection against the six cardinal sins.

sharp blows the tooth is usually so loose that it can be removed with the fingers. To stanch the flow of blood, stems of certain plants believed to have styptic properties are heated over embers and then packed into the wound.

In the mountainous regions of Vietnam live the Montagnards, who consider normally shaped incisor teeth too "doglike." Therefore, at puberty they knock out the upper incisors or file them down even with the gum. All the lower incisors they file to points. The practice originated as part of a ceremony of initiation into manhood; the custom is continued today for its esthetic effect alone.

In Vietnamese villages, the local sorcerer acts as healer. He conducts certain rituals to invoke the help of beneficial spirits and other rituals to control the evil ones. He wears a special costume that includes large wooden plugs in the earlobes, but to insure that his appearance is entirely proper for his incantations and rites, his four upper incisors are filed down to the gum line.

Mutilation, as has been noted, is often done for esthetic reasons. Thus, the Atayal aborigines, who live in the secluded mountain villages of Taiwan, extract the back teeth for beauty's sake. Perhaps the ensuing collapse of the bite and protrusion of the front teeth is really the effect they are seeking.

Sometimes, mutilation is confined to the soft tissues of the oral regions, again for ritual purposes. Thus, when a Sara woman of the African nation of Chad becomes betrothed her lips are pierced by her intended husband. He then inserts a wooden peg into the incision and keeps exchanging smaller pegs for larger ones until finally the opening is large enough to allow a flat disc to be inserted.

Other methods of adornment practiced today by primitive people are very similar to those of the Incas and Aztecs. Natives living in remote areas of Malaysia today inlay their teeth with bits of brass wire and with semiprecious stones, believing it enhances their beauty.

By contrast, the Fulani, who inhabit the Sudan, admire white, even teeth, and to emphasize them they blacken their lips and surround their eyes with black pigment. The effect is quite startling.

Many more examples of oral mutilation and deformation exist. It is interesting that such a variety of people, who have had no contact with each other and whose cultures are in other respects very different have developed such similar customs.

About 1955 an Australian aborigine had his teeth examined and treated by a traveling public-health dentist.

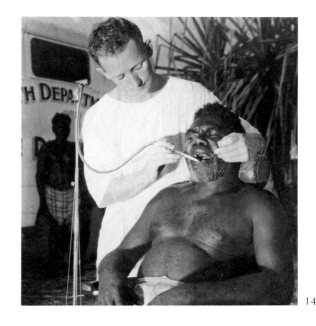

14

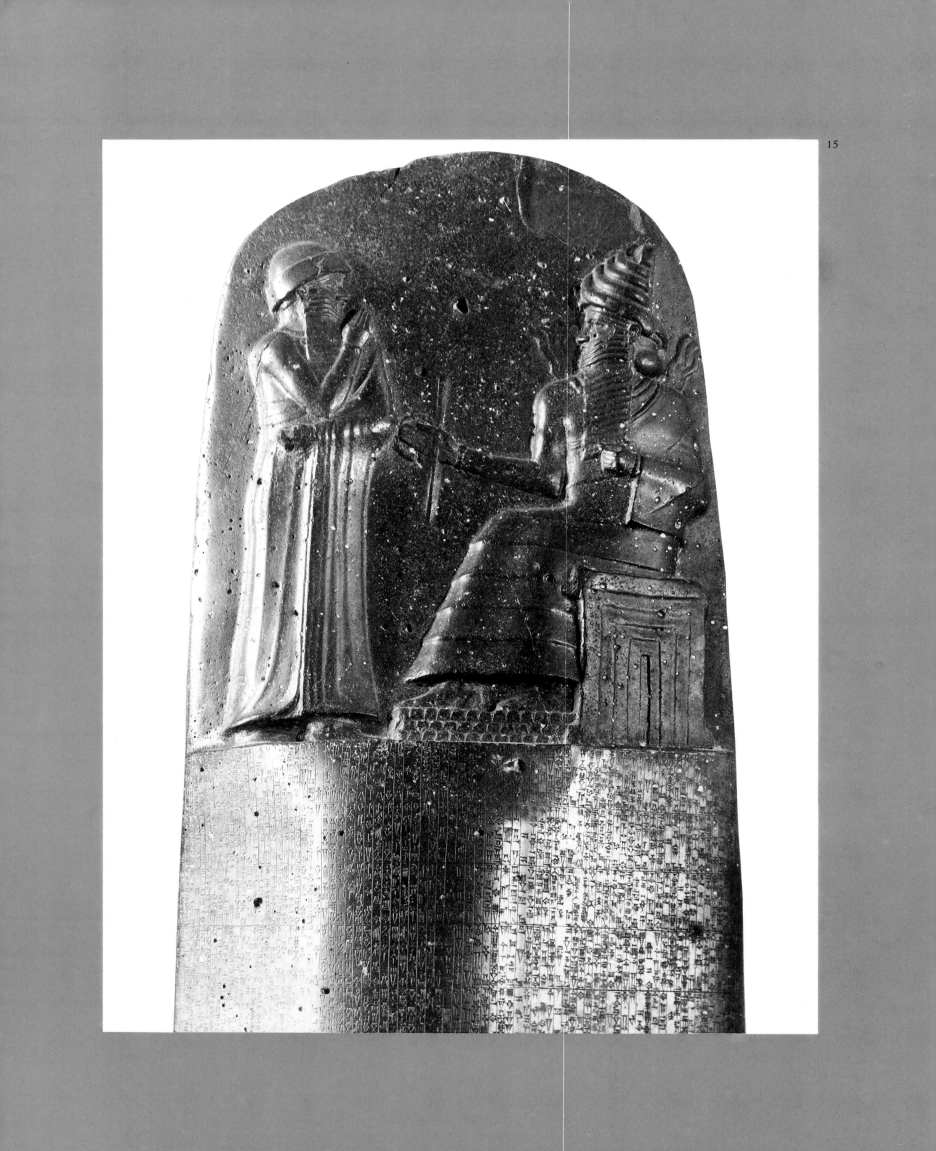

II
THE ANCIENT NEAR EAST

Mesopotamia

Between 3500 and 3000 B.C., on the fertile plain between the Tigris and Euphrates rivers the Sumerians developed an advanced civilization. Many of their wedge-shaped, or "cuneiform," scripts on clay tablets have survived in the ruins of the royal library of the Assyrian king Ashurbanipal, who lived in the seventh century B.C. It is from these tablets that much of our knowledge of Mesopotamian medicine and dentistry is derived. As in primitive societies, the medicine practiced in Mesopotamia was largely magical or religious in nature. Great emphasis was placed on auguries and divination, especially by examination of the liver of a sacrificed sheep. It was believed that demons inhabiting the body were responsible for disease, and filthy and disgusting remedies concocted from worms and insects were used to sicken and drive out these evil spirits.

A high point for medicine and surgery came during the empire of Babylonia. For the first time, physicians of a true sort treated diseases by drugs and by simple surgery. Handsomely rewarded if successful, they stood in risk of severe punishment if tragedy followed their ministrations. The code of laws drawn up during the reign of Hammurabi (1792–1750 B.C.) has come down to us on a stele of black diorite, now preserved in the Musée du Louvre (fig. 15), and here the punishments and rewards due practitioners of medicine were clearly spelled out:

> Law 196: If someone injures the eye of an equal
>   his own eye is destroyed.
> Law 198: If someone injures the eye of an inferior
>   he is fined a *mina* of silver.
> Law 200: If someone knocks out the tooth of an equal
>   his own tooth is knocked out.
> Law 201: If someone knocks out the tooth of an inferior
>   he is fined a third of a *mina* of silver.

It is interesting to note that, although an eye was clearly considered more valuable, nevertheless a substantial sum was placed on the value of a tooth.

Among the clay tablets in Ashurbanipal's library are a number devoted exclusively to diagnosis and prognosis, and the state of the teeth was used as a means of determining the course and source of an illness:

> If he grinds his teeth the disease will last a long time.
> If he grinds his teeth continuously and his face is cold he has
>   contracted a disease through the hand of the Goddess Ishtar.

Since grinding the teeth was considered both very dangerous and pathognomonic, a remedy was proposed. A human skull was placed upon a chair, and for three days, morning and night, sacrifices were placed before it. Then conjurations were to be spoken seven times into the skull, and the skull was kissed seven times seven by the patient before retiring, and then he would become well.

The royal libraries yielded an intriguing letter written by the court physician of the Assyrian king Essarhaddon (ruled 681–669 B.C.), which reads, in part, "As regards the cure of the [aching] teeth about which the king wrote to me, I will [now] begin with it; there is a great lot of remedies for [aching] teeth." Unfortunately, the letter does not tell us what those remedies were. Another letter, in response to a king's inquiry about his son's illness, states, "The inflammation wherewith his head, hands, [and] feet are inflamed is due to his teeth. His teeth must be drawn . . . then he will be well."

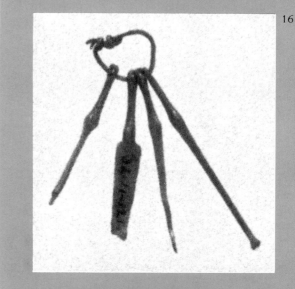

16

At the site of Tepe Gawra, about twenty miles from ancient Nineveh, archaeologists found this four-thousand-year-old set of toilet articles, which includes a makeup applicator, an ear scoop, and a finely crafted toothpick. © The University Museum, University of Pennsylvania, Philadelphia.

15

The seven-foot-tall stele of Hammurabi, dating from the eighteenth century B.C., contains 282 paragraphs regulating the practice of medicine and dentistry in Babylonia. A relief at the top, about two feet in height, shows on the left the king himself standing before the sun god Shamash, who holds in his hand a staff, symbol of power. Musée du Louvre, Paris.

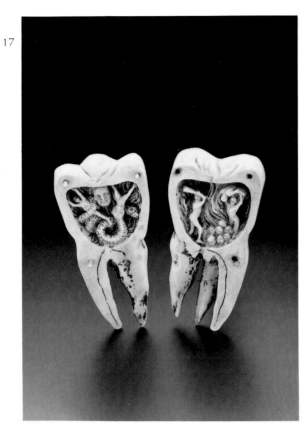

17

About 1780 an artist in southern France carved an ivory replica of a human molar tooth, about four inches high, which can be opened to reveal on the left a toothworm devouring a man. On the right, the torment of toothache is equated with the tortures of hell. Collection Deutsches Medizinhistorisches Museum, Ingolstadt.

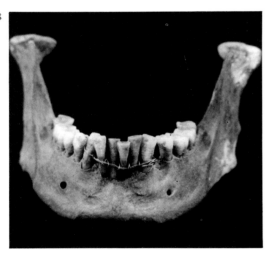

18

The owner of this mandible from ancient Sidon (Lebanon) suffered some twenty-five hundred years ago from a common modern dental problem, and the treatment received would not seem outdated today. The gums and bone receded from the base of the teeth and the incisors were bound in place by gold wire. Archaeological Museum, American University of Beirut.

The belief (stubbornly clung to until the eighteenth century A.D.) that a toothworm causes dental caries was first documented in Babylonia. A clay tablet found in the royal library recounts the myth with poetic starkness:

> *After Anu [had created heaven] . . .*
> *The earth had created the rivers,*
> *The rivers had created the canals,*
> *The canals had created the marsh,*
> *The marsh had created the worm.*
> *The worm went weeping, before Shamash,*
> *His tears flowing before Ea:*
> *"What wilt thou give me for my food?*
> *What wilt thou give me for my sucking?"*
> *"I shall give thee the ripe fig and the apricot."*
> *"Of what use are they to me, the ripe fig and the apricot?*
> *Lift me up and among the teeth*
> *And the gums cause me to dwell!*
> *The blood of the tooth will I suck,*
> *And of the gum will I gnaw the roots!"*

The Phoenicians

The Phoenicians, a people contemporary with the ancient Egyptians and Hebrews, lived in what is modern-day Lebanon. They carried on extensive trade with the other nations of the Mediterranean basin; King Solomon purchased the famed cedars of Lebanon for his temple in Jerusalem from Hiram, king of Tyre, then the principal Phoenician city. Besides cedar wood, Phoenician exports included a highly prized purple linen from Tyre and Byblos, embroidered cloth from Sidon, as well as glass, pottery, and wine. Much of the metalwork and jewelry they exported was copied from examples produced in Greece and Egypt as well as Babylonia, and even today when a piece of metalwork is found in Greece or North Africa it is difficult to know whether it is of Greek or Phoenician origin. Though lacking originality, Phoenician artisans were nevertheless exceptionally skillful, and their goldsmith's work was known and prized throughout the Mediterranean area.

Although not a great deal of material has been unearthed through archaeological excavations, enough has been found to justify the conviction that among these people were skilled practitioners and artificers who constructed sophisticated dental restorations.

In 1862 Charles Gaillardot, digging at a grave site near the ancient city of Sidon, discovered a prosthetic appliance dating from about 400 B.C. (fig. 19). It consisted of four natural lower teeth holding between them two carved ivory teeth that replaced two missing incisors. The artificial teeth were bound to the neighboring teeth by strands of gold wire.

A spectacular find in 1901, also at Sidon, was a mandible of about 500 B.C. whose anterior teeth, severely loosened by periodontal disease, had been intricately bound together with gold wire (fig. 18). The wiring is similar to that found on teeth in contemporary Egyptian tombs, indicating that there was an exchange of knowledge, perhaps of practitioners, between the two countries. Egypt had established suzerainty over Phoenicia by the sixteenth century B.C., but as the result of a great political upheaval in the fourteenth century, they lost control of the land. Nevertheless, the cultural influence of Egypt was strongly stamped upon the products of Phoenician craftsmen.

The Hebrews

Sound, healthy teeth were highly valued by the early Hebrews. There are numerous references to the importance of healthy teeth in the Old Testament, much of which deals with the period antedating 1000 B.C. Sound teeth were considered objects of beauty. In the Song of Solomon (2:2) the lover states, "Thy teeth are like a flock of sheep that are even shorn, which came up from the washing; whereof every one bears twins; and none is barren among them." Moreover, teeth were considered symbols of strength, and loss of them was equated with weakness and infirmity. The physical requirements for the role of high priest, as stated in Leviticus, prevent anyone from serving who is not a whole person, and the rabbis have interpreted this to include one who has even a single tooth missing!

In Lamentations (3:16) Jeremiah cries out, "God hath broken my teeth with gravel stones"; and Jewish tales relate that Esau wept at his encounter with Jacob after twenty years because his teeth were loose and painful. The Psalms of David often equate sound teeth with strength. In Psalm 3 David implies that his enemies have been rendered powerless by the loss of theirs: "Arise, O Lord, save me, O my God: for thou hast smitten all mine enemies upon the cheek bone; thou hast broken the teeth of the ungodly" (3:7). In the Proverbs of Solomon bad teeth symbolize weakness: "Confidence in an unfaithful man in time of trouble is like a broken tooth" (in an early Latin translation the tooth is described as *putridus*, or "decayed," rather than broken). The Bible even sets forth the punishment to be meted out to those who cause others to lose teeth: "Thou shalt give life for life, eye for eye, tooth for tooth, hand for hand, foot for foot . . . And if a man smite the eye of his servant, or the eye of his maid, that it perish; he shall let him go free for his eye's sake. And if he smite out his manservant's tooth, or his maidservant's tooth; he shall let him go free for his tooth's sake" (Exodus 21:23–27). Clearly, the early Hebrews considered the destruction of a tooth grave indeed if a bonded servant was to be given his freedom as compensation for the offense. It is therefore quite surprising that the Hebrews themselves apparently practiced no form of surgical or restorative dentistry. Instead, as we learn in the Talmud, they availed themselves of the services of Phoenician or Greek practitioners who had developed dental care to a high degree of excellence.

In addition to the written laws cited earlier, which were contained in the Torah, or Five Books of Moses, as well as in the other books of the Bible, much Jewish law is embodied in the Talmud, which consists of the law transmitted by oral tradition (Mishna) and the varying interpretations and commentaries upon this oral law (Gemara). This mass of information began to accumulate after the Babylonian captivity of 586 B.C. and was codified in the Jerusalem Talmud (A.D. 370–90) and the Babylonian Talmud (A.D. 352–427). The latter has become the standard reference source, for the yeshivas, or academies, that existed in Babylonia in the second and third centuries of the Christian Era were held in exceptionally high esteem, and the pronouncements of their rabbis were given the status of law. Many references to medicine appear in the Talmud, almost always in order to bring out a religious point or settle a religious dispute. Nevertheless, we can gain from these books insight into the status of dental care at that time and learn who delivered that care.

One of the most intriguing disputations deals with the question of what a woman might "go out" with on the Sabbath without violating a ban against carrying on that day, for the Jews consider carrying a form of work, and work was prohibited on the Sabbath. She might leave with a peppercorn in her mouth (as a breath sweetener) but not with a gold crown. The Jerusalem Talmud says, "It is clear that in the case of a gold tooth, which is valuable, she should not go out, for if it should fall [out] she would [probably] put it back," which would obviously constitute work. In addition, the tractate also forbids going out with a less costly artificial tooth, but in this case the reason given is that if it should fall out the woman would probably be too embarrassed to ask the artisan who made it for her to construct another.

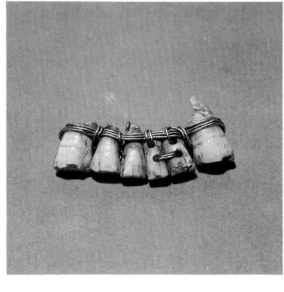

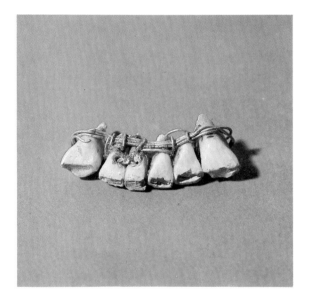

Shown here are front and back views of a mandibular fixed bridge—four natural human incisor teeth and two carved ivory teeth bound with gold wire—found in Sidon, chief city of ancient Phoenicia. The prosthesis dates between the fifth and the fourth centuries B.C. Musée du Louvre, Paris.

A study of this tractate and others of a similar nature have led to certain inferences. First, since only women are mentioned in the Talmud as having either gold crowns or artificial (single) tooth replacements, it is likely that these restorations were done for cosmetic purposes only. (One story in the Babylonian Talmud, dating from the first century A.D., concerns a maiden lady who was rejected by a man to whom she was betrothed because she displayed an unsightly artificial tooth. Rabbi Ishmael arranged to have a new one made for her of gold, and it so improved her appearance that the man accepted her in marriage.) Second, since the crown and artificial tooth mentioned in the disputation quoted above were capable of falling out, we must conclude that they were not cemented in. Third, specific craftsmen referred to as *nagra*, a category that included a variety of artisans, made the artificial teeth and crowns.

The Talmud is also rich in references to treatment supposed to be efficacious in either remedying or preventing oral problems. One was admonished not to take too much vinegar since it was "harmful to the teeth as smoke is to the eyes." However, if the gums were wounded then vinegar was recommended, as was wine. Sour fruit juice was held to be helpful for toothache and not injurious to healthy teeth. Prolonged exposure to the vapors of the bathhouse was said to result in blackened teeth, as was prolonged fasting. Spleen chewed and spit out was considered by the rabbis to be good for the teeth, leeks were considered harmful, and unripe grapes were said to make the teeth blunt.

An unusual remedy for toothache appears in a commentary by Rabbi Bar Rab Huna: he recommends placing a garlic clove ground with oil and salt on the left or right thumbnail, depending on which side of the head is the aching tooth, and putting a rim of dough around it, taking care that it not touch the flesh, for that would cause leprosy! Long lists of remedies for toothache appear throughout the Talmud, including the most blatant old wives' tales and highly repugnant "medicines." But we must assume the intent was always good, for a certain Rabbi Yochanan expressed the general belief that the person who whitens the teeth of his neighbor is better than the person who gives him milk to drink.

Tooth extractions were dreaded by the ancient Jews, much as they were by their Gentile contemporaries. One section of the Talmud advises that one ought not "make a habit of taking medicines. Do not take long strides. Avoid having a tooth extracted." Rabbi Chananel justifies avoiding an extraction, saying, "When an eyetooth is painful, do not extract it, because your eyes must suffer instead"— the inference being that the extraction would unnecessarily endanger the eyes!

An interesting aspect of the Talmudic disputations concerns the ills that might be treated on the Sabbath. In accordance with the Jewish belief in the sanctity of human life, one might violate the Sabbath when a life-threatening situation existed. Which conditions were life-threatening and which were not was determined by dividing illnesses into those that were inward and those that were outward, the latter generally being considered of a less serious nature. But into which category did toothache fall, since it was usually not life-threatening yet was an "inward" condition? One answer was reached by considering who performed the treatment. If an "expert" practitioner had to be called upon (that is, a physician, most often a pagan) then obviously the condition was a serious one. A certain rabbi consulted a pagan female practitioner on the Sabbath for the relief of a severe toothache. She is described in the Talmud as an expert, and the treatment she rendered was intricate and involved. The rabbi was thus absolved by his colleagues of any wrongdoing. By contrast, those who resorted to the ministrations of itinerant practitioners, whose work probably consisted solely in drawing teeth, would have been held to be at fault.

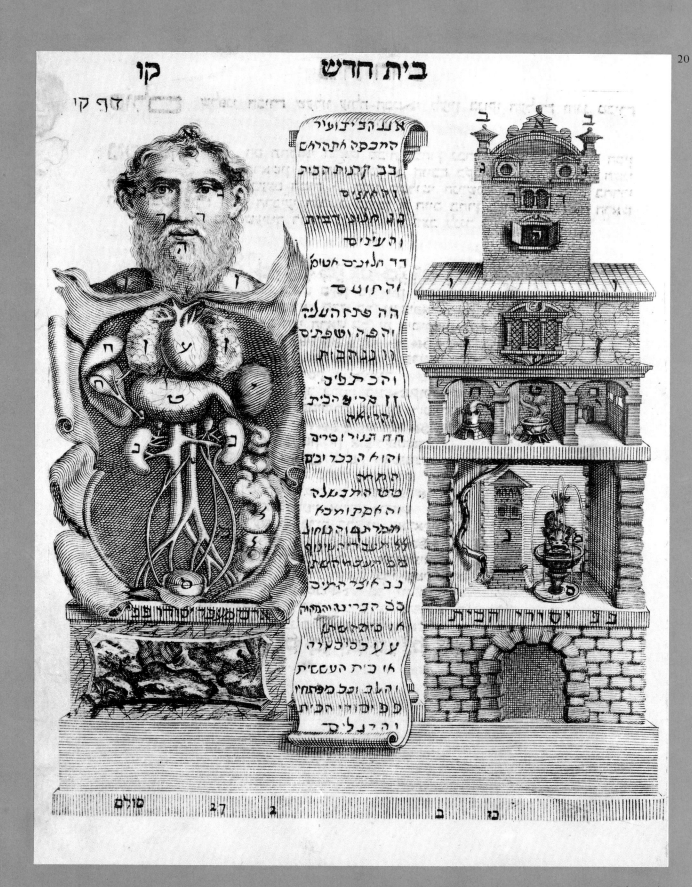

This illustration from the Hebrew book *Sefer Haols-mot o Maaseh Tovia* by Tobias Kohn, published in 1717 in Venice, compares the human body to a house. The reader is cautioned that the doorway (the mouth) must be kept scrupulously clean to protect whatever enters from contamination. Jewish Theological Seminary of America, New York.

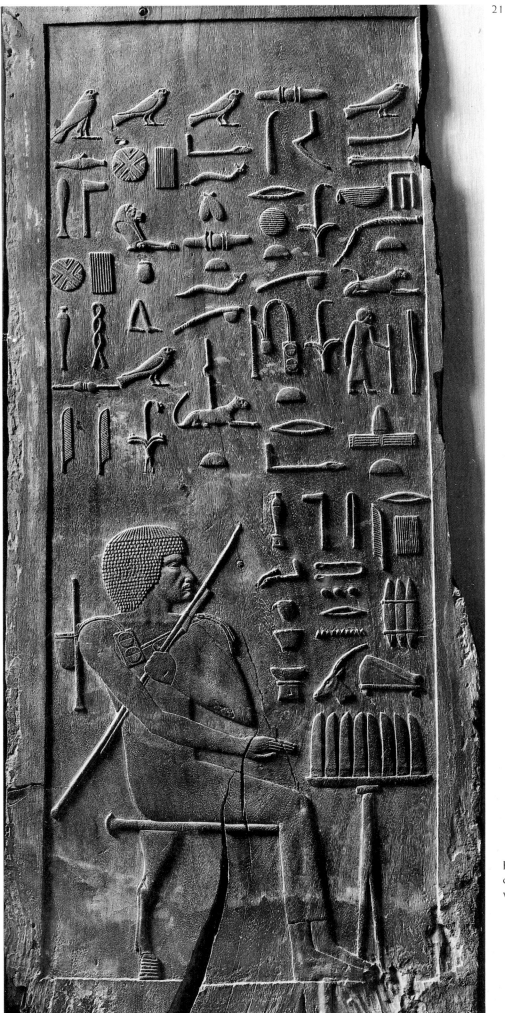

Hesi-Re, "Chief of the Toothers and the Physicians," was an Egyptian doctor of about 3000 B.C. who specialized in dentistry.

The Egyptians

About 3100 B.C., the kingdoms of Upper Egypt and Lower Egypt were united by King Menes. During the period that followed, known as the Old Kingdom (3100–2181 B.C.), there reigned a pharaoh named Zoser. About the year 2600 he ordered to be built at Saqqara one of the most enduring of all ancient edifices, the great Step Pyramid; he commissioned as architect a most versatile scholar, knowledgeable in astronomy, literature, art—and what we know him best for—medicine. This was Imhotep, who in time became venerated as the god of healing and whom the Greeks later equated with their own god Asclepius. It was to Imhotep that ill persons turned for healing. In fact, the pharaoh placed such high value upon his knowledge that he had him buried near his own tomb in the necropolis of Memphis.

The practice of medicine in Egypt was thus clearly established as long as 4,600 years ago. Soon doctors began to specialize in healing certain parts of the body and certain organ systems. More than 2,000 years later Herodotus, a Greek historian of the fifth century B.C., described this same specialization from his own observation: "The practice of medicine is so divided among them that each physician is a healer of one disease and no more. All the country is full of physicians, some of the eyes, some of the teeth, some of what pertains to the belly and some of the hidden diseases."

The earliest dentist whose name we know is Hesi-Re, who lived during the reign of Zoser and who is described on the plaque illustrated in figure 21 as "the greatest of the physicians who treat the teeth." Further evidence that dental treatment was distinct from other aspects of medical treatment is found in the stele ordered by the Pharaoh Sahura as a gift to his favorite physician, Ny-Ankh-Sekhmet. At the bottom of the stele, identified by a hieroglyphic inscription, is a small figure characterized as Men-Kaoure-Ankh, a "man of the tooth."

The Egyptians suffered from a variety of dental diseases, and even the pharaohs were not immune to their ravages. It appears that extraction was the principal remedy for the relief of dental distress. It is also probable that early dentists drilled holes through the cortical plates of the jawbones in order to relieve the pressure of the purulent exudate associated with an abscessed tooth. A number of skulls thus drilled have been found; one of the earliest, dating from the period of the Old Kingdom, is now in the collection of the Peabody Museum of Harvard University.

An intriguing similar find in a burial field near Saqqara dates from the time of the New Kingdom (1570–1085). It is a man's skull with a severely carious lower first molar. At about the level of the apices of the roots of this tooth are two perfectly cylindrical holes, each exactly five millimeters deep and exactly two millimeters in diameter (fig. 22), leading downward to the root apices. They are not at all like fistulas that might have occurred naturally, being too perfectly matched. This skull now reposes in the Musée de l'Homme in Paris. It is apparent that the Egyptians were skilled in the use of the drill, as can be seen in many of their tomb paintings.

One of the principal causes of dental disease among the early Egyptians was the coarse diet consumed by rich and poor alike. Grain for bread, a principal staple, was ground on rough stones, and during the process numerous small particles of grit became incorporated into the flour. In addition, since the early Egyptian diet was principally vegetarian, and since the soil was very sandy, much grit was consumed in the main dishes as well. Severe wear of the occlusal surfaces of the teeth resulted, with consequent pulp exposure and abscess or cyst formation. Many studies have been done on the connections between diet and dental disease in early Egypt. F. Filce Leek, an English scholar, has written extensively on such linkages.

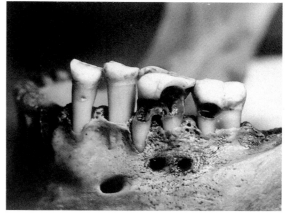

22

This close-up view of a mandible found at Saqqara, dating between 1570 and 1085 B.C., shows two cylindrical holes of exactly the same diameter and depth to the right of the mental foramen. Presumably they were drilled to relieve pressure from pus accumulated at the distal root of a severely carious first molar. Musée de l'Homme, Paris.

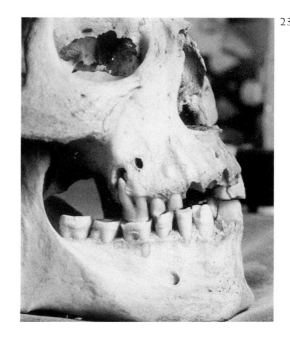

23

The crude millstones of the early Egyptians shed quantities of abrasives into the flour they ate. The occlusal surfaces of the teeth of this New Kingdom skull, found at Deir el Bahari, show signs of extreme attrition, probably the result of consuming the staff of life three times a day for many years.

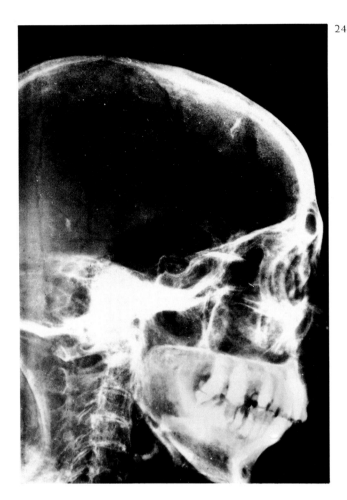

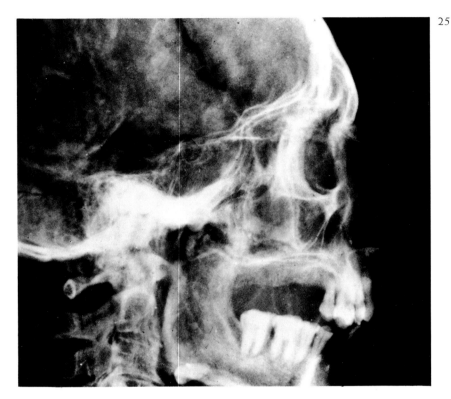

The radiograph of the skull on the left shows that Thuya, mother-in-law of Pharaoh Amenhotep III, suffered from periodontal disease and extremely broken-down dentition. Pharaoh Merenptah, who lived about two hundred years after Thuya, in the thirteenth century B.C., lost all his posterior upper teeth when the gums receded. The radiograph of his skull (right) indicates, in addition, that a considerable part of his lower jaw was also destroyed by periodontoclasia.

Many ancient skulls show evidence of trauma to the teeth due in part to the generally precarious nature of life in those days as well as to incessant warfare. Avulsion of teeth due to trauma was not uncommon. Malocclusion was also prevalent, with the pharaonic skulls showing particularly striking evidence of severe protrusion of the upper front teeth.

There is considerable disagreement as to the nature of dentistry in ancient Egypt. Oral medicine was indeed practiced; however, it is likely that the teeth were not operated upon, for even pharaonic mummies show no evidence of such care but rather exhibit severe natural dental destruction. It is fortunate for us that the Egyptians learned to make writing paper from the papyrus plant, for the extremely dry climate of the land has preserved these papyri for thousands of years. The principal documents dealing with medical treatment are the Hearst, the Edwin Smith, and the Georg Ebers papyri. The last, in the library of Leipzig University, is the most voluminous and the best preserved. Dating from about 1550 B.C. it is not an original work but merely a compilation of many medical texts of still earlier times, some written as early as 3500 B.C. It contains numerous references to dental ills, including gingivitis, erosion, pulpitis, and toothache. Among the treatments cited is one to cure "the throbbing of bennet blisters of the teeth," probably some type of swelling of the gum. In order to "cure the tooth that gnaws unto the upper part of the flesh," one was advised to use this recipe: "Reduce to a paste and apply on the tooth one part cumin, one part incense, one part onion."

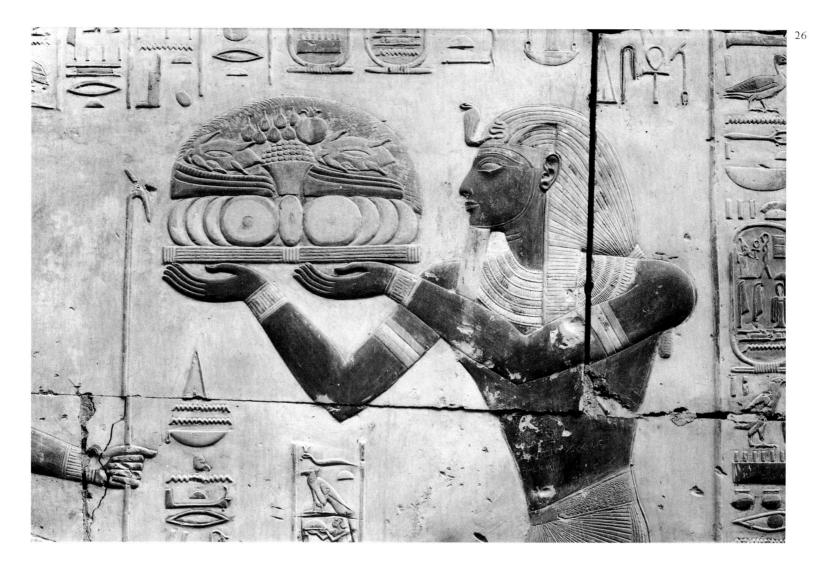

In this carved limestone relief Pharaoh Sety I gives food to the goddess Isis. Prominent on the tray are the round loaves of coarse bread that were the chief staple of the Egyptian diet. The goddess was in no danger, but both royalty and commoners in time suffered the results of chewing Egyptian bread with its high grit content, as can be seen in figure 23.

Although the Ebers Papyrus makes no mention of surgical intervention for dental ills, the Edwin Smith Papyrus, of the seventeenth century B.C., cites numerous operations of fractures and dislocations of the mandible; compound, comminuted fractures of the maxilla; perforation of the zygoma; and laceration of the lip. Since forceps are so prominently pictured in various stela and wall carvings, we can assume that extractions were indeed carried out.

Oral hygiene seems to have been given no thought by these ancient people. Though thousands of toilet and cosmetic articles have been excavated or found in tombs, no toothbrush or similar cleaning device has yet been discovered. Many skulls show severe accretions of tartar, with consequent periodontal breakdown and bone loss. No attempt seems ever to have been made to remove these noxious accumulations from the teeth.

Two intriguing finds have created much speculation and argument among dental historians. One is a pair of molar teeth bound together with gold wire, dating from about 2500 B.C. (fig. 28). Some scholars have concluded that the wiring was done during the patient's life to strengthen a periodontally weakened tooth by attaching it to a stronger one. When the teeth were found by Hermann Junker in 1914 in a burial chamber at Gizeh the wire had what appeared to be calculus adhering to it, and this would support their theory; however, the looser tooth may have been bound to its neighbor postmortem to prevent its loss during the embalming and burial of the corpse.

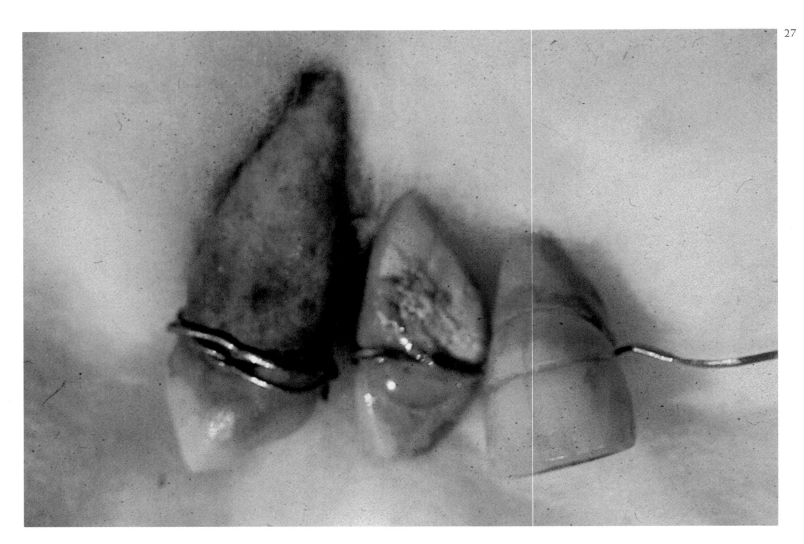

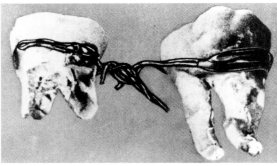

In 1952 Shafik Farid found at El Qatta, near Cairo, an upper right canine tooth bound twice with gold wire and two right incisor teeth fastened to each other with wire threaded through the central incisor and wound once around the lateral incisor. This Old Kingdom fixed bridge was probably inserted in the mouth of a corpse after death, though some scholars have claimed it was a prosthesis for a living person.

Working at Gizeh in 1914, Hermann Junker found these molar teeth dating from about 3000–2500 B.C. They were bound together with gold wire either during life or possibly after death, while the corpse was prepared for burial. Roemer-Pelizaeus Museum, Hildesheim.

Still more intriguing remains were discovered by Shafik Farid in 1952: three teeth bound together by gold wire (fig. 27). Although they have studied the prosthesis extensively, dental historians have been unable to agree on the type of treatment involved. Some have claimed it represents an early example of tooth replacement, with the right central incisor as the pontic, supported by the teeth on either side. However, since this incisor has a complete root it is difficult to see how it could have been placed in the mouth without impinging on the gum in the area of the missing tooth. A more reasonable explanation is, once again, that the tooth was replaced postmortem. The Egyptians did their very best to inter a corpse in as complete a state as possible, for they firmly believed that the body must be kept intact to house the soul in the afterworld. Nevertheless, the find offers still further proof that the ancient Egyptians had a drill capable of cutting a fine hole through the body of a tooth.

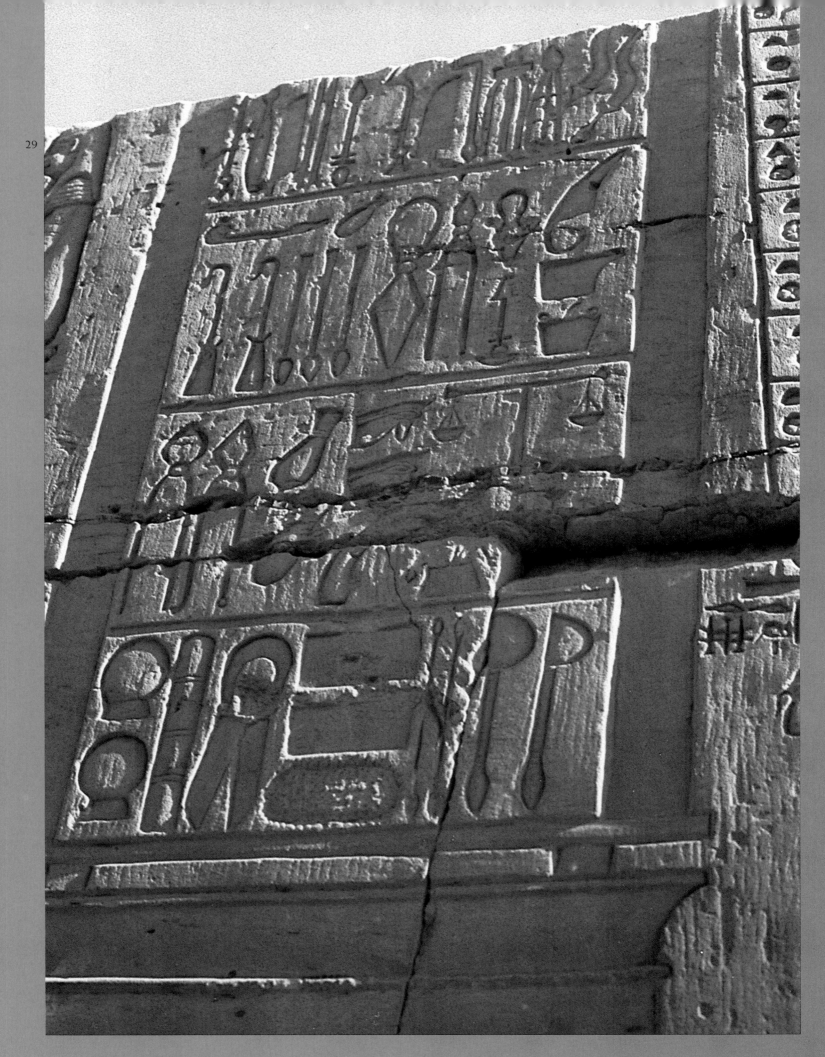

29

This carving on the wall of the Ptolemaic temple
(304–30 B.C.) at Kom Ombo, just north of Aswan,
shows many surgical instruments, including knives
and several kinds of forceps.

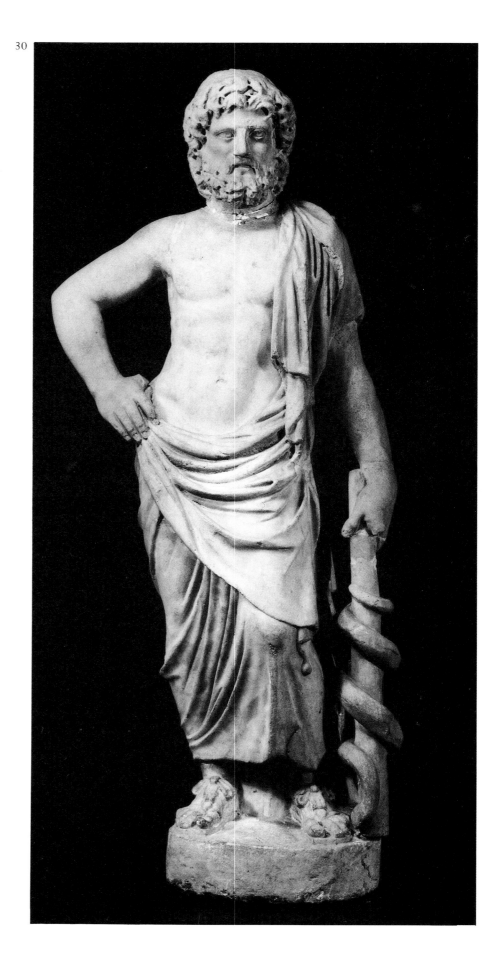

Asclepius, the Greek and later the Roman god of healing, is usually represented holding a staff encircled by a snake, which is the emblem of medicine. Another, very similar Roman statue in the Borghese Museum includes at the god's left a small deity called a *telesphoros*, associated with life, death, and sleep. The little figure expresses the close relationship between the cult of Asclepius and the practice of temple-sleep. Wellcome Institute Library, London.

III
THE CLASSICAL WORLD

Greece

The origins of classical Greek culture lie in the displacement by Dorian invaders of the Achaeans, the first Greek peoples, who had built a great Bronze Age civilization in Greece and later in Crete. Crete—which at that time enjoyed the most advanced European civilization—had long been the home of a chthonic religion, one in which worship of the underworld was a central feature. Fundamental to this worship was the symbolic snake, and probably it is this creature that became the emblem associated with the Greek god of healing, Asclepius. Using his symbol, doctors invoked divine assistance in their healing. About 1200 B.C. the Achaeans were pushed south by the Dorians into small pocket strongholds on the mainland, and about 1100 B.C. they moved out to islands in the seas bordering their land as well as to the coast of Asia Minor. The Dorians, who swept after them, seized much of the mainland and settled in Crete and also on the islands of Cos and Cnidus.

Gradually the inhabitants of Greece, Ionia, and the Aegean Islands began to think and act as a cultural unit. Toward the beginning of the sixth century B.C., they developed a comprehensive philosophical system of thought, and the natural sciences and medicine were an outgrowth of this system. Medical schools came into being at Cos and Cnidus and they were flourishing by the middle of the fifth century B.C. The earliest of the Hippocratic writings can be traced to about the fifth century B.C., but rational medicine, as advocated by the Hippocratic school, existed side by side with sacerdotal medicine, based on the worship of Asclepius. The cult had numerous centers called *asklepions*, and the most prominent was at Epidaurus.

The general method of treatment at the *asklepions* was fairly formalized. The patient first relaxed in the holy precincts, took in the beauty of the surroundings, and enriched his soul by attending theatrical performances. Then he would present himself to the priest, who would give him a sleeping potion and direct him to a mat on the floor or to a bed, where he would fall into a fitful sleep. The priest, often carrying sacred snakes, would visit the patient while he was in this state of mixed sleep and wakefulness, and it is likely that the patient mistook the priest for the god himself. The priest would advise the semihypnotized patient as to the course of his treatment. If the patient was cured it was customary for him to make a temple offering of a stone tablet carved in the shape of the affected part of his body and inscribed with thanks to the god for granting recovery from the illness. Many of these votive tablets have been found at Epidaurus and at other sites, and among them are representations of teeth and jaws, evidence that dental maladies were treated.

In contrast to this system of practice is the Hippocratic method. Probably the work of numerous early physicians at Cos and Cnidus, the extant writings are known collectively as the Hippocratic Corpus.

Of the father of medicine, Hippocrates, little is known. He was born at Cos about 460 B.C. and died between 377 and 359 B.C. He practiced and taught not only at Cos but also at Thasos, Athens, Thrace, and elsewhere. Central to Hippocrates' teaching was the rational approach to disease; treatment was based on careful observation of the patient, with an attempt—albeit primitive—to treat observable problems *rationally*.

In an attempt to explain states of disease and health, Hippocrates postulated the existence of four principal fluids in the body, the cardinal humors: blood, phlegm, black bile, and yellow bile. He also suggested that there were four elemental conditions—cold, hot, dry, and moist—and that a state of health existed when these humors and qualities were in balance. Disruption of the natural balance would result in disease: for example, too much phlegm made the body too

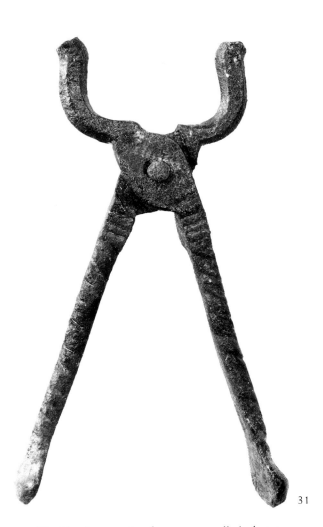

31

The Greek extraction forceps was called *odontagra*. National Archaeological Museum, Athens.

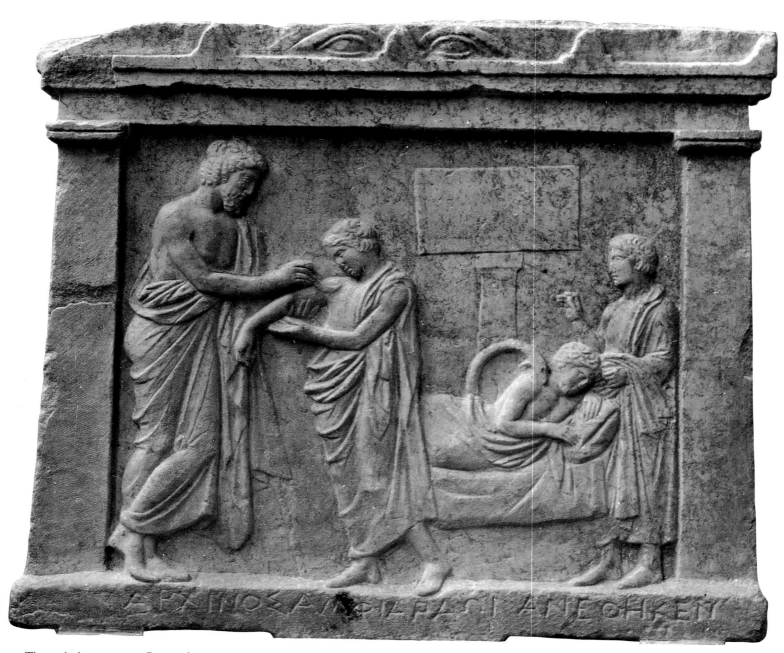

This stele from ancient Greece shows a scene in an *asklepion*, a center of healing based on the worship of Asclepius. One suppliant is being treated by a votary of the god in the foreground. A priest visits another patient lying on a bed while a sacred snake coils around him. National Archaeological Museum, Athens.

cold and too wet, as when the patient suffered from the common cold and "excess" phlegm exuded from the nose.

Scattered through the Hippocratic writings are numerous references to the teeth, their formation, and their eruption; and to maladies of the teeth and mouth and methods of treatment. They show awareness of the way teeth developed: "The first teeth are formed by the nourishment of the fetus in the womb, and after birth by the mother's milk. Those that come forth after these are shed are formed by food and drink. The shedding of the first teeth generally takes place at about seven years of age, those that come forth after this grow old with the man, unless some illness destroys them." *On Dentition*, written in the form of brief sentences or aphorisms, contains much in the way of folk belief concerning tooth eruption; for example, "Other conditions being equal, those children who cut their teeth in the winter get over the teething period best," and "Those who during dentition do not get thinner and who are very drowsy run the risk of becoming subject to convulsions."

A basic, mistaken Hippocratic premise was that cold creates spasms in the blood vessels, causing the blood to stagnate and turn to pus. Specific parts of the body were believed to be more susceptible to cold, and thus we read, "The bones, the teeth, and the tendons have cold as an enemy, warmth as a friend; because it is from these parts that come the spasms . . . that cold induces, heat removes."

Hippocrates confused the accumulation of fluid where there was inflammation and consequent edema with the cause of the inflammation itself. In his book *On Affections*, he observes: "In cases of toothache, if the tooth is decayed and loose it must be extracted. If it is neither decayed nor loose, but still painful, it is necessary to dessicate it by cauterizing. Masticatories also do good, as the pain derives from mucus insinuating itself under the roots of the teeth. Teeth are eroded and become decayed partly by the mucus, and partly by food, when they are by nature weak and badly fixed in the mouth."

Book Seven of *Epidemics* cites numerous case histories, many of which explain the importance Hippocrates attached to toothache and dental disease: "At Cardias, the son of Metrodoros after a toothache had gangrene of the jaw; terrible overgrowth of flesh on his gums; he gave a moderate amount of pus; the molar teeth and the jaw fell out."

Hippocrates believed that problems with the teeth arose from a natural predisposition or an inherited weakness. Extraction was to be considered only when a tooth was loose, for the operation was regarded as fraught with danger. But, "as to the pincers for pulling out teeth," he says, "anyone can handle them, because evidently the manner in which they are to be used is simple."

The dental forceps he refers to, made of iron and known as *odontagra*, have been discovered in various excavated sites in Greece. One, said to have been kept by the priests in the temple of Apollo, god of healing, at Delphi, is made of lead, a metal too soft to be used in extracting a firmly rooted tooth. Perhaps it was meant to hammer home a message: do not extract a tooth unless it is loose enough to be taken out with a lead forceps.

Many more references to the teeth, jaws, and other oral structures are to be found in the Hippocratic writings, spread throughout the many books. Apparently, whatever dental practice existed was performed by the general physician. This point is brought out even more clearly by Aristotle, the greatest philosopher of antiquity, who was born nearly a century after Hippocrates, in 384 B.C., and who died in 322 B.C. He wrote widely and is considered the father of comparative anatomy. In his book *History of Animals* he deals extensively with the differing dentitions of different classes of animals. He also wrote on human teeth and their afflictions. Although he believed that theory should follow demonstrable fact, he made many incorrect assumptions, such as that men have more teeth than women and that teeth continue to grow throughout a person's lifetime. The following passage from *Mechanics* gives a clue to the status of dentistry in his day. Discussing extractions, Aristotle says:

> Why do doctors extract teeth more easily by adding the weight of the *odontagra* than by using the hand only? Can it be said that this occurs because the tooth escapes more easily from the hand than from the forceps? Ought not the irons to slip off the tooth more easily than the fingers, whose tips, being soft, can be applied around the tooth much better? The dental forceps is formed by two levers. . . . By means of this [double lever] it is much easier to move the tooth, but after having moved it, it is easier to extract it with the hand than with the instrument.

Thus, we may conclude that, contrary to Hippocratic teaching, extracted teeth were no longer exclusively loose teeth. And those who extracted the teeth are specifically referred to as "doctors."

Greek culture spread throughout much of the known world in the wake of Alexander the Great, and one of the prime centers for study came to be the city named for him, Alexandria. Here the arts and sciences flourished and here during the third century B.C. lived the noted physicians Erasistratus and Herophilus.

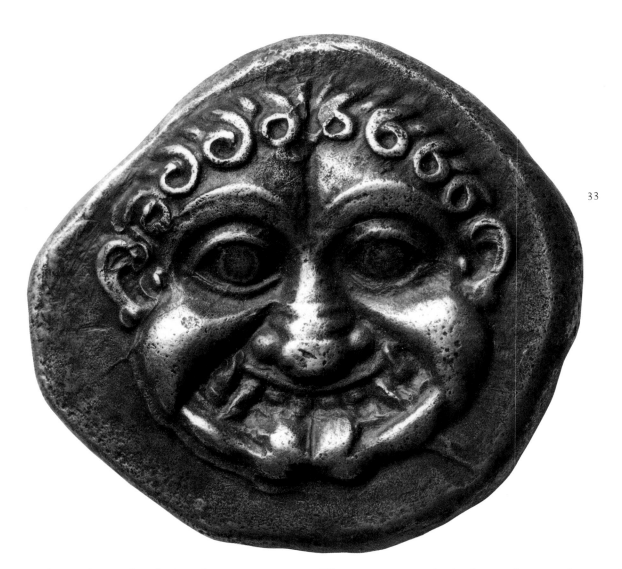

Animals bare their teeth to frighten their enemies, and men of primitive tribes sharpen their teeth in imitation of beasts of prey. On this Greek coin of the sixth century B.C. the grotesque teeth of the mythical Gorgon are an important symbol of her power to dispel evil influences.

They were apparently the first to dissect cadavers and probably also the bodies of condemned criminals. Although little remains of their writings, they were described in later centuries as having discussed the blood supply to the teeth as well as cases of persons who had died from the extraction of a tooth.

The practice of oral hygiene was slow in coming to Greece. A disciple of Aristotle, Theophrastus (died c. 287 B.C.), wrote that it was considered a virtue to shave frequently and to have white teeth; yet regular dental care was not known until Greece became a Roman province. Under Roman influence, the Greeks learned to use a multitude of materials as tooth cleansers, among them pumice, talc, emery, ground alabaster, coral powder, and iron rust. Diocles of Carystus, an Athenian physician of Aristotle's time, admonished, "Every morning you should rub your gums and teeth with your bare fingers and with finely pulverized mint, inside and outside, and remove thus the adherent food particles."

Although the Greeks considered strong teeth indicative of good health, large teeth were for them a symbol of ferocity. Gorgons, mythical creatures described by Homer as "frightful phantoms of Hades," were in every aspect terrifying and unnatural. Their heads were entwined with serpents, their hands were of brass, and their bodies were covered with impenetrable scales. Their teeth were said to be of brass and as long as the tusks of a wild boar. Yet, with all these horrible accouterments to choose from, the artist who designed an archaic Greek coin of about 450 B.C. emphasized only the elongated teeth to portray the creatures' frightful power (fig. 33).

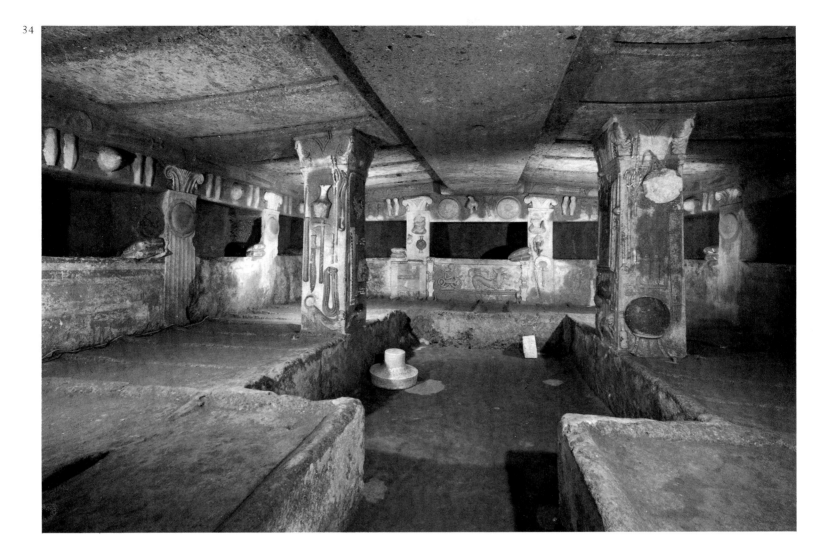

Etruria

The Etruscans probably emigrated from Asia Minor to the Italian peninsula and settled there in prehistoric times. They first occupied the central region between the Arno on the north and the Tiber on the south; later they spread north into the Po valley. At the end of the seventh century the Etruscans conquered the small settlement of Rome. In the sixth century the Romans revolted, overthrew their Etruscan masters, and conquered them in turn. However, in typical fashion they adopted and expanded on much of the Etruscans' highly developed culture and many of their skills, including their advanced dental practices.

In truth, we know very little about the mysterious Etruscans. They were so effectively integrated into Roman life that almost all traces of their civilization disappeared, save their burial grounds. We are certain, however, that on their arrival in Italy, like other nations of the Middle East, the Etruscans practiced cremation (as did the Romans until about 200 B.C.); about 500 B.C., with the introduction of inhumation, both methods of burial were resorted to. Their tombs have yielded a rich harvest for dental historians, for even if the rest of the corpse was reduced to ashes its teeth remained. Principal among the finds are a variety of bridges made to replace one or more missing teeth. The usual practice was to devise bands of soft, pure gold to surround remaining teeth. Bands were also constructed to carry the artificial replacements, and all these bands were soldered together. In some cases human teeth, cut off at their necks, were fastened to the gold band by rivets or pivots. In most cases, however, the teeth of calves or oxen were used to simu-

The Etruscan Tomb of the Reliefs at Cerveteri, about twenty miles north of Rome, looks much as it did in the fourth century B.C. It resembles a room in an Etruscan house and is decorated with stucco replicas of household utensils and surgical instruments.

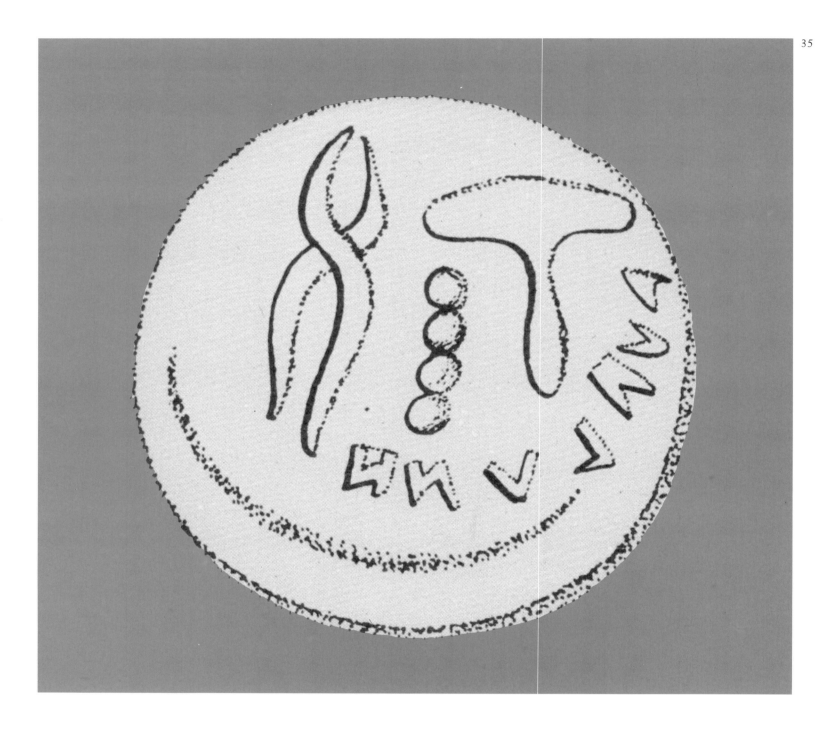

A forceps for extracting teeth appears on the Etruscan coin of about 300 B.C. shown in this modern drawing.

late the missing natural ones. In some cases a groove was cut down the middle of a wide ox's tooth to give the appearance of two teeth. Most of these teeth were probably removed from the jaws of young animals before they had erupted since few show signs of wear or attrition on their biting edges.

Some tombs have yielded clay tablets with an entire set of teeth carved on them; these served as votive offerings to the deities who might be expected to heal diseases of the mouth and aching jaws or teeth.

36

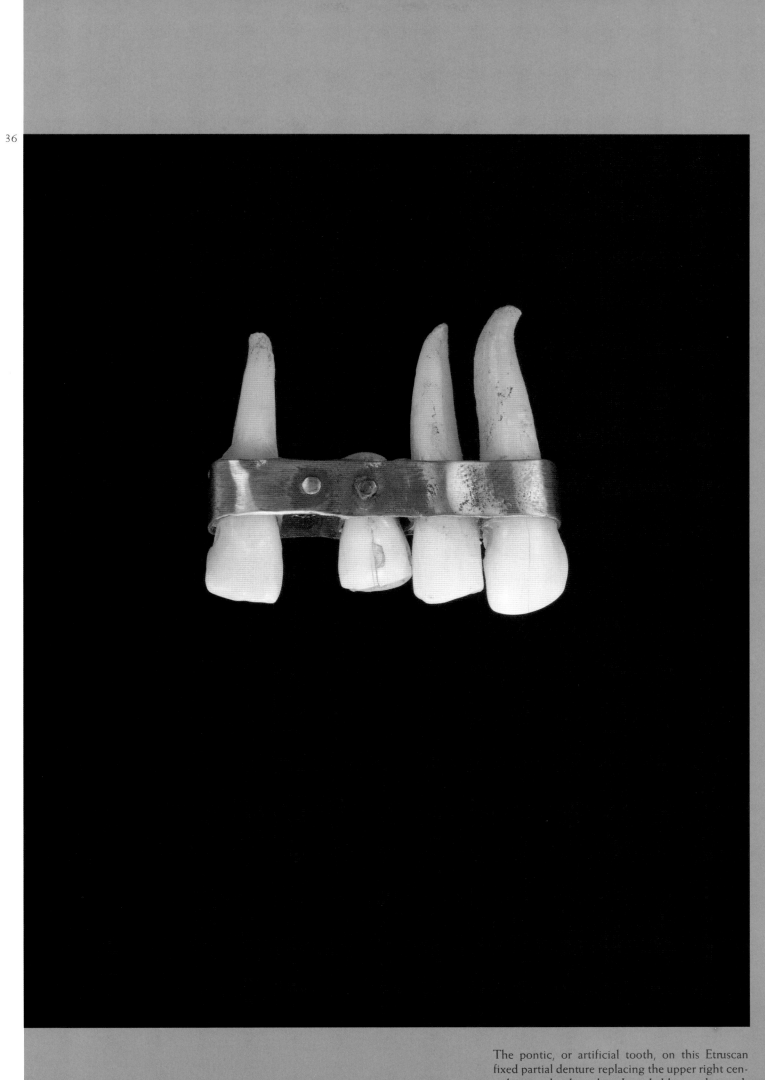

The pontic, or artificial tooth, on this Etruscan fixed partial denture replacing the upper right central incisor has been lost. It probably was the tooth of an ox riveted to the gold strap. Musée de l'Ecole Dentaire de Paris.

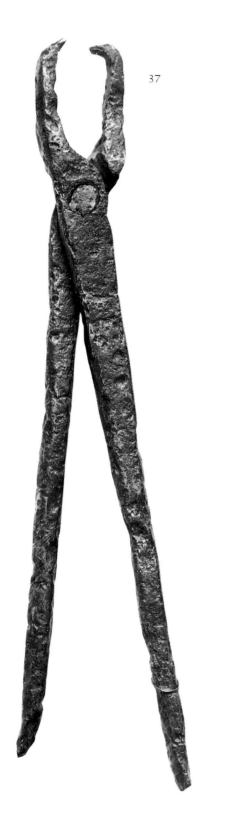

37

This Roman bronze pincers or forceps is of the type carved on the right side of the gravestone shown in figure 38. Magyar Nemzeti Museum, Budapest.

Rome

When the medical profession was in its infancy in Rome, dentistry was being practiced there. About 450 B.C. a commission of magistrates was empaneled to write a body of laws for the nation, later known as the Laws of the Twelve Tables. At that time the wealthy customarily burned or buried their dead with gold ornaments in order to honor them. But gold was scarce and the elders feared that this practice would weaken the state economically; thus, one of the new laws specifically forbade the burial of gold with a corpse—with the specific exception of dental devices: "It shall not be unlawful to bury or burn [the corpse] with the gold with which the teeth may perchance be bound together."

Who was it who "bound the teeth" with gold? In order to answer that question, we must briefly discuss higher education, including professional education, in Rome. Higher education was open only to the limited number of freeborn members of society who could afford it. Even after close contact with Greece had popularized training in philosophy and science, the Roman ideal of the liberally educated person remained the complete orator. To excel in public affairs was the goal of the freeborn citizen. Education began with the teaching of the fundamentals of reading and writing, and then the child was ready for the rhetoric master. "Besides oratory, all knowledge should be pursued," said Cicero. But for the Roman citizen this would not include the pursuit of medical knowledge. Men of wealth like Cicero found it natural to believe that liberal studies should not be directed toward making money. Asked to clarify his views on liberal studies, the renowned Stoic philosopher Seneca said, "No study is to be included among the good which results in money-making. . . . It is the study of wisdom that is lofty, brave, and great-souled. All other studies are puny and puerile."

Yet the Romans had need of practitioners of the healing arts, and these came from three major groups: foreigners, especially Greeks; slaves; and freedmen. Cicero in his book *Duties* (1:42) listed medicine as an honorable profession for people of a certain social station, that is, slaves or freedmen—not native Romans.

The first foreign physician in Rome we know of was a Greek who practiced there about the year 219 B.C. However, the first of the renowned Greeks to win fame and fortune in Rome as a physician was Asclepiades, a native of Bithynia in Asia Minor, who arrived in Rome in 91 B.C. Although he had no formal medical training, he achieved marked success in his chosen field and founded what may be considered the first medical school of ancient Rome. This laid the groundwork for the establishment of the first true medical school, albeit a primitive one, the Schola Medicorum, founded about the year A.D. 14. Under the emperor Vespasian its teachers became civil servants.

Women, too, were found in the ranks of the medical practitioners. (They had little reason to strive for "professional" learning, for the rhetoric schools trained orators and pleaders, and women never gained the right to practice law in ancient Rome.) The earliest women doctors were Greeks who combined midwifery with magic and probably also beauty treatments. However, in the second century A.D. the famous physician Soranus of Ephesus declared that women wishing to enter medical practice should have the "ability to write, a good memory, health, an even temper, discretion, a knowledge of dietetics, of pharmacy and, to some extent, of surgery"—a not unimpressive list of qualifications. Women physicians were ultimately recognized as the equals of their male colleagues, for the code of the emperor Justinian, promulgated in the sixth century, refers to "physicians of either sex."

There is no word for dentist in the early Latin language, for dentistry as a separate profession did not exist among the Romans but was included as part of medical practice, and Roman physicians made no distinction between diseases affecting the mouth and teeth and those affecting other parts of the body. Nor did nonprofessionals specialize in dentistry; although we have extensive knowledge of the services performed by Roman barbers, no mention is ever made of

A Greek surgeon in Rome named Chelerino died there about A.D. 4. That he practiced dentistry may be deduced from the forceps and extracted tooth carved on his tombstone in the cemetery of the Basilica of San Lorenzo Fuori le Mura.

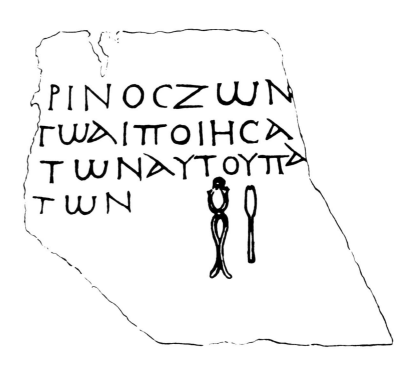

their extracting teeth. Indeed, the encyclopedist Celsus, writing about the time of Tiberius, described in detail the surgical instruments used by the physicians of his day and included among them forceps and a special instrument known as *tenaculum* for the extraction of the roots of the teeth.

An astute observer, Celsus (c. 25 B.C.–c. A.D. 50) wrote one of the most authoritative compendiums of medical knowledge in ancient times, yet he is believed not to have been a physician. In *On Medicine*, which has served as a basic text until recent times, he discusses numerous aspects of dentistry. While references to simple oral hygiene and basic treatment of such problems as teething difficulties are scattered throughout the various chapters—a prescription in Chapter Twenty-five of Book Five, composed of ten ingredients to be used to produce sleep in persons tormented by toothache, for example—the whole of Chapter Nine in Book Six deals with toothache. This affliction, which Celsus describes as "among the worst of tortures," was to be treated with a variety of hot poultices, mouth rinses, steam applications, purgatives and laxatives, and a variety of other remedies. He advised the owner of a decayed tooth to be in no haste to extract it; and if certain remedies previously cited were of no use, he suggested that other, more powerful ones ought to be tried. If the tooth was finally to be drawn, he suggested filling the cavity with linen thread or lead so that the crown would not fracture when the beaks of the forceps were applied to it.

Numerous other subjects were taken up in Celsus's book: the use of the file to smooth fractured crowns; the repositioning of malposed newly erupted permanent teeth; the treatment of jaw fractures; the ligation of loose teeth to stabilize them. He also considered the need for oral hygiene: black stains on the teeth were to be scraped off and the teeth rubbed with a mixture of pounded rose leaves, gallnuts, and myrrh, after which the mouth was to be rinsed with pure wine.

Another famed Roman physician who wrote extensively on dental treatment was Scribonius Largus, personal doctor to the emperor Claudius (about A.D. 47). Among his various suggestions for treating toothache was the following passage, which gave further credence to the ancient notion that a toothworm was responsible for dental caries: "Suitable against toothache are fumigations made with the seeds of the hyoscyamus [probably belladonna or henbane] scattered on burning charcoal; these must be followed by rinsings of the mouth with hot water; in this way, sometimes, as it were, small worms are expelled."

In spite of the attempts of Celsus and others to put the treatment of disease on what they believed to be a rational basis, it was difficult to root out myths like that of the toothworm and the old wives' tales that were generally relied on for the relief of physical distress. Early medicine at Rome was in fact a combination of the primitive magic of the Italic peoples mingled with the priestly lore of the Etruscans and superstitions of Greek origin. Belief in magic cures is reflected in an ancient fragment, a magic charm for "footache" repeated "thrice nine times" while one spat and touched the ground:

> Earth take the pest to thee!
> Health, tarry here with me!

The great naturalist Pliny the Elder (who died during the eruption of Vesuvius in A.D. 79) described a cure for toothache that consisted of finding a frog in the light of the full moon, prying open its mouth and spitting into it, and uttering some such formula as "Frog, go, and take my toothache with thee!" He mentioned an even more bizarre toothache preventive—to bite off the head of a live mouse twice a month—although he was careful to add that he would not vouch for the efficacy of the treatment.

The most concrete evidence that it was the physician who practiced dentistry in Rome can be found in the works of Galen, who lived in the capital from about 166 until his death in about 201. He had a tremendous reputation and served as physician to the emperor Septimius Severus. He was a voluminous writer who gathered all the medical knowledge of his time, and his work continued to be the authoritative account of the science until Renaissance times.

At first Galen followed Hippocrates' recommendation to observe and study and then make a diagnosis and a plan of treatment. In time, however, as his reputation grew, he abandoned this course, basing his theories as well as his practice upon beliefs and assumptions rather than observations. He stopped dissecting corpses, studying animals instead, and many times his inferences were incorrect. The physicians of the Middle Ages slavishly followed Galen, and not until the Renaissance, when great advances were made in anatomy, were his ideas questioned.

Galen based his theory of pathology upon the Hippocratic concept of the four cardinal humors, wary of upsetting their balance lest disease result. Although in the following passage from On Hygiene Galen is in error as to the causative factors involved in caries, pyorrhea, and other diseases of the mouth, he is quite clear as to who treated these conditions and that they *were* treated.

> When the head becomes disordered in nature it produces many excrements from which lesions of the lower organs occur, because the excrement passes to them. Now most readily their passage is to the mouth. . . . It is obvious also that uvulitis, tonsillitis, and gingivitis, and cervical adenitis, and dental caries, and ulcers, and pyorrhea in the mouth are due to the catarrhal ichors descending to them from the head. And the great majority of doctors either incise the uvula or give drugs to promote expectoration of what has flowed down through the trachea into the lung. But some doctors treat the stomach, some the teeth and mouth or even the conditions in the nose. . . . But it were better, I think, to remove the source of trouble by strengthening the head.

In addition to the treatment of oral diseases and the extraction of teeth, the Romans were skilled in restoring carious teeth with gold crowns and replacing missing teeth by means of fixed bridgework. Reference to gold wiring in the Laws of the Twelve Tables suggests that prosthodontics was practiced in the early Republic. By the Christian Era, dental restorations had become quite sophisticated, and full and partial dentures were not uncommon.

The satirists of the empire made reference to practitioners who grew rich supplying artificial teeth and other prosthetic devices and in the same context they

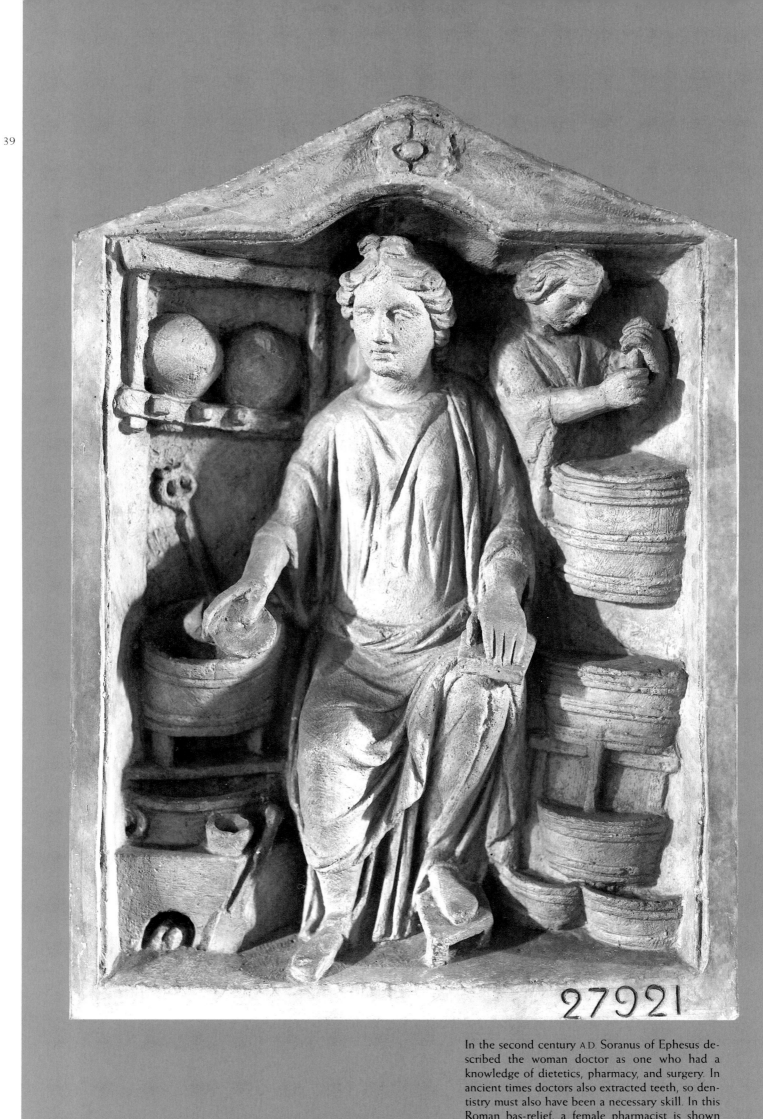

27921

In the second century A.D. Soranus of Ephesus described the woman doctor as one who had a knowledge of dietetics, pharmacy, and surgery. In ancient times doctors also extracted teeth, so dentistry must also have been a necessary skill. In this Roman bas-relief, a female pharmacist is shown among the instruments of her calling. Musée des Antiquités Nationales, St. Germain-en-Laye.

mention physicians who have amassed tremendous wealth. Thus, it is not unreasonable to assume that prosthetic appliances were fashioned by goldsmiths or other artisans and that they were then placed in the mouth by the physician, just as dentists and laboratory technicians share responsibilities today.

Much of what we know of Roman dentistry (indeed of most aspects of Roman life) comes from the writings of the satirists, principal among whom were Martial and Juvenal. Martial's writings (he died about A.D. 103) are replete with references to dental appliances:

> Lucania has white teeth, Thaïs brown. How comes it?
> One has false teeth, one her own.
>
> And you, Galla, lay aside your teeth at night
> Just as you do your silken dress.

In one of his epigrams a dentifrice powder speaks to an old woman who has false teeth: "What have you got to do with me? Let a girl use me. I am not accustomed to clean bought teeth." Yet another passage preserves for us the name of a prominent Roman dental practitioner:

> Gallus, I'm at your service all the day
> Trudging the Aventine three times each way;
> Cascellius draws bad teeth or does repairs,
> Hyginus burns from eyelids worrying hairs.
> A knifeless Fannius docks lax uvulas,
> Eros removes from slaves degrading scars.
> Hermes, like Podalirius, ruptures cures;
> Who, Gallus, heals an injury like ours?

In another writing he again mentions Cascellius, who, he says, "has grown rich like a senator among the grandes and belles dames and who cures the dental diseases, and how he can pull teeth!"

The Romans had a high regard for oral hygiene. Although they did not have soap, they did use water freely for washing. The daily ablutions made in the fourth century were described in verse by Ausonius, a scholar from Bordeaux, in his ode "Ephemeris: The Occupations of a Day": "Come, slave, up! Give me my slippers and my muslin mantle. Bring me the garment [amictus] you have got ready for me, for I am going forth. And pour out the running water that I may wash my hands, my mouth, my eyes. . . ."

The use of tooth-cleaning powders was apparently widespread, and the more involved their preparation and the more numerous their ingredients, the more highly were they regarded. A variety of substances were used for this dentifricium—bones, eggshells, and oyster shells. Having been burnt and sometimes mixed with honey, they were reduced to a fine powder. Although fancy and superstition dictated the choice of ingredients, the addition of such astringents as myrrh or niter suggests a desire not only to clean the teeth but to strengthen them when loose. References have been found to a substance that the Romans called nitrum, probably either potassium carbonate or sodium carbonate, which was burnt and rubbed on the teeth to restore their color.

In one regard at least, upper-class Romans outdid hygiene-conscious people of today: when guests were invited to dinner they were provided not only with spoons and knives but also with elaborately decorated toothpicks of metal, often of gold, which they took home with them. And it was considered quite proper to pick the teeth between each course of the meal!

Apollonia, Patron Saint of Dentists

In the early days of the Roman Empire, the newly formed Christian sect enjoyed many privileges and immunities, but during and after the reign of Nero it suffered a series of repressive persecutions. By 225 the Church was growing rapidly, and this disquieted the government since the Church refused to recognize the state religion and the divinity of the emperor. Many of their practices and attitudes were viewed with suspicion by non-Christians, and there were uprisings against them in many cities of the empire during the third century.

The Church Fathers of those early days kept in touch with each other by letter. In one communication to Fabius, bishop of Antioch—reported by the chronicler Eusebius (265–339[?]) in his *Church History*—Dionysius, bishop of Alexandria, recounted the story of Apollonia. Daughter of a prominent magistrate in Alexandria, she had been arrested and offered the choice of renouncing Christianity and professing faith in pagan beliefs or being burned at the stake. When she refused to recant, said Dionysius, "a mob seized this marvelous aged virgin, Apollonia, broke her teeth and threatened to burn her alive." Seeing the pyre lit, and recognizing that death was near, Apollonia asked to be untied so that she might kneel and say her prayers. When this was done she leaped into the flames, thereby demonstrating that she died of her own free will, a martyr to her faith. Legend has it that as she was being consumed by the fire she called out that those who suffered from toothache and invoked her name would be relieved of their suffering. Apollonia was canonized a saint in the year 249, and her feast day is February 9.

A cult associated with Saint Apollonia developed relatively quickly in Europe, most probably because of the ubiquitousness of dental ills. Almost every church and cathedral on the Continent contains a likeness of the saint, in sculpture, stained glass, fresco, or needlework. Her martyrdom has also been the subject of numerous paintings by artists ranging from the most renowned masters to the simplest folk painters. And in spite of the fact that Dionysius specifically referred to her as an elderly woman, she is almost universally depicted as young and comely.

Study of the saint's iconography has yielded a rich harvest of information about earlier dental practices. Apollonia is always shown holding a forceps (frequently with a tooth grasped in its beaks), and these instruments are of many different types, some not much different from those used today, others almost a foot long and strongly resembling a blacksmith's tongs.

By chance, the cult of Saint Apollonia has also enriched our knowledge of the theater during the Middle Ages, when miracle plays depicting the lives of the saints were popular. These theatrical performances were often given in the courtyards of inns, with the audience looking on from the tiered balconies of the rooms surrounding the stage. In the mid-1400s a wealthy man named Etienne Chevalier commissioned a book of hours (a devotional work containing the prescribed daily prayers) from Jean Fouquet, one of Europe's greatest painters. Fouquet placed a tiny representation of a religious scene at the bottom of each page, and one of these depicts an audience watching players enacting the martyrdom of Saint Apollonia (fig. 40). It is the only contemporary representation of a medieval miracle play that has come down to us.

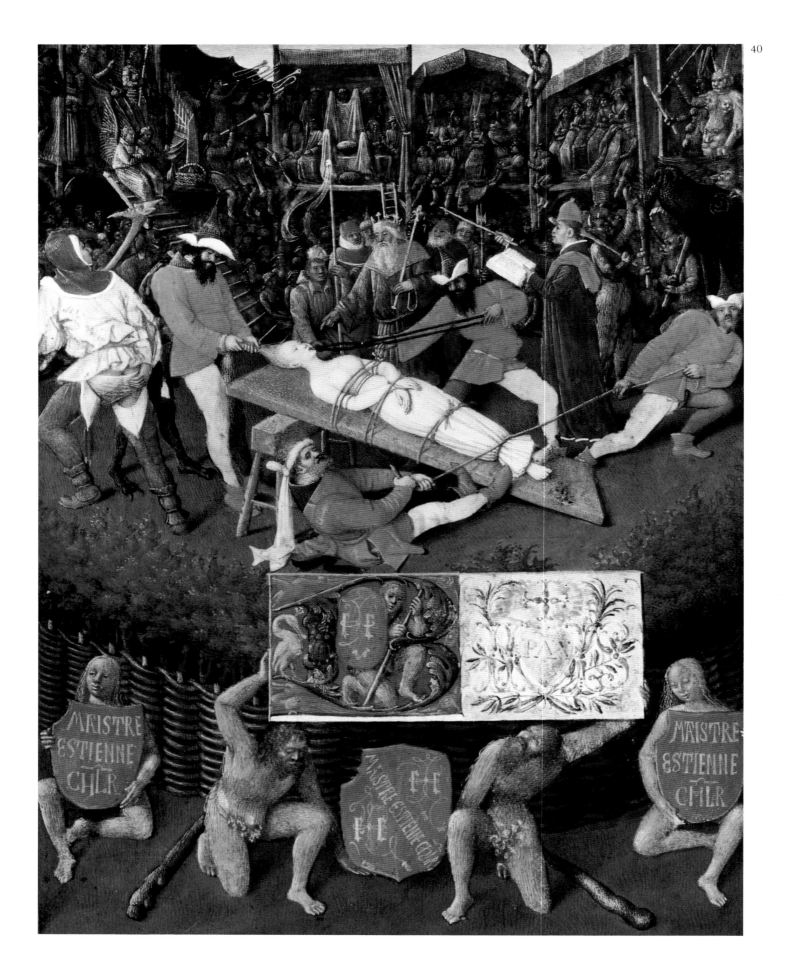

41

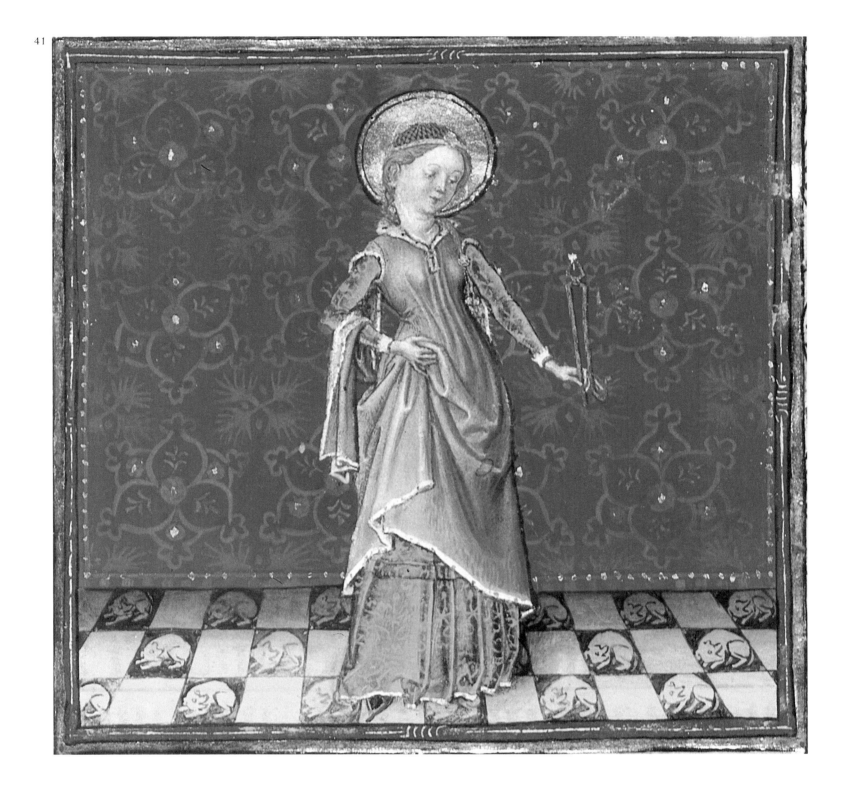

40

The martyrdom of Saint Apollonia is the subject of this mid-fifteenth-century illumination from the *Hours of Etienne Chevalier* by Jean Fouquet. Though after her death in A.D. 249, she was described as an aged deaconess by the bishop of Alexandria, the saint is usually depicted as young and beautiful. Fouquet shows her as her tormentors are extracting her teeth, with an audience such as might have attended a medieval miracle play looking on. The actor on the left exposes his *derrière* in an act of disrespect. Musée Condé, Chantilly.

In a fifteenth-century illumination from the *Hours of Catherine of Cleves*, Saint Apollonia is shown, dental forceps in hand, on a pavement of white and black tiles ornamented with the heads of dogs, symbol of fidelity. Pierpont Morgan Library, New York (Ms. 917).

IV
THE EARLY MIDDLE AGES

The Byzantine World

The demise of the Western Roman Empire occurred about A.D. 476, after repeated onslaughts by the barbarian tribes of the north. However, the fabric of Roman society had been undergoing continuing degeneration for several centuries. A multitude of reasons have been cited for this decay: the overwhelming number of slaves in the empire, the support of whom became an impossible burden on the economy; the rise of Christianity, which weakened the power of the state by denying the divinity of the emperor; and the need to devote a disproportionate share of the national wealth to the armed forces because of continuing depredations of the Germans and other tribes upon borders of the empire.

Foreseeing the transfer of power to the East, the emperor Diocletian in 285 divided the empire into eastern and western regions. The major city of the East was the ancient metropolis of Byzantium, and in 330 Constantine the Great changed its name to Constantinople and made it the official capital of the Eastern Empire. As such it remained for more than a thousand years, until its conquest by the Ottoman Turks in 1453.

No advances in medical or scientific thought were made during the Byzantine era. Byzantium simply went on marking time in the past. The only contribution the Eastern Empire made to medicine was to preserve some of the language, culture, and literary texts of the earlier Greek and Roman worlds. The principal activity of the Byzantine medical workers was the compilation of earlier knowledge, and in this regard four individuals stand out.

Oribasius (c. 325–c. 403), physician to Emperor Julian the Apostate, authored a monumental compendium of seventy volumes entitled *Collectiones medicae*, much of which has been lost. This was essentially a rewriting of the works of Galen, and the references to dentistry are those of the earlier master.

About two hundred years later the principal medical encyclopedist was Aëtius of Amida, physician to the emperor Justinian I (ruled 527–565). He left an extensive compilation, the *Tetrabiblion*, which contained detailed descriptions of the diseases and treatment of the mouth and teeth.

Alexander of Tralles (525–605) was the sole Byzantine compiler to display any special originality. Author of twelve books on medicine, he too reflected the fears of his predecessors regarding the use of forceps for extractions, advising practitioners instead to loosen the affected tooth until it could be removed with the fingers by applying under the edge of the gum a mixture of rose oil, flesh of the crabapple, cracked alum, sulfur, pepper, cedar resin, and wax. This concoction was intended to inflame the gingiva, making the tooth unstable.

The last of the Greek eclectics who wrote on dentistry was Paul of Aegina (625–690), and by his own admission he added little that was new to the subject. Yet he capably summarized the basic medical knowledge of the ancients, including (in his *Epitome*, of seven books) a clear picture of the status of dental surgery in his time. In a chapter "On Affections of the Mouth," he made a sharp distinction between an inflammatory parulis and a tumorous epulis, and described the method of dealing with each type of growth. His comprehensive description became the basis for understanding these diseases until very recent times. He also discussed teething and described extractions in detail (repeating Celsus's advice to fill a carious tooth with linen thread before proceeding in order to minimize the danger of fracturing the crown). Paul explained how to use a file to reduce the height of a tooth that projected above the level of its neighbors, and he was probably the first to write of the need to scale the teeth, removing incrustations of tartar with chisels or other instruments. He advocated proper oral hygiene at all times, warning about foods that might cause vomiting and foods that might leave a sticky residue upon the teeth. He insisted that the teeth should never be used to break hard things, and that the most important time to clean them was after the last meal of the day.

With Paul of Aegina, progress in dentistry came to a halt, and few prosthetic restorations were even attempted. Ascetic Christianity, with its fundamental contempt for the welfare or beauty of the human body, dominated the Western world. Dentistry thus sank into the torpor of the Dark Ages, a sleep that was to last until the Renaissance, some seven hundred years later.

Western Europe: Fifth to Twelfth Centuries

With the fall of Rome, the Western world gradually sank into a mire of ignorance, superstition, and intellectual passivity. The transition was not sudden and catastrophic, but gradual. Continual incursions by the barbarian Germanic tribes of the north devastated great tracts of land and destroyed not only lives but cities, artworks, cultural treasures, and the mechanisms of commerce. Countries were split up into small, isolated city-states, and trade with the flourishing world of Byzantium all but ceased. People fell back upon agriculture as the sole means of earning a livelihood, and there was little incentive to pursue the finer things in life, let alone to make scientific discoveries. Seeking protection against hostile forces, people put themselves under the protection of the Church, which became the only institution that exercised restraint upon the barbarian lords.

Wherever the Muslims made inroads in Europe—the Iberian peninsula and the islands of the western Mediterranean—Arabic language and culture became dominant and remained so for seven hundred years. But in those areas under the sway of Christendom, Latin became the official language of cultural expression. Under the aegis of the Church, the knowledge of the earlier classical writers was compiled, translated, and paraphrased, and the writings of the Byzantines were copied as well. Cassiodorus (490–575), after serving as chancellor to the Ostrogothic king Theodoric, in 540 retired to Squillace in Calabria and founded a monastery, where he devoted the last thirty-five years of his life to learning. It is due primarily to Cassiodorus's efforts that so many ancient Latin writings have been preserved.

By the sixth century the gradual transfer of learning into the hands of the clergy had been accomplished. With Christian control of thought and learning came monastic medicine, which was no longer based on rational principles. Refusing to accept the fact that man is ruled by natural law and subject to the natural forces about him, and reluctant to admit its own impotence in the face of natural calamities, the Church persecuted those who sought to establish rational conceptions of nature's processes. Almost all progress in medicine came to a halt; indeed, all the sciences disappeared as schools of secular learning crumbled, and the vacuum was filled by religious dogma.

Some "scientific" compendiums were written, but these were merely a hodgepodge of excerpts from Pliny, Galen, and other Roman scholars, whose authorship was not acknowledged, however. In addition, many new works (today called pseudepigrapha) were produced and falsely attributed to earlier authorities. Thus, we have Pseudo-Pliny, Pseudo-Soranus, and many others. Some original writing was done, but it was of doubtful merit.

The most learned man of his time was Bishop Isidore of Seville (570[?]–636), who compiled an enormous *Etymologies*, an encyclopedia of origins, the fourth book of which contains a survey of medical terms, with many false and far-fetched derivations. He described the dentition, using the term *praecisores* (precutters) for the incisors, since this was the designated term of Saint Augustine. He repeated Aristotle's false statement that men had thirty-two teeth and women only thirty. In addition, he mistakenly ascribed to the gingiva the task of tooth formation.

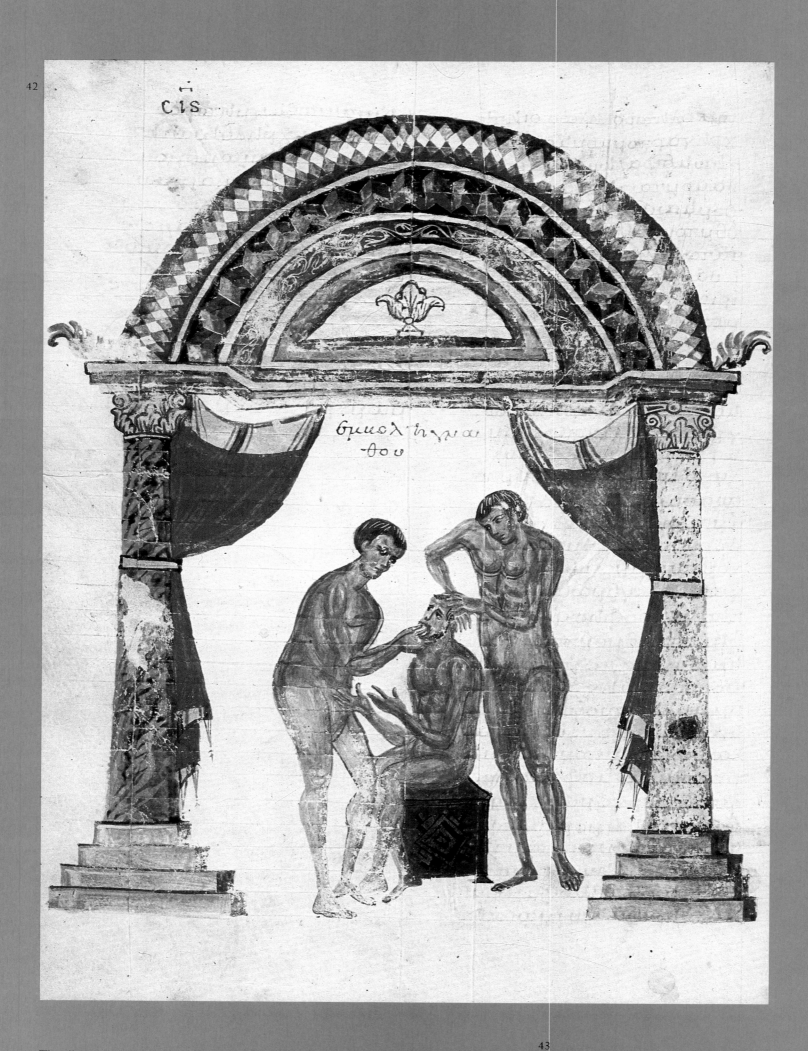

43

This illustration in a ninth-century Byzantine copy of an earlier commentary by Apollonius of Citium on Hippocrates shows the recommended method of reducing a dislocation of the lower jaw. Biblioteca Medicea Laurenziana, Florence.

A late-medieval practitioner extracts a patient's tooth in this watercolor painting from a fifteenth-century German *Schachzalbuch*. Landesbibliothek, Stuttgart (Cod. poet. 202, fol. 59).

43

Oder ob sy wart gewar
Vnd sy es verswieg so gar
Lang das sie jms seitte me
Vor scham jch must sagen hie
Von einer die tet der vngliich
Als jch hort wan jch
An dem buch mit fant
Es wart mir von sagen erkant
Ein kischafft wie ein frowe jren man dar
Zu broht das er ließ den sierden zan vß brechen

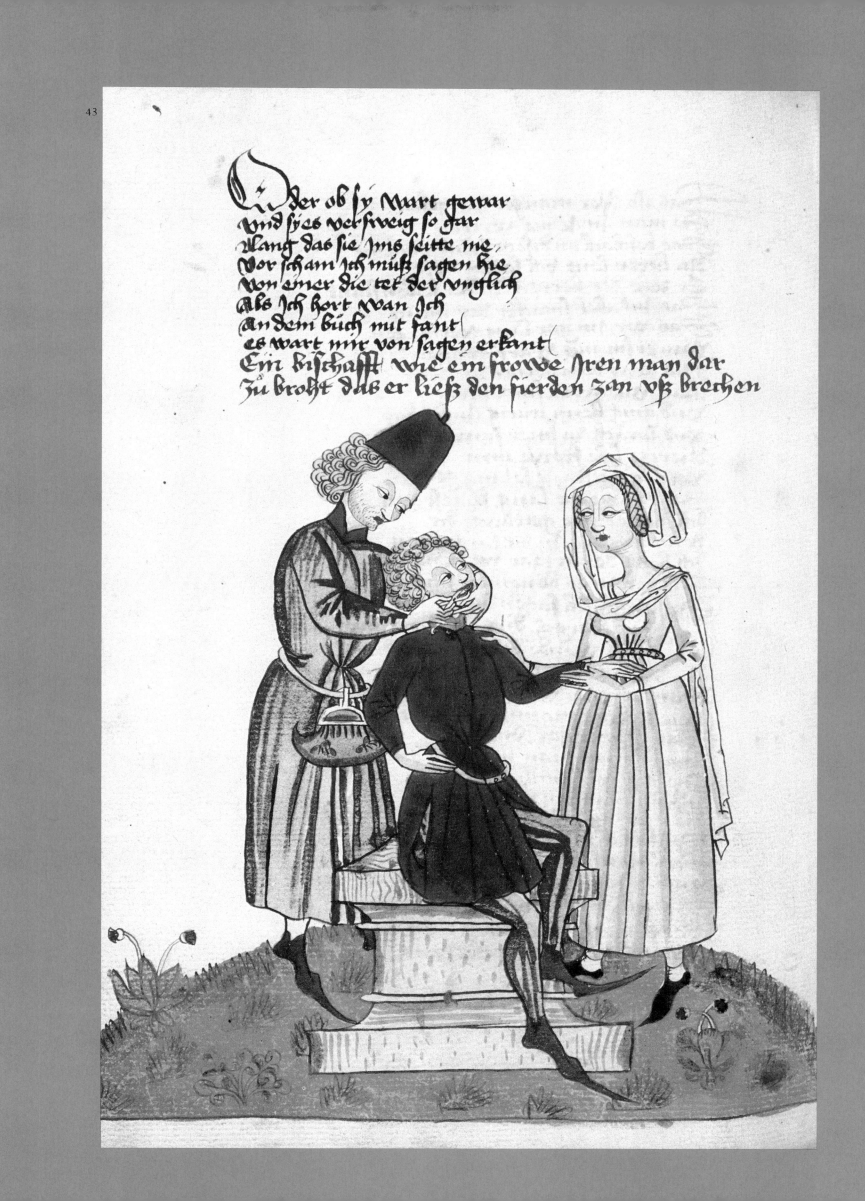

In England the Venerable Bede (673–735) wrote an ecclesiastical history in which is incorporated some discussion of medical treatment common in his day. He mentions remedies for toothache, mostly concoctions of many drugs. He also recommends letting blood from a vein beneath the tongue as a cure for the toothache.

Vindician, writing in the seventh century, reiterated the Hippocratic doctrine that toothache originates in the head and travels down to the tooth, ultimately ending at its root. He repeated numerous "cures," among them henbane root, asparagus cooked in vinegar, pellitory, and the sap of ivy instilled into the ear. Indeed, most medical remedies of the period were derived from herbs, grasses, roots, and other parts of plants, and thus the popular botanicals—which list plants with curative powers and their method of usage, preparation, and administration—became the principal type of medical books.

However, still greater reliance was placed upon wonder cures offered by strolling surgeons and mountebanks, upon the healing power of holy relics, upon prayers for saintly intercession, and upon exorcism of evil spirits that had caused illness in the first place. In times of epidemics, great crowds passed the nights in churches, a practice reminiscent of the "temple sleep" of the earlier Greeks.

What little surgery was practiced was fraught with the gravest danger, and surgeons were frequently put to death if it was a lord who had failed to survive his operation. Little wonder then that Pope Gregory II counseled prayer and endurance of pain rather than submission to the knife. Even tooth extraction was generally avoided, except as a last resort, and then only when the tooth was loose. An anonymous writer of the seventh century mentions a patient who died after a firm tooth was removed—for along with the tooth its "connection" to the brain and lung was also ripped out!

The most important documentation of dental practices of the time was provided by Saint Hildegard, abbess of Bingen, in Germany (1099–1179). She wrote of the healing power of plants, meats, and minerals in her book *Physica*, giving their German names. Her information on the teeth was Aristotelian, for she ascribed toothache to the presence of decaying blood in the arteries that supply the teeth. She also mentioned the toothworm and advocated the smoke of burning aloe and myrrh to drive it out. She lists numerous remedies for toothache, including rinses with hot concoctions of such plants as nightshade and wormwood. Poultices of various preparations applied to the jaw, and powders of burnt salt and pulverized bone she recommended as cures for loose teeth.

Hildegard also believed in simple preventive measures, maintaining that the toothworm flourished because the mouth had not been rinsed with clear, cold water. This she recommended doing each morning upon arising and several times later in the day in order to preserve the health of the teeth. However, her only reference to oral surgery is lancing an abscess of the gum to facilitate the drainage of pus.

It was in the little seaside town of Salerno, near Naples, that the earliest changes in medieval medical thought and practice began to take place. There, in the tenth century, independent schools where medicine was taught and studied were established. Although anatomy at these schools was based on study of swine, and physiology followed Galen, an attempt was made to study disease in a straightforward and rational manner. The Salernitan masters were the first to cultivate medicine as an independent branch of science. Four mainstreams of culture contributed to the formation of the school, as they did to so many other scholarly endeavors of the period: Greek, Arabic, Jewish, and Latin. The oldest Salernitan medical documents are compilations in barbarous Latin of writings by Roman authors and pseudo-authors. One of the most prolific writers at Salerno was Constantinus Africanus (1020–1087), who claimed earlier writings as his own, but who also may have brought to the institution stimulating new medical knowledge from Arabic sources.

The Edict of the Council of Tours

In Italy during the twelfth century medicine was advancing slowly out of the Dark Ages, but a long step backward was taken when the Church restricted the practice of medicine in the monasteries. During the early Middle Ages, medicine in Europe was practiced almost entirely by Jewish and Muslim physicians, who were the inheritors of the learning of the ancients. The only other professional healers were traveling doctors, usually quacks and humbugs, whose ministrations were strongly frowned upon by the Church Fathers, who felt it was far better to fast and pray for healing than to come to believe in the curative power of pagan amulets. Gradually, however, monks began to practice medicine, in some cases to the neglect of their regular clerical duties. Consequently, the Church began promulgating edicts to limit such secular activities. The first two were issued at Clermont in 1130 and at Rheims in 1131; the Lateran Council published a third in 1139; and the most important, announced at Tours in 1163, declared that henceforth the practice of surgery by monks was forbidden.

Hippocrates and later Greek and Roman doctors had included surgery as part of their legitimate practice—a tool to confirm diagnosis and to cure internal maladies. The Arabs, interpreting Galen's dictum that "surgery is only one mode of treatment," conceived the profession of surgery as separate from and inferior to the profession of medicine. Obsessed with the idea that it is unclean to touch the human body, much more so to cut into it, and fortified by the Koran's interdiction against dissection, these Arabic commentators on Galen spread their doctrine among all medieval practitioners. Thus, when in a famous dictum—*ecclesia abhorret a sanguine*—the Council of Tours declared that shedding blood was incompatible with the clergy's holy office, the effect spread far beyond the walls of the monasteries. Henceforth, all surgeons—not the unskilled, peripatetic surgeon alone but his competent colleagues as well—came to be treated as inferior to practitioners of general medicine. The faculties of the newly emerging medical schools did little to alter this unfortunate attitude, and thus the schism between medicine and surgery widened, much to the detriment of medicine.

44 (page 60)

Richard of Acerra was wounded at the siege of Naples in 1194. In an illustration from Peter of Eboli's *De rebus siculis carmen* (c. 1196) he is shown with the arrow still embedded in his cheek. He is being treated by a surgeon attended by two nurses, who bear salves and dressings. Wounds of the face and mouth were common on the medieval battlefield since these areas were not protected by armor. Burgerbibliothek, Bern (Ms. cod. 120, fol. 10).

45 (page 61)

Charles I, who ruled the Kingdom of the Two Sicilies from 1266 to 1285, asked the Prince of Tunis for a manuscript of the compendious work by the Arabic doctor Rhazes entitled *Kitab al-Hawi*. In this three-part initial capital from a south Italian manuscript written in 1282, the story of the translation and delivery of the book is depicted. At upper right, the prince is consigning the manuscript to three Neapolitan envoys. At upper left, the envoys deliver it to Charles. Below, in the upper section of the initial letter *E*, Charles hands the manuscript to the Jewish scholar Faraj bin-Salim, who is seen below hard at work on a translation, which he eventually entitled *Liber continens* (*Compilation*). Bibliothèque Nationale, Paris (Ms. Lat. 6912, fol. 1).

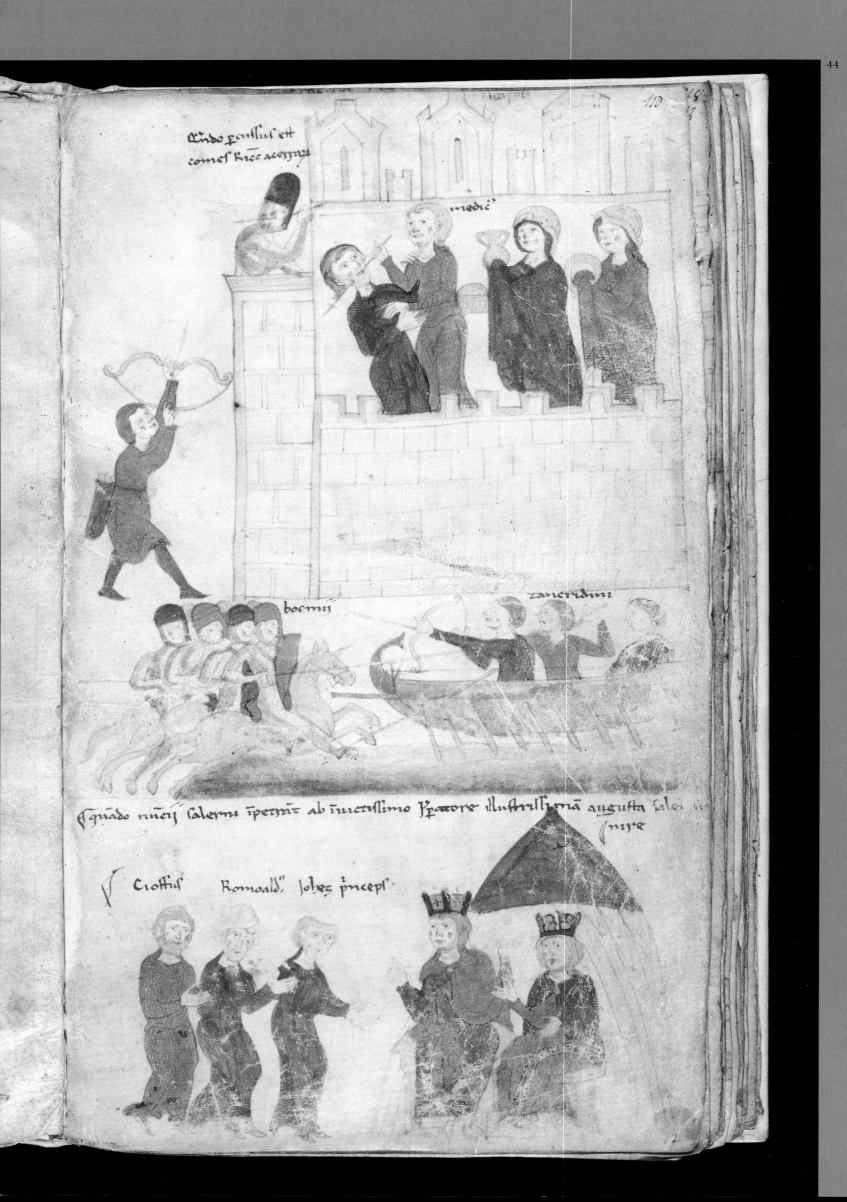

Quando gensslus est
comes Ricc acersan

medic̄

bocmij   zancridini

Aquando nuncii salerni impetruit ab inuictissimo ῑperatore illustrissima augusta salel
snize

Crossus   Romoald̄   Iohes̄ p̄nceps̄

Jnapit phemium libri elhauy ad
honorem dei cuius nomen sit bene
dictum inseaula seaulorum amē.

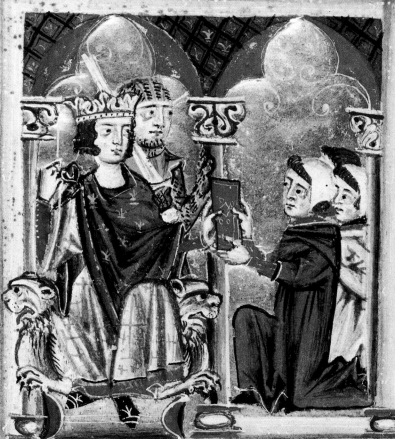

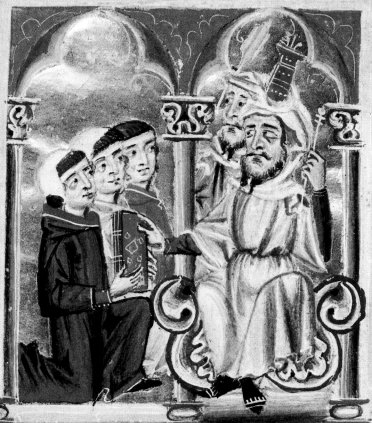

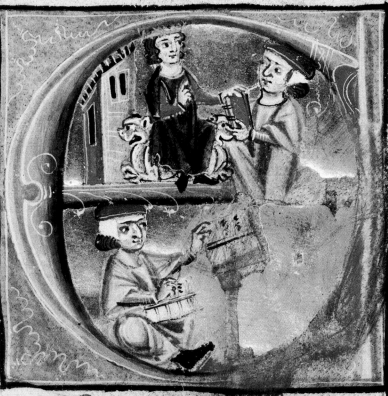

velulis pa
sius omni
um uanis
et uarijs
phylosofo
rum erro
ribus om
niq3 huma
no intellec
tu meorū

perscriptax fidne que totam nature
faculta tem excedunt penitus capti
uato veritati puime firmites inhere
tes catholice fidei lumine perlustrati
vnisita tem machine mundialis in

46

لا يشتهي الطعام او من كانت قوته تحلل وصفته على هذه الصفه

ومما العيون جزر يؤخذ من العسل جزو فيخلطونه بالعصار ويطحونه على الصفه الى الذهب

اللتين ثم يرفعونه ع ع ع ع وقد به تحت ذراب

نقال له ابوما لي على هذه الصفه يؤخذ ثمع الشهد فيغسل

بالماء ويؤخذ ذلك الماء ويرفع ه وينبغي اذا شرب هذا الشراب ان

يصرف ومن الناس من طبخه وبنوع غير موافق للارض لكثره ما فيه من

In the thirteenth century an artist of the Baghdad School illustrated a translation of Dioscorides' *De materia medica*. This leaf depicts a drugstore of the time. The pharmacist prepares a potion containing honey for his customer, who has decided to wait for it. Metropolitan Museum of Art, New York. Bequest of Cora Timken Burnett, 1957.

V
THE ISLAMIC WORLD

After the turbulent Bedouin tribes, united into a cohesive fighting force by the caliph Omar, successor as head of Islam to the Prophet Muhammad, burst out of the Arabian peninsula around the year 635, the character of world politics, culture, and learning underwent a profound change. By the end of the seventh century all of the Middle East and North Africa and almost all of Spain had come under their sway.

Arabic Scholarship

During the early years of conquest and conversion, the fanatical and fatalistic Umayyad caliphs, whose court was at Damascus, ignored all matters of the mind, but by the middle of the eighth century the ruling Abbasids, established at Baghdad, had become friends of learning, and science and medicine flourished in their eastern caliphate.

In 756 the western caliphate was founded by Abd-er-Rahman, a scion of the Umayyad dynasty who had escaped the massacre of his relatives and managed to flee to Spain, where he established his court at Córdoba. By the tenth century this city called itself the most civilized in Europe, with seventy libraries, nine hundred public baths, fifty hospitals, and an outstanding university.

When we speak of the writers of this period as Arabic, we are referring to the language in which they wrote, the lingua franca of Islam. The majority of them were Persian- or Spanish-born, and many of them were Jewish. One of their most beneficial contributions was to preserve and translate into Arabic and Hebrew the works of such classical writers as Aristotle, Galen, and Pliny. The earliest European medical schools, at Salerno in Italy and Montpellier in France, relied on these texts, which had been translated back from Arabic or Hebrew into rude Latin. In fact, the translation of Greek works into Arabic was one of the most important intellectual ventures carried out under the aegis of the caliphs at Baghdad. Without their patronage most classical knowledge would have gone into oblivion during the Dark Ages.

In remarkable contrast to the Umayyads, who were extremely insular in their outlook, was the great Abbasid caliph Harun al-Rashid. Spurred by a passionate interest in foreign learning, Harun encouraged scholars to make translations into Arabic from Greek, Latin, Persian, Assyrian, and the Indian languages. In 791 he wrote to all his provincial governors, ordering them to encourage learning, to hold state examinations, and to offer financial rewards to those students who passed them. He appointed a Syrian Christian, Yuhanna ibn-Masawayh, to translate ancient medical texts into Arabic. Another celebrated compiler was Hunain ibn-Ishaq (c. 809–877), who translated into Arabic from the original Greek the scientific texts of Galen, Oribasius, Paul of Aegina, Dioscorides, Hippocrates, Plato, Aristotle, and Archimedes, as well as the Old Testament.

Although the body of Islamic literature devoted to health and healing is extensive, it contains no work dealing solely with dentistry. Most medical treatises recapitulate the works of the ancients, adding here and there observations based on contemporary experience and practice. One of the oldest surviving is *Firdaus al-hikma (Paradise of Wisdom)*, written by Ali ibn-Sahl Rabban at-Tabari about 850, which deals briefly with dentistry—offering an explanation for the origin of the teeth, treatment for fetid breath, and recipes for dentifrices. Only in the tenth century do we find extensive writings on stomatology, by the four great luminaries of Islamic medicine.

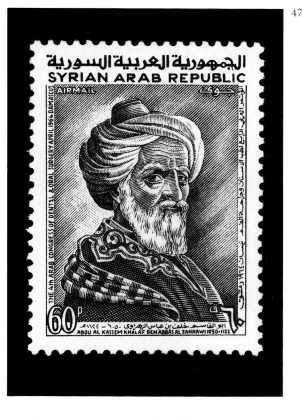

This Syrian stamp issued in 1964, commemorating the Fourth Arab Congress of Dental and Oral Surgeons, honors Albucasis, the great tenth-century Arabic surgeon.

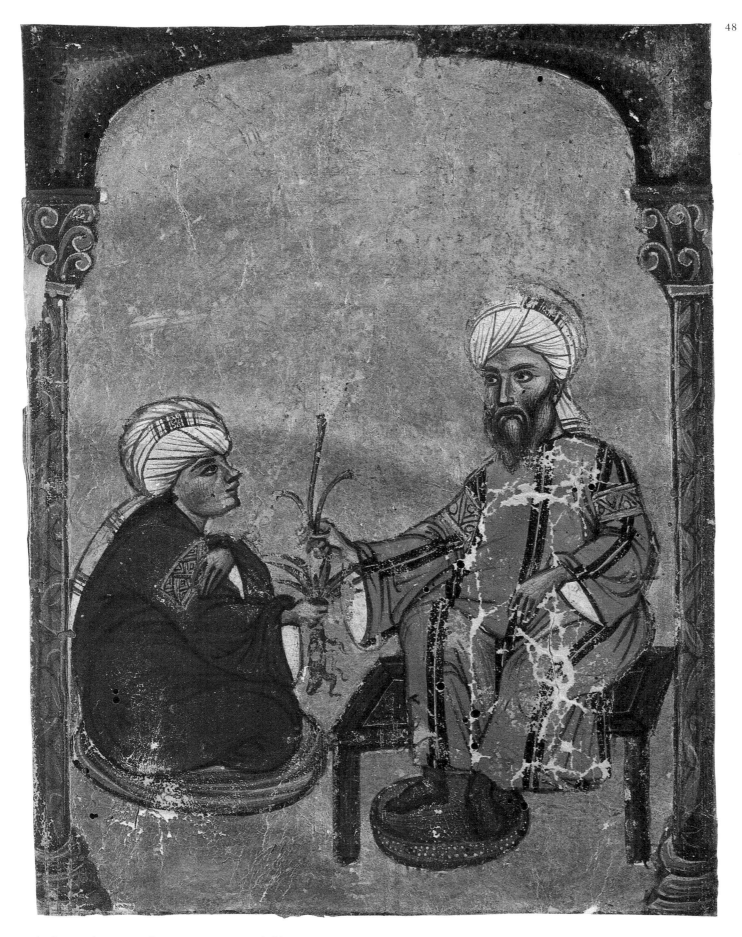

A thirteenth-century Byzantine artist, probably
from the region of present-day Iraq or Syria, drew
this posthumous portrait of the Roman herbalist
Dioscorides discussing a medicinal plant with a
student. Arabic therapy relied heavily upon drugs
of all kinds, and Dioscorides' first-century herbal
De materia medica was closely studied. Library of the
Topkapi Sarayi Museum, Istanbul (Ms. Ahmet III,
2127, fol. 2).

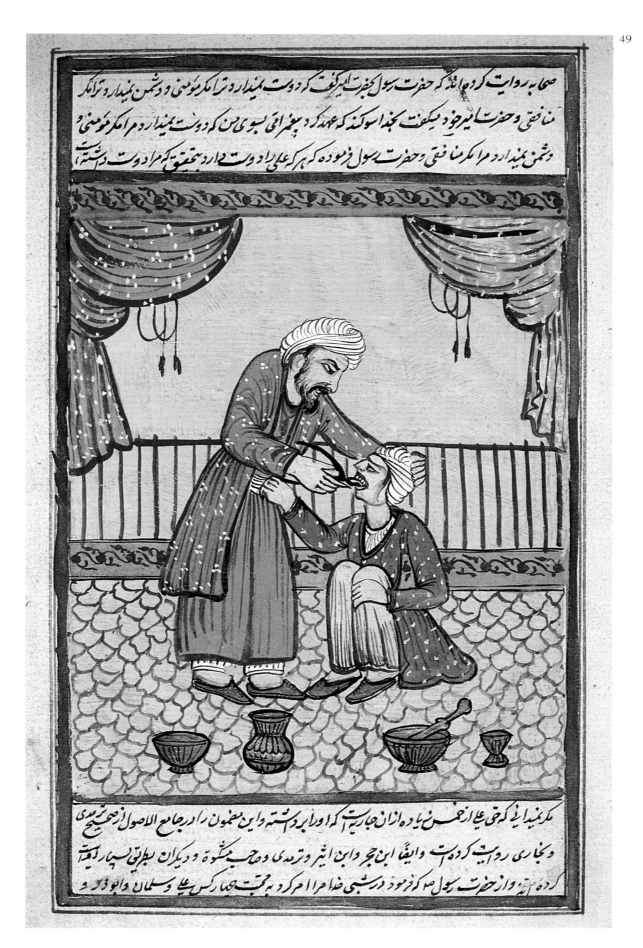

A Persian dentist of the late eighteenth century extracts a tooth. The text that fills this hand-painted page is derived from the Koran and stresses the need to deal kindly with one's fellow man.

Rhazes

Abu-Bakr Muhammad ibn-Zakariya al-Razi (841–926), known in the West as Rhazes, wrote many books, most of which have been lost and only a few of which have been translated. His greatest achievement, *Kitab al-Hawi*, or *Liber continens (Compilation)*, is a selection of classical works to which Rhazes appended his own observations and also those of his contemporaries (see fig. 45). It provides us with an excellent survey of Islamic dentistry from the seventh to the tenth century. *Kitab al-Mansuri* (dedicated by Rhazes to the Persian sovereign al-Mansur) is probably the first book since ancient times to discuss dental anatomy in detail. Rhazes correctly identifies not only the individual teeth but the mode of action of the mandible.

Rhazes's ideas on dental therapy were, for the most part, primitive. He suggested a host of worthless remedies, including instilling various tinctures into the ears to prevent toothache. He relied on red-hot cautery via a cannula, or tube, to prevent toothache, and fumigation and the application of boiling oil to treat carious teeth. He advocated fillings made of alum and mastic and believed in astringents to tighten loose teeth. Like most of his contemporaries, he strongly advised against extraction. When this was unavoidable, he suggested first smearing arsenic paste around the tooth to loosen it.

Ali Abbas

Shortly after Rhazes died, another Persian physician, Ali ibn'l-Abbas al-Majusi (died 994), published an excellently organized work known in the West as *Royal Book*, which covered the entire spectrum of Arabic medicine, including one chapter on diseases of the teeth. He, too, relied on cautery with red-hot needles to prevent odontalgia. If this treatment failed to relieve the pain, Ali Abbas advised extraction.

Albucasis

The greatest physician of the western caliphate was Abul Kasim (abu-al-Qasim Khalaf ibn-'Abbas al-Zahrawi, called Albucasis in the West), who was born in Córdoba in 936 (fig. 47). He received his education at the university there, and there he also taught. He became physician to Emir Hakam II and authored the great treatise *Al-Tasrif (The Method)*, an encyclopedia of medicine and surgery, the first to depict an array of several hundred surgical instruments, whose use Albucasis described in detail. This portion of *Al-Tasrif*, translated into Latin as *De chirurgia*, brought him the greatest fame and entitles him to recognition as the first important oral surgeon.

Albucasis's contributions to dentistry are among his greatest achievements. He understood that calculus on the teeth is a major cause of periodontal disease and gave explicit instructions for scaling the teeth, describing the instruments—of his own devising—that were to be used (fig. 50). The following excerpt from the chapter "On the Scraping of the Teeth" indicates how important he considered this treatment.

> Sometimes on the surface of the teeth, both inside and outside, as well as under the gums, are deposited rough scales, of ugly appearance, and black, green or yellow in color; thus corruption is communicated to the gums, and so the teeth are in process of time denuded. It is necessary for you to lay the patient's head upon your lap and to scrape the teeth and molars, on which are observed either true incrustations, or something similar to sand, and this until nothing more remains of such substances, and also until the dirty color of the teeth disappears, be it black or green or yellowish, or of any other color. If a first scraping is sufficient, so much the better; if not, you shall repeat it on the following day, or even on the third or fourth day, until the desired purpose is obtained.

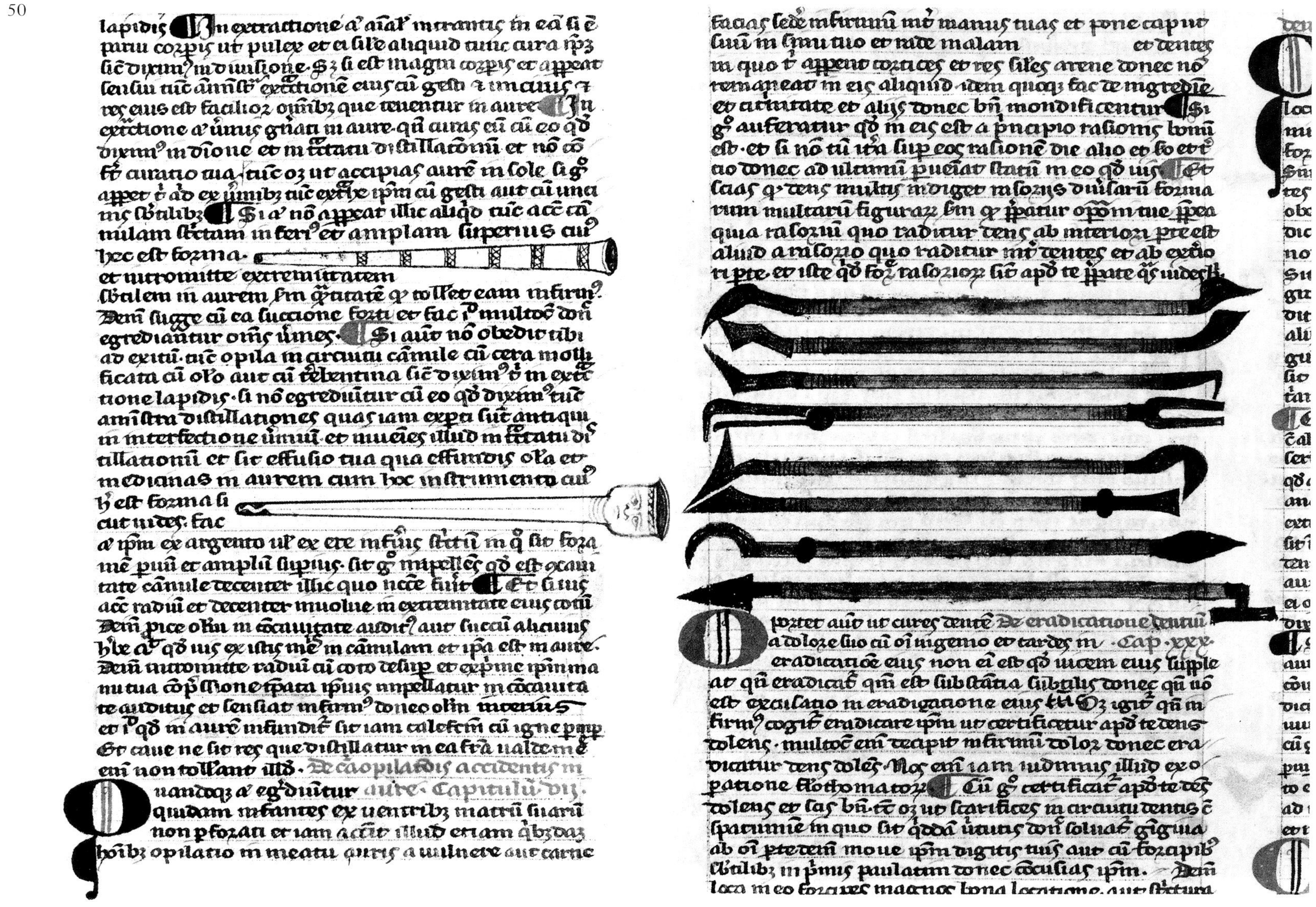

Albucasis stressed the importance of protecting adjacent structures when cauterizing with hot iron, and minutely described how a copper tube might be used as a cannula, advising, "After the cauterization, the patient should keep his mouth, for an hour, full of good butter."

Though Albucasis advised that one should be very slow in deciding to remove a tooth, "as this is a very noble organ, the want of which cannot in any way be perfectly supplied," he made a considerable contribution to the methodology of extraction. At the outset, he warned, pains should be taken to determine which tooth was at fault, since very often a patient is deceived by pain and asks to have removed what proves to be a sound tooth (this, he said, frequently occurs when a barber is the surgeon). He then advised:

> It is necessary to detach the gum from the tooth, all around with a sufficiently strong scalpel; then either with the fingers or a light pair of forceps the tooth must be shaken very gently until it is loosened. Then the surgeon, keeping the head of the patient firmly between his knees, applies a stronger pair of forceps and extracts the tooth in a straight direction, so as not to break it. . . . When the tooth is corroded and hollow, it is necessary to fill the cavity with lint, compressing it hard inside with the end of a probe, so that the tooth may not break under

Illustrating facing pages of a twelfth-century Latin translation of Albucasis's *Al-Tasrif* are drawings of dental scalers and a cannula and cautery bearing the likeness of a human face. Staatsbibliothek, Bamberg (Ms. 91, fol. 75).

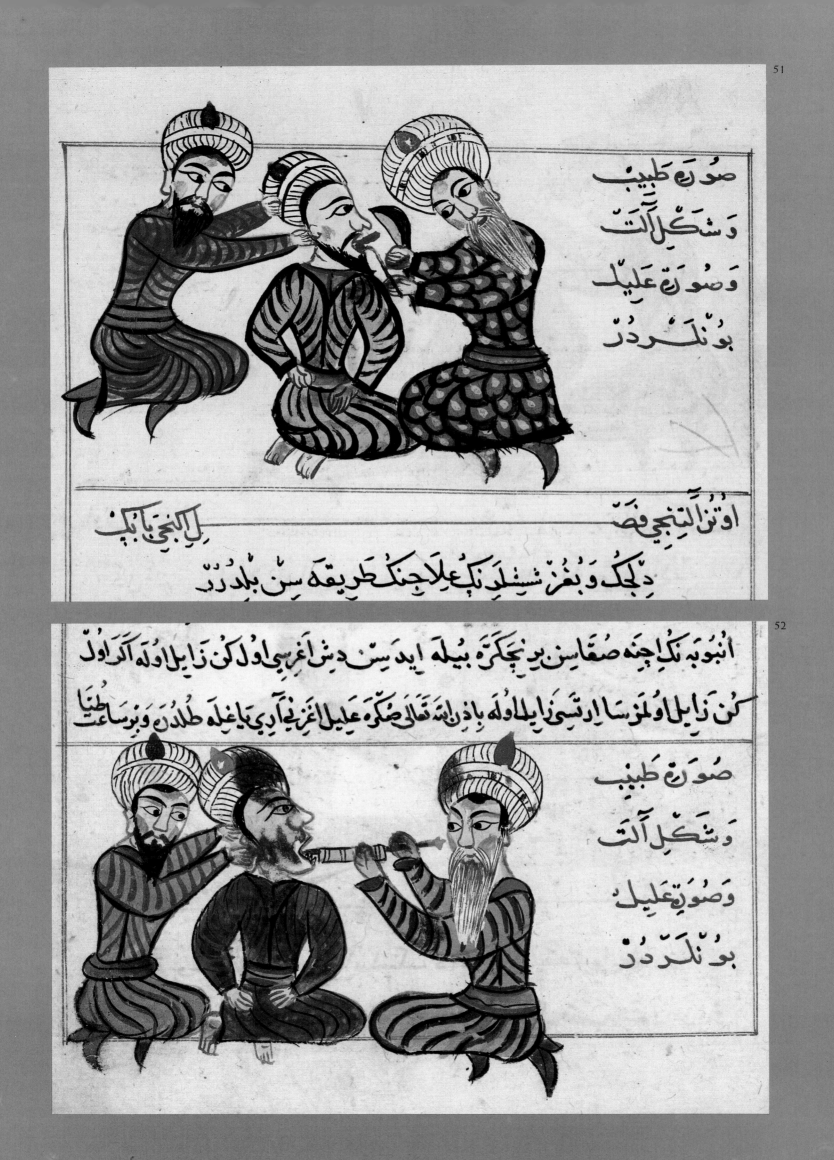

صورة طبيب
وشكل آلت
وصورة عليل
بو نلردُرْ

اوتزالتنجي فصل

الثجي يابك

دلكك وبغز شيشلرنك علاجنك طريقه سن بلدردز

انبوبه نك اچنه صقاسن بر نجكره بيله ايد سن دشاغربى اولكن زايله اده اود
كن زايله اولمز سا ادتسه زايله اده له باذن تعالى صكره عليل اغزنى آچدرى ياغله طلدن وبرساعت نا

صورة طبيب
وشكل آلت
وصورة عليل
بو نلردُرْ

51 An Arabic surgeon operates to remove a cyst under his patient's tongue. Bibliothèque Nationale, Paris (Ms. suppl. turc 693).

52 An Arabic dentist is cauterizing the dental pulp with acid, using a protective cannula, in this illustration from a Turkish translation of *Imperial Surgery*, a twelfth-century Persian manuscript. Bibliothèque Nationale, Paris (Ms. suppl. turc 693).

This frontispiece of a lost Arabic manuscript of the thirteenth century shows a dentist caring for a patient with toothache. He has prescribed the medicinal plant growing at his feet for her relief.

53

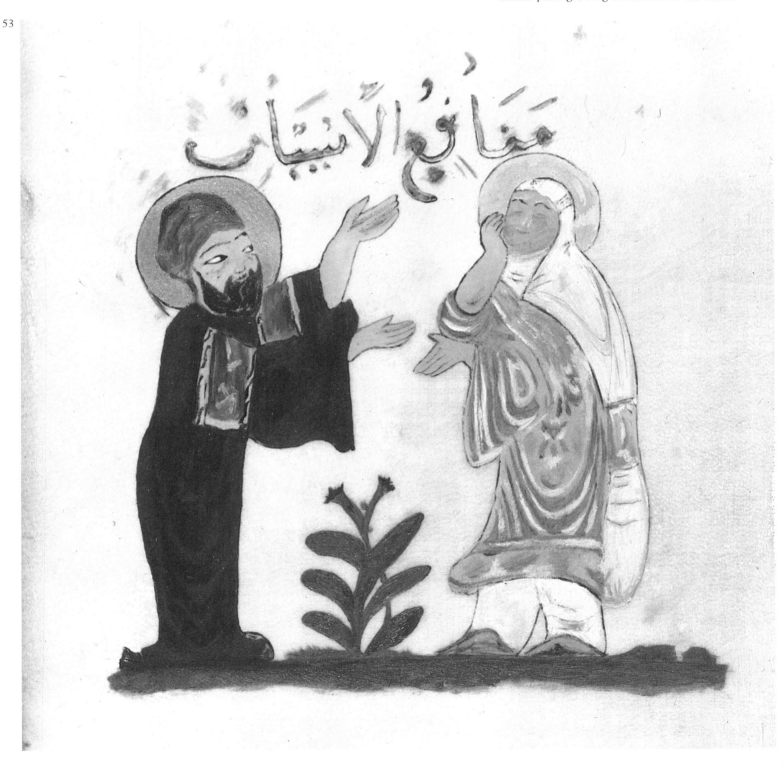

pressure of the instrument. . . . It is necessary, therefore, to avoid acting like the ignorant and foolish barbers, who in their temerity do not observe any of the above-mentioned rules, and therefore very often cause the patients great injuries, the least among which is the breaking of the tooth, the root being left in the socket, or else the taking away, together with the tooth, of a piece of maxillary bone, as the author often happened to see.

This passage provides us with interesting information about the types of practitioners who provided dental services: the barber (probably also a charlatan) and the better-trained surgeon or physician.

Albucasis also recommended ligation for loose teeth, even going so far as to suggest replanting loose teeth that had fallen out and wiring them to their neighbors to stabilize them. He also advised that when teeth were missing they should be replaced with artificial ones made of ox bone and ligated to sound teeth.

Another of this great physician's contributions was his description for surgically removing an epulis: One should, he said, take it up "with a hook or grasp [it] with a forceps and cut it at its root and let the pus or blood flow out." Styptic powders were then to be used to stanch the wound. Albucasis added that if the growth returned after treatment it should be cauterized; then it would not return.

Avicenna

One of the greatest of the Islamic physicians was abu-'Ali al-Husayn ibn-Sina (980–1037), whom we call Avicenna (fig. 54). The scope of his attainments is almost unbelievable. Probably the greatest intellectual of Islam, he mastered the Koran at ten. Soon after, he had absorbed the science of logic and read Euclid and Ptolemy and, indeed, almost all the literature available to him. By the age of sixteen he had completed the study of medicine, for, as he said in his biography, "Medicine is not a difficult science, and naturally I excelled in it in a very short time." At twenty-one he had composed an encyclopedia of all the sciences except mathematics.

His literary output was enormous, and it is said that he wrote fifty pages each evening. Of all his works, the most famous is his *Al-Qanun* (*The Canon*). Probably the best known medical text of all time, it earned for him the title prince of doctors.

Concerning dental treatment, however, Avicenna wrote little that was new. He stressed the importance of keeping the teeth clean, and recommended for this purpose a number of dentifrices such as meerschaum, burnt hart's horn, salt, and burnt and powdered snail shells. He discussed teething, suggesting that fats and oils, as well as the brain of a hare or the milk of a bitch, might be smeared on the gums in difficult cases.

Avicenna examined in detail the causes of toothache, and in his texts we again find mention of the toothworm, for which he prescribed fumigation: "Take four grains each of henbane and leek seeds and two and one-half onions; knead these with goat fat until smooth, and from this paste make pills with a weight of one dirham; burn one pill in a funnel under a covering of the patient's head."

The use of a file to reduce the height of an elongated tooth and of arsenic for fistulas and "foul ulcers" of the gums are among the many subjects discussed by Avicenna.

One of the most significant sections of *The Canon* deals with the treatment of fractures of the jaw. Avicenna emphasized that it was important to determine if a fracture had been correctly reduced. This could best be done, he said, by observing whether the teeth were brought into proper occlusion after the reduction. This accomplished, he advised putting a supportive dressing around the jaw, head, and neck and a light splint along the teeth. Then, if necessary, gold wire might be used to reinforce the stability of the bandage. This rational and sound procedure was notably advanced for the eleventh century, not very different from the treatment recommended today. It formed the basis for treatment by the surgeons of the later Middle Ages.

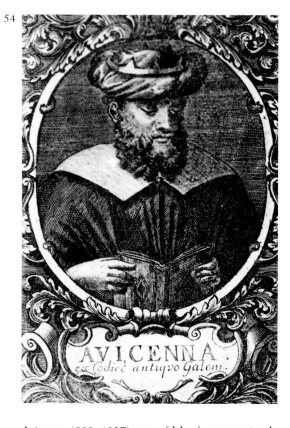

54

Avicenna (980–1037), one of Islam's greatest intellects, authored *Al-Qanun* (*The Canon*), probably the most influential medical text of all time. In his great treatise Avicenna discussed the treatment of dental problems extensively.

Advances in Pharmacology and Oral Hygiene

Despite the learned investigations of scholars like Avicenna, no progress in the study of anatomy was made in the Islamic world. The Koran strictly forbade dissection—a reflection of the Near Eastern taboo against touching a dead body—and, in addition, the Arabic aversion to blood made doctors reluctant to undertake surgical operations—a bias that extended to tooth extraction, except as a last resort. A British physician who traveled in the Middle East in the late 1700s was struck by the gaps in Islamic anatomical knowledge. Commenting on discussions he had had with Muslim physicians and on their medical texts, he observed pithily, "They change the site of viscera, vary the distribution of nerves and blood vessels, at pleasure, and, when necessary to their demonstration, can even create new bones, unknown in the European skeleton."

As a result of the prohibition against surgery, Muslim doctors explored other methods of healing. Intensive study of plants to determine their medicinal value yielded a rich store of pharmaceutical knowledge, which eventually was incorporated into the medicine of the West. Some basic concepts of chemistry, and the Arabic words used to describe them—*alcohol, alkali, alembic,* and *elixir*—permeated European civilization after the Crusades. In the Arab world, pharmacy became a respected profession, separate from medicine. As long ago as the tenth century, Muslim pharmacists ran their own drugstores and dispensed drugs as prescribed in writing by physicians.

The Prophet Muhammad and Oral Hygiene

Muhammad, who was born in Mecca about 570, introduced basic oral hygiene into the Arab world by incorporating it into the Muslim religion. Islam teaches the importance of cleanliness of the body as well as of the mind. Among other duties required by the Koran, ritual ablution five times a day before prayers is a compulsory obligation. This ablution includes rinsing the mouth three times, or fifteen times a day! An English traveler who lived for some time in the city of Aleppo, in Syria, in the late 1700s, described the end of a dinner in a Muslim household where he was an invited guest: "After getting up from the table, everyone resumes his place on the Divan and waits till water and soap be brought for washing out the mouth and hands."

The Prophet also recommended cleansing the teeth with a *siwak* (or *misswak*), a twig of the *Salvadora persica* tree, whose wood contains sodium bicarbonate and tannic acid as well as other astringents that have a beneficial effect upon the gums (fig. 55). A *siwak* twig about half an inch in diameter is soaked in plain water for twenty-four hours until the fibers have separated. Then a small portion of the bark is peeled off, exposing the fibers, which are dense and moderately stiff. When these fibers of "nature's toothbrush" wear down, a new section can be prepared by cutting off the worn portion. It is said that Muhammad was so fond of cleaning his teeth that he asked for his *siwak* on his deathbed and expired a few minutes later.

There are many more traditions of oral hygiene attributed to the Prophet, including the use of a toothpick to remove food debris from interproximal spaces and massaging the gums with a finger. To this day, those who prepare bodies for burial wrap a clean piece of rough cloth around a forefinger and carefully clean the teeth of a corpse before interment.

Many other hygienic practices of Muhammad's time are still observed and the *siwak* is still commonly used on the five occasions described by ibn-Abdin, a Muslim theologian of the last century: 1) when the teeth become yellowish; 2) when the taste of the mouth changes; 3) after arising from bed at any time; 4) before prayer; and 5) before ablutions.

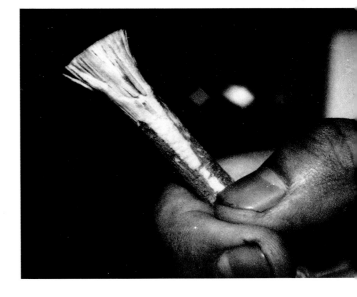

The Middle Eastern toothbrush, called *siwak* or *misswak*, is a twig of the *Salvadora persica* tree soaked in water for a day to separate the fibers.

56

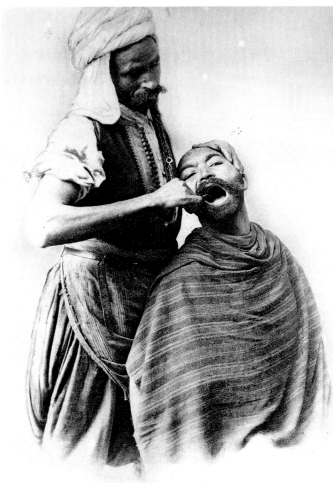

Algérie. — *Dentiste arabe*

In this photograph of about 1910 an Algerian dentist is seen extracting a tooth with a European instrument called a key.

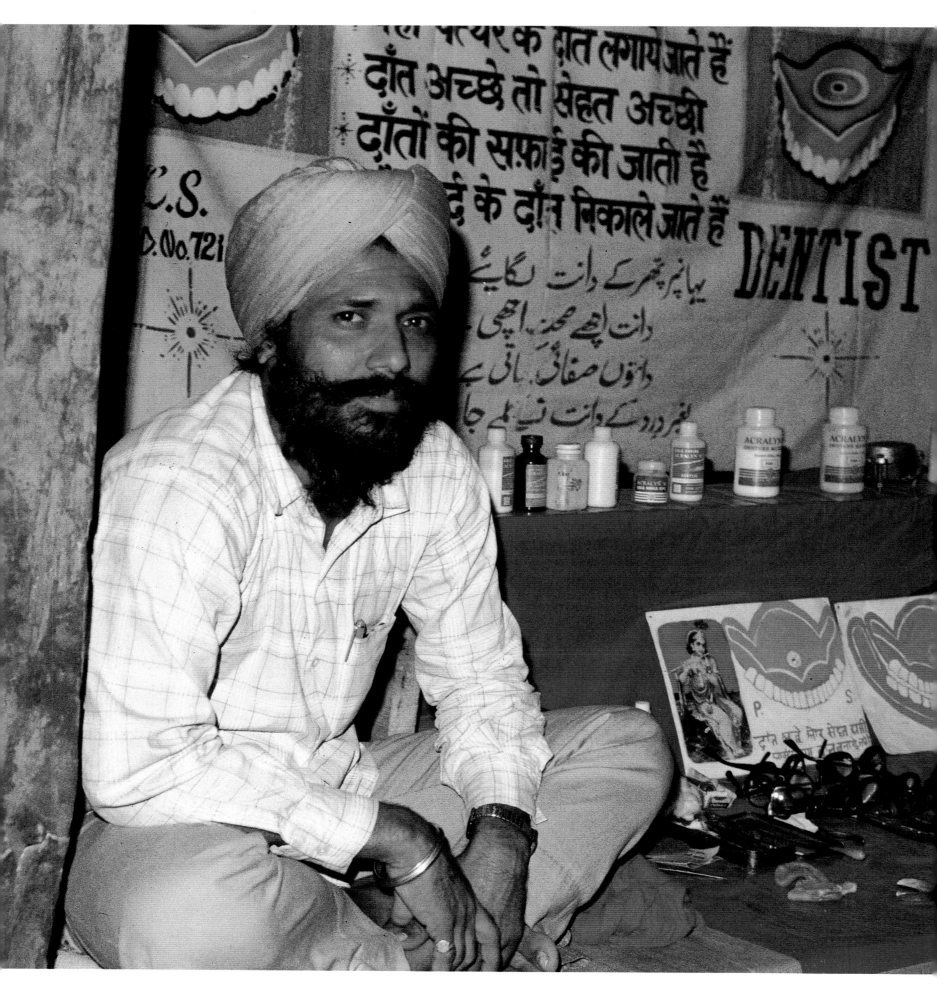

A contemporary Indian dentist waits for customers beside his street stall in Amritsar. His salves, potions, and instruments are ranged prominently on the stand beside him, as are the spectacles that form part of his stock-in-trade.

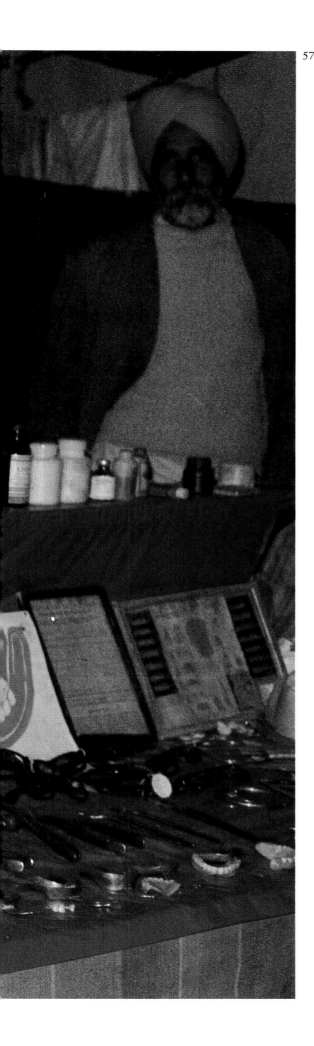

VI
THE FAR EAST

India

About 1500 B.C. the native population of India was overrun by the Aryans, a nomadic people, probably from present-day Iran. Their language, which they imposed upon the land, belonged to the same Indo-European family as Greek and Latin, and from it evolved the tongue called Sanskrit, a word meaning "perfected" or "elegant"—indicating, among other things, that it was the language of the elite.

In the large body of literature brought with them by the conquerors were four sacred books, the Vedas. (*Veda* has the same root as "wisdom," as does the Sanskrit word for physician—*vaidya*, "he who knows.")

The fourth book, *Atharva Veda*, was a collection of magical spells representing the lore of the Atharvan priests. As a companion to this Veda there developed a system of medicine eventually called *ayurveda*, or "science of life." Ayurvedic medicine is based essentially on two treatises, in prose and verse, of the first half of the first millennium A.D. These two great treatises were based on material taught probably hundreds of years earlier by two practitioners, Charaka, who wrote on medicine, and Sushruta, who wrote on surgery.

Indian medicine is based on the notion that the seven hundred vessels of the human body carry, in addition to blood, three basic *doshas* (principles), similar to the cardinal humors of Greek medicine. Any derangement of these *doshas*—*pitta* (bile), *kapha* (similar to phlegm), and the most capricious, *vayu*, or "wind"—would result in disease. An example of the dangerous nature of *vayu*: a dislocated jaw was attributed to an inrush of air rather than to having opened the mouth too wide.

In addition to these three basic *doshas* were numerous *dhatus* of the body—chyle, blood, muscle, fat, bone, marrow, semen, urine, and sweat—and if any of them increased or decreased significantly from the norm, distinguishable clinical symptoms would be detected.

In early times, surgery was regarded as the most important branch of medicine; in the *Ayurveda* it is accorded first place and heads the eight divisions of medicine. Later, the practice was much hampered by Buddhist proscriptions against handling the dead as well as against dissections. The field was divided into *salya*—devoted chiefly to the extraction of foreign objects such as fragments of wood, earth, and iron, and arrows—and *salakya*, the treatment of diseases of the ears, eyes, mouth, nose, and all other bodily parts above the clavicle.

No surgical operations were performed without paying strict attention to an elaborate system of religious rituals. First, the heavenly auspices had to be favorable. Then, the god of fire was propitiated with offerings of curdled milk, rice, drinks, and jewels. Finally, the patient was seated facing the east, the surgeon the west.

Sushruta advocated that the patient be given a good meal and strong wine before his operation. "The effect of the meal . . . will be to sustain [his] strength . . . while the effect of the wine will be to make him unconscious of the pain." Before operations on the mouth, however, the patient was advised against eating. After surgery, the doctor recited a series of incantations: "May the god of fire protect your tongue . . . may Brahma and the other gods bless you . . . may your life be prolonged . . . may you be free from pain."

Dentistry was held to be of divine origin in India, as it was in much of the ancient world. Tradition dating from as early as 5000 B.C. has it that the Ashvins, twin sons of the sun, imparted their holy knowledge to Indra, and Indra handed down the science of life to Dhanvantari, deity of medicine, who imparted the light of truth to Sushruta and Charaka.

Most of our knowledge of early Indian dental treatment comes from the *Sushruta Samhita* (*samhita* means "collection"). Sushruta prescribed excision for "fleshy

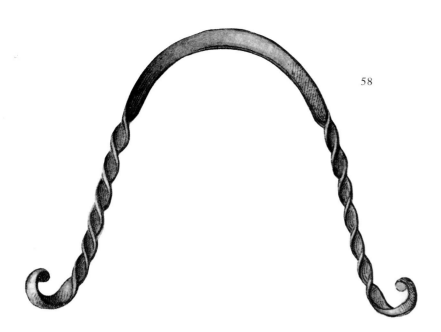

58

For centuries in India the daily ritual of oral hygiene has included scraping the tongue as well as brushing the teeth, usually with the chewed end of a twig of the mango tree, and rinsing the mouth with concoctions of aromatic herbs and spices. The early Hindu tongue-scraper shown here is made of silver.

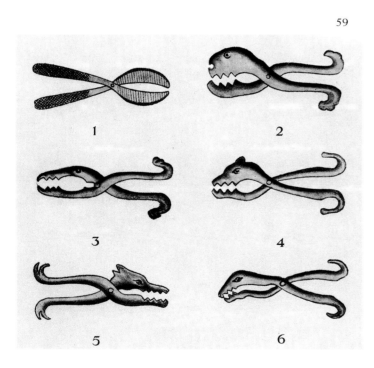

59

1 2
3 4
5 6

These ancient Indian forceps are each named for a resemblance to the head of an animal. For example, the fourth is called "cat," the fifth "jackal." The forceps were used to extract not only teeth but also foreign bodies such as arrowheads.

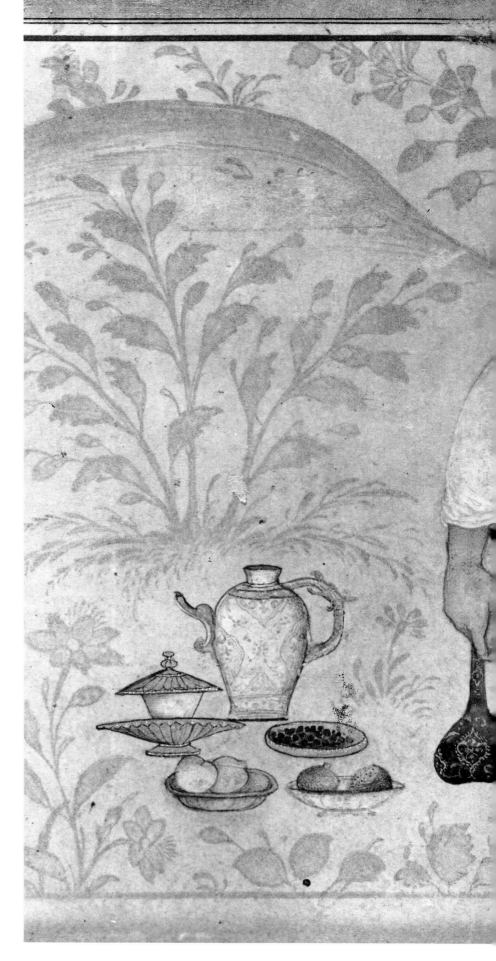

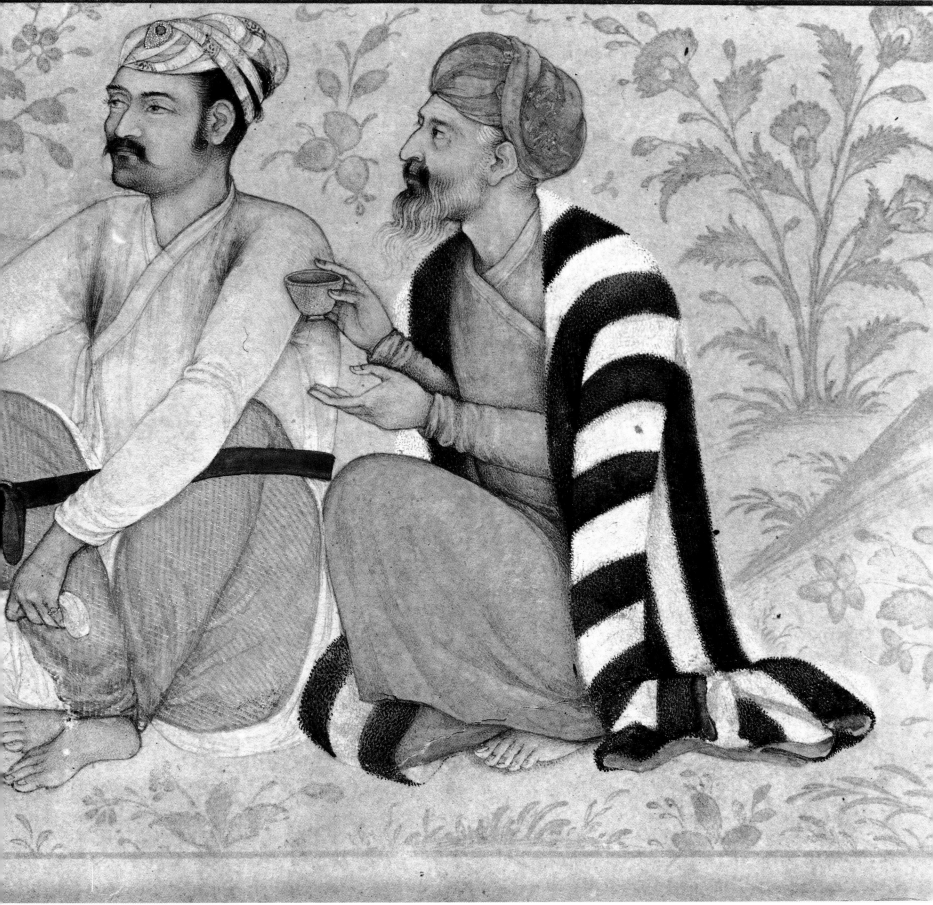

A Mughal prince is served a dish of sweetmeats by a servant in this detail of a leaf from *Album of Jahangir* (c. 1590–1615). A high incidence of caries among the Indian upper classes resulted from a diet rich in sugar. Los Angeles County Museum of Art. The Nasli and Alice Heeramaneck Collection, Museum Associates Purchase.

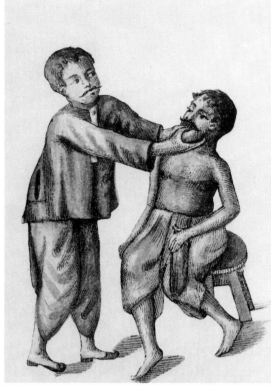

An Indian surgeon of the mid-nineteenth century reduces a dislocation of the mandible. His very ancient method is quite similar to the modern procedure.

Once the pain and indignity of the most recent visit to the local tooth-drawer was only a memory, people of past eras were amused by caricatures of such experiences. In this Indian bas-relief from the Temple of Bharhut, an artist of the second century B.C. has depicted an elephant pulling on a cable to draw a giant's tooth. One monkey encourages the elephant by biting its tail and other monkeys look on with interest. Indian Museum, Calcutta.

growths of the palate . . . red tumors of the palate . . . and tumors over the wisdom teeth." If a tumor grew on the gums or tongue it was scarified or cauterized rather than excised.

Cautery was often the preferred remedy, especially in diseases of the mouth. The surgeon used a specially designed iron, whose flattened ovoid end was heated red hot. Hot fluids might also be used—honey, oil, or wax, brought to the boiling point.

Like his Greek counterpart, the Indian surgeon might recommend bloodletting with leeches because "bad blood causes diseases of the mouth." The maximum amount to be withdrawn at a time was one *prastha*, or "handful."

Fractures of the jaws were treated by complicated bandaging, and the method of reducing mandibular dislocations was as follows: the region around the joint was heated, the jaw brought into its correct position, a tight bandage applied under the chin, and a drug administered to help drive out the evil wind. (In the *Sushruta Samhita* this latter treatment is not discussed in the section concerning luxations in general, but rather in the portion entitled "Diseases of the Teeth Proper.")

The diet of the upper classes was especially rich in fermentable carbohydrates, including honey and such sticky fruits as figs and dates. Consequently, we may assume that this group suffered a high incidence of dental caries; indeed, there are numerous remedies for aching teeth in Indian literature. Complicated potions were prescribed for toothache, but there were also other forms of treatment, including scarification, enemas, and bleeding; the use of mouthwashes, ointments, gargles, and sneeze-inducing materials (such as pepper mixed with cow's urine); and the ingestion of foods that would drive out the bad wind.

Vagbhata, a surgeon active about A.D. 650, collected many of Sushruta's teachings and added to them his own. He discussed killing a toothworm by filling the cavity in a carious tooth with wax and then burning it out with a heated probe. If this failed to relieve the pain, he recommended extraction with a specially designed forceps, the beaks of which were shaped like an animal's head.

Sushruta described two kinds of surgical instruments: *yantra*, or "blunt," and *sastra*, or "sharp." One hundred one *yantras* are described in his work, and among them is the *dantasanka*, a special forceps for extracting teeth. However, Sushruta disapproved of extracting firmly rooted teeth, preferring to remove only those that were loose, using for the purpose a specially designed lever, much like the modern dental instrument called an elevator, but whose tip was flattened and shaped like an arrow.

Unlike Sushruta or Charaka, Vagbhata accords teething some attention in his consideration of diseases of children. He felt that diseases of many kinds, including fever, diarrhea, coughing, and cramps, could be caused by difficult teething. As a treatment he advocated applications of ground pepper in honey, or ground-partridge or quail meat in honey. But he cautioned against too strenuous measures because "the diseases of eruption fade away by themselves." This advice is far sounder than the barbarous custom of lancing a child's gums, so freely practiced in the Western world in the eighteenth and nineteenth centuries.

Both medical and religious beliefs have done much to focus the attention of the Indian upon his teeth. The Hindus consider the mouth the gateway to the body and therefore insist that it be kept scrupulously clean. The Brahmins, or priests, rub their teeth for about an hour while facing the rising sun, reciting their prayers and invoking heaven's blessing on themselves and their families. No devout Hindu will breakfast without first cleaning his teeth, tongue, and mouth, for he believes that many ailments are caused by bad teeth.

Both Charaka and Sushruta discuss proper deportment and the daily regimen, giving special attention to oral cleanliness, and both Sushruta and Vagbhata speak of the need for removing calculus from the teeth, using for the purpose a special instrument with a flat, diamond-shaped end. Sushruta begins his chapter on general hygiene with the admonition, "Early in the morning a man should leave his bed and brush his teeth."

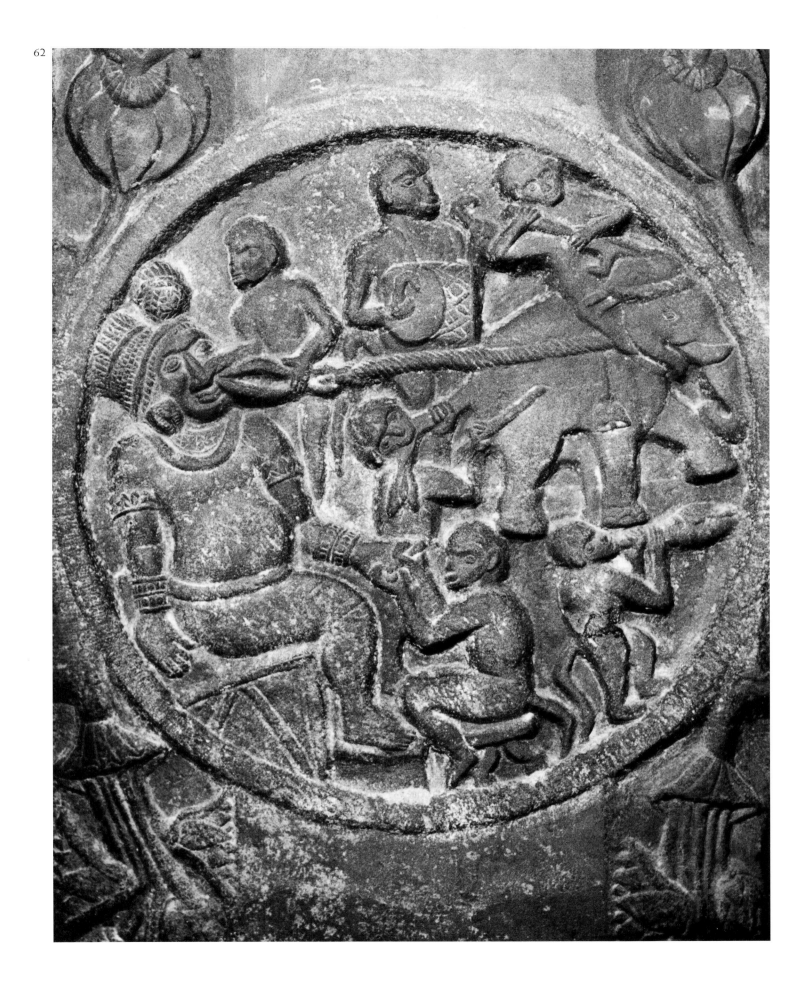

Indians consider the idea of using a toothbrush with animal-hair bristles as little short of barbaric. Their toothbrush is made from a fresh twig whose end is frayed into fibers. The tree from which it is taken varies according to the time of the year and the user's temperament. It generally has a bitter taste and an astringent quality.

The daily ritual is not confined to brushing the teeth. After the regular ablutions and evacuation, the tongue is scraped with a specially designed instrument (fig. 58) and the body is anointed with aromatic oil. Finally, the mouth is rinsed with concoctions of betel leaves, camphor, and cardamon, or other herbs. More than two millenniums ago, Greek doctors were familiar with Indian mouthwashes for bad breath. In *On Diseases of Women* Hippocrates describes an "Indian preparation" made by pounding together anise, dill, and myrrh in white wine.

The Sacred Tooth of Buddha

Of all the sacred relics in the world, none is more highly venerated than the sacred tooth of Buddha, enshrined at the Dalada Maligawa, or Temple of the Tooth, in Kandy, Sri Lanka (Ceylon), the most sacred place of the Buddhist religion. There, once each year, is held the Festival of the Sacred Tooth, during which an elephant clad in scales of shimmering gold parades down paths strewn with rose petals, with a golden casket on his back containing the revered relic while hundreds of thousands of devout pilgrims bow in worship. Yet the venerated tooth is but an ivory carving, and therein lies a fascinating story.

When Gautama Buddha died, about 483 B.C., one of his disciples, Kemo Thoro, extracted a tooth before the body was consumed on the funeral pyre. Thoro took the tooth to the town of Kalinga, which became known as Dantapura, the Town of the Tooth.

In A.D. 411 the Buddha's tooth was brought to Ceylon; about the year 1315 it was captured there by the Malabars, who took it back to India. But through the prowess of Prahrama Bahu III, a Buddhist priest, it was recovered and returned to Sri Lanka. During the troubled times that followed, the tooth was hidden in various parts of the land. But in 1560 it was discovered by the Portuguese, carried to Goa by Don Constantine de Braganza, and burned in the presence of the Governor of India and his court.

At this point a resourceful Buddhist, Vikrama Bahu, carved a new tooth out of ivory, and this is today enshrined in the temple in Kandy. Buddhists everywhere readily accept it as a worthy successor to the original one.

The Temple of the Tooth is a small, unimposing granite building, but the riches it contains are incalculable. Cervantes once remarked, "Every tooth in a man's head is more valuable than a diamond," but the Buddha's surrogate tooth is worth the king of Spain's ransom—as Lord Frederic Hamilton's description indicates. (Hamilton was given the opportunity to view the tooth by the British Colonial Secretary who was, in 1920, the official protector of the relic.)

> At the conclusion [of a prayer] eight men staggered across the room, bearing a vast bell-shaped shrine of copper, about seven feet high. This was the outer case of the tooth. The Hereditary Keeper produced an archaic key, and the outer case was unlocked. The eight men shuffled off with their heavy burden, and the next covering, a much smaller bell-shaped case of gold, stood revealed. All the natives present prostrated themselves, and we, in accordance with our orders, bowed our heads. This was repeated six times, the cases growing richer and more heavily jeweled as we approached the final one. The seventh case was composed entirely of cut rubies and diamonds, a shimmering and beautiful piece of work.... When opened, this disclosed the largest emerald known, carved into the shape of a Buddha, and this emerald Buddha held the tooth in his hand. (*Here, There, and Everywhere*, New York, 1921)

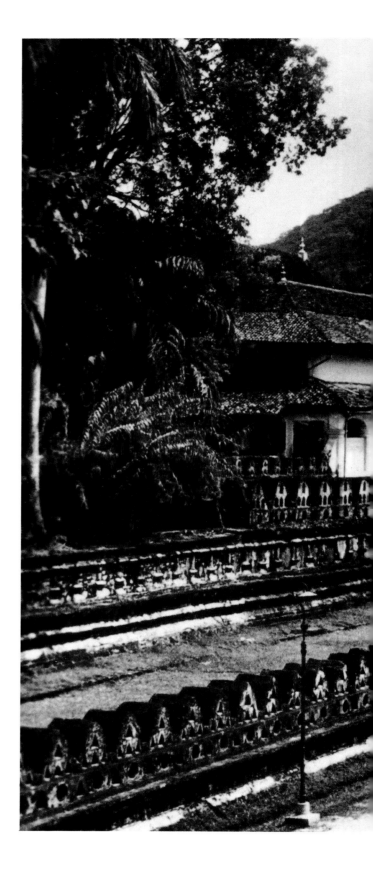

One of the holiest shrines of the Buddhist religion is the Temple of the Tooth in Kandy, Sri Lanka. Here is housed a replica of a tooth of the Buddha himself, which was destroyed by the Portuguese in 1560. Once a year the sacred replica is carried in a procession on the back of a bejeweled elephant before hundreds of thousands of the faithful.

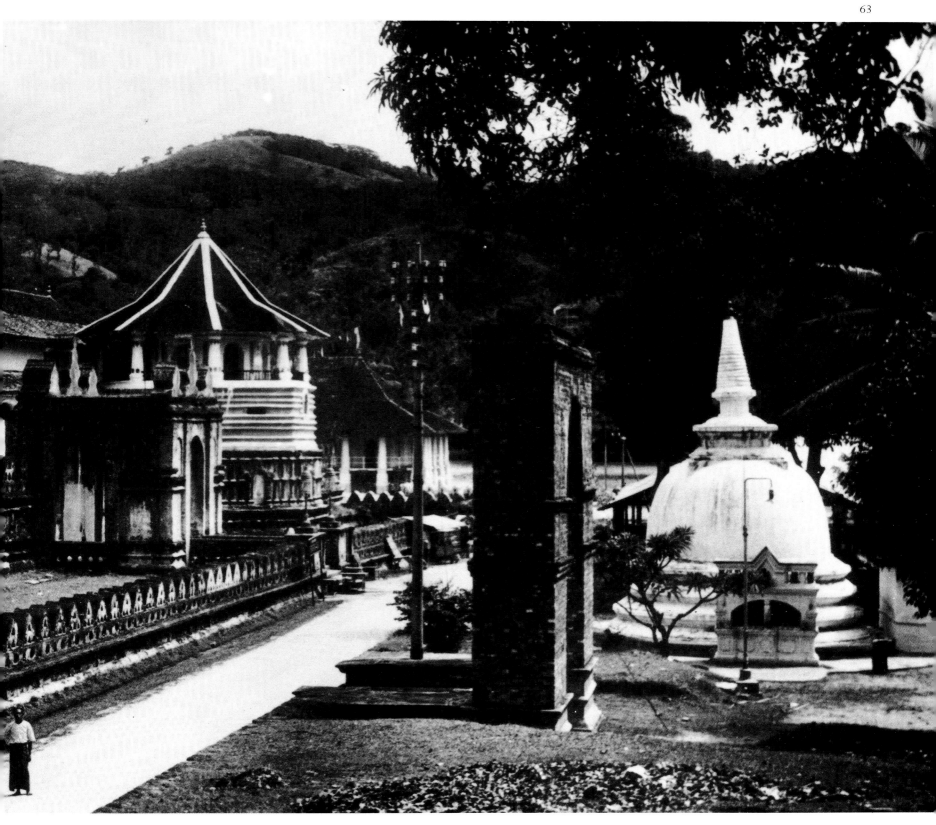

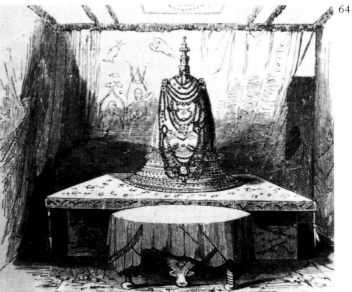

Inside this golden container are several smaller ones which, when removed, disclose an emerald figurine holding the sacred tooth of Buddha, venerated at the Temple of the Tooth, Kandy, Sri Lanka.

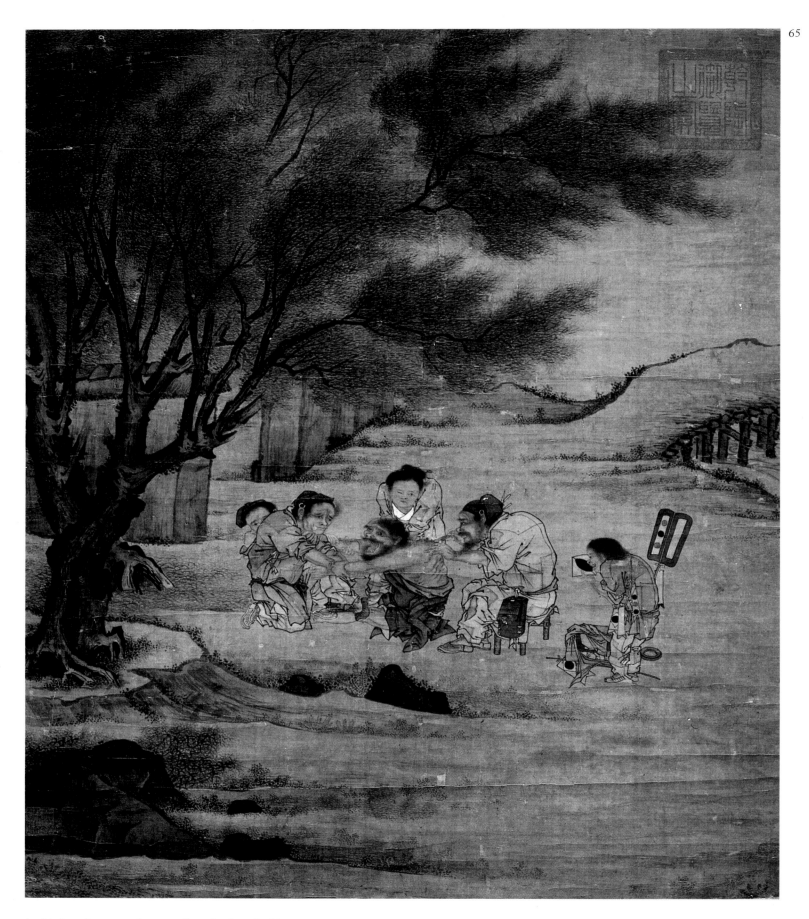

In this bucolic scene, the great Sung landscapist Li
T'ang depicts a country doctor cauterizing a patient's arm by burning it with the powdered leaves
of an aromatic plant. "Moxibustion," as the treatment is called, is still resorted to by the "barefoot"
doctors and dentists who serve the mass of the rural Chinese people. National Palace Museum, Tai-
pei, Taiwan.

China

The Chinese were making significant contributions to human progress as early as 2000 B.C. By that time they had not only domesticated the dog, pig, goat, sheep, and horse but had developed the potter's wheel; by 1500 B.C. they were weaving textiles of silk. When Moses was leading the Israelites through the Sinai desert, the Chinese were writing with brush and ink on paper made of bamboo strips. By Buddha's day, about 500 B.C., they had adopted a law code, issued coinage, and invented a game like football. And in the ensuing thousand years this enterprising people introduced to the world true paper, gunpowder, the compass, the abacus, spectacles, paper money, and, most important of all, the art of printing with wood-block type.

It is not surprising, therefore, that dentistry was practiced early in China. There is evidence that the Chinese used arsenic to treat decayed teeth—probably to kill the pulp and relieve the pain of toothache—about the second century A.D., and they developed a silver amalgam for fillings more than a thousand years before dentists in the West. "Silver paste" is mentioned in the *materia medica* of Su Kung (A.D. 659) and again about 1108 in the *Ta-kuan pen-ts'ao* by T'ang Shen-wei. During the Ming period, in their *materia medicas*, Liu Wen-t'ai (1505) and Li Shih-chen (1578) discuss its formulation: 100 parts of mercury to 45 parts of silver and 900 parts of tin. Trituration of these ingredients produced a paste said to be as solid as silver. Other early writings indicate that full dentures were being constructed by the Chinese as early as the twelfth century.

When Marco Polo traveled to China in the 1270s, he found in the province of Kardandan that "both the men and women of this province have the custom of covering their teeth with thin pieces of gold, which are fitted with great nicety to the shape of the teeth, and remain on them continually." Whether these gold plates served a cosmetic or a therapeutic purpose we do not know. Certainly, however, the technical ability to practice restorative dentistry existed in China in the thirteenth century.

In the field of oral medicine the Chinese also made definite contributions as long ago as the 1300s. One of their great diagnosticians, Hua Shou, in his commentary on the *Nan Ching*, a very early medical work written during the Later Han dynasty (A.D. 25–220), described the whitish spots in the mouth that are the premonitory symptom of measles.

In the eleventh century T'ing To-t'ung and Yu Shu described the entire process of mastication and deglutition. Although their description of the stages of the process that were visible to them—chewing and swallowing—were accurate, they were wrong in their conception of what happened to the food once it reached the stomach, ascribing digestion to the action of vapors arising from the spleen.

Oral surgery also has a long history in China. We read in an ancient monograph that a cleft lip was repaired in an operation performed during the Ch'in dynasty (255–206 B.C.), the earliest report of such surgery anywhere in the world. By the seventeenth century A.D., Chinese surgeons were familiar with many diseases of the mouth and throat and undertook the treatment of such conditions as tonsillar abscesses and epitheliomas of the lip. And during the eighteenth century further advances were made in understanding oral disease and oral anatomy. Between 1784 and 1826 Chao Wen-tsin compiled a major work on surgery in which numerous instruments for operations in the mouth were depicted.

An important medical treatise containing an extensive description of oral anatomy, *Illustrated Notes of Symptoms and Treatment in Laryngology*, appeared in 1822. It contains a detailed description of the oral structures and defines the division between the oral cavity and the pharynx. The work also includes articles on mouth and throat abscesses as well as tumors of the tongue, lips, and chin.

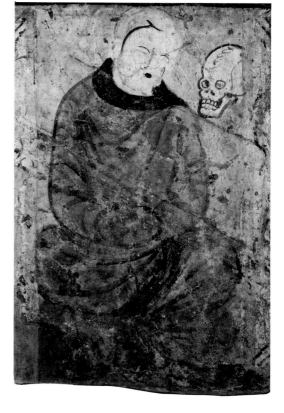

This early sixth-century wall painting from the Cave of the Navigator, Qizil, Afghanistan, depicts a Buddhist monk in meditation before a skull. The early Buddhist missionaries helped to introduce oral hygiene and dental therapy in China. Museum für Indische Kunst, Staatliche Museen, Berlin.

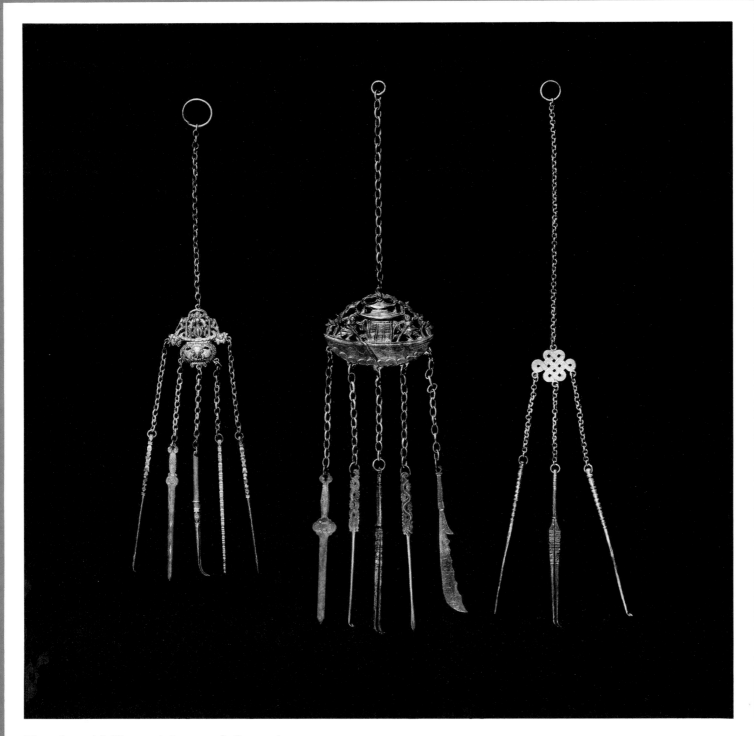

These beautiful Chinese toilet sets of silver and ivory include toothpicks as well as tweezers and ear scoops. American Museum of Natural History, New York.

Traditional Medicine

Throughout their long history the Chinese have clung to several beliefs that run counter to the tenets of modern medicine, and although great strides have been made in medical and dental education, the great majority of the Chinese people are still treated by traditionalist doctors. At the basis of their therapeutics lie the principles of *yang* and *yin*. The former is identified with masculinity, the sun, and the sun's light and heat. The feminine *yin* is identified with moistness, darkness, and cold. Good health is the result of maintaining *yang* and *yin* in proper balance. These forces are thought to circulate throughout the body along twelve meridians whose exact course is not known, yet whose approximate position has been established. When the balance of *yang* and *yin* in the body is incorrect, a needle is inserted into the proper spot on one of the meridians, permitting morbid forces to escape and wholesome ones to enter, thus restoring balance and arresting the course of illness.

This theory of disease and its cure is akin to the Hippocratic theory of the cardinal humors and their relation to disease processes. But whereas the Greeks drew blood to restore physiological balance, the Chinese relied upon a vital principle called *ch'i*—something like the Greek *pneuma*, or "spirit." *Ch'i* could be either drawn out or replenished simply by puncturing the right "vessel" with a needle.

More than 360 points on the surface of the body that are thought by the Chinese to be directly linked with internal structures have been charted. A number of these points—116 in all—are believed to be connected with the teeth and other oral structures, and acupuncture treatment of oral ailments has proven singularly effective in spite of the fact that no reason convincing to Western science has been offered for its efficacy. It is used widely in multiple tooth extractions as well as in the treatment of gingivitis, stomatitis, and glossitis.

As a supplement to acupuncture, traditional Chinese doctors turn to moxibustion, which is akin to cautery, but which results in a localized inflammation such as that brought about by cupping. A preparation of the powdered leaves of *Artemisia vulgaris*, a relative of wormwood, is piled on a precisely designated spot on the skin and then set afire. It is allowed to smolder until only ashes—and frequently a blister—are left. Today a slice of onion, garlic, or ginger is often placed beneath the smoldering cone, or else the cone is removed before being completely consumed, in order to avoid blistering the skin. The rationale for the practice may be that fire, being *yang*, will counter an excess of *yin*. Moxibustion is used widely, along with acupuncture, for treatment of toothache and other oral ills.

Herbal medicine is also a mainstay of the traditionalists. Much of their stock in trade dates back to 1578, when the great pharmacologist Li Shih-chen published in fifty-two volumes his monumental work, *Pen-ts'ao kang-mu*, in which roughly 1,900 drugs and 8,000 prescriptions are listed. One of the most frequently prescribed herbs is ginseng. Long believed to be effective for a variety of ailments, this aromatic root is dispensed in the form of powders, pills, and teas, and is often taken in combination with other herbs.

Inspection of the tongue is a diagnostic tool peculiar to old-fashioned Chinese medicine. Changes in the appearance of the tongue are believed to reflect disease and to indicate the severity and suggest the prognosis of the condition. Tongue examination was first described in the *Nei Ching (Canon of Medicine)*, a body of lore committed to writing about 300 B.C. The technique used today remains essentially unchanged: color, coating, and moistness of the tongue are all carefully noted as an aid to diagnosis.

The traditional explanation for caries and toothache is the ubiquitous toothworm, or *chong ya*. The Chinese assume that its destructive action can be prevented by removing food debris from the mouth after eating, so rinsing the mouth after meals remains a common practice, as does brushing the teeth. The toothbrush as we know it today, with the bristles perpendicular to the handle, was invented by the Chinese in the 1490s.

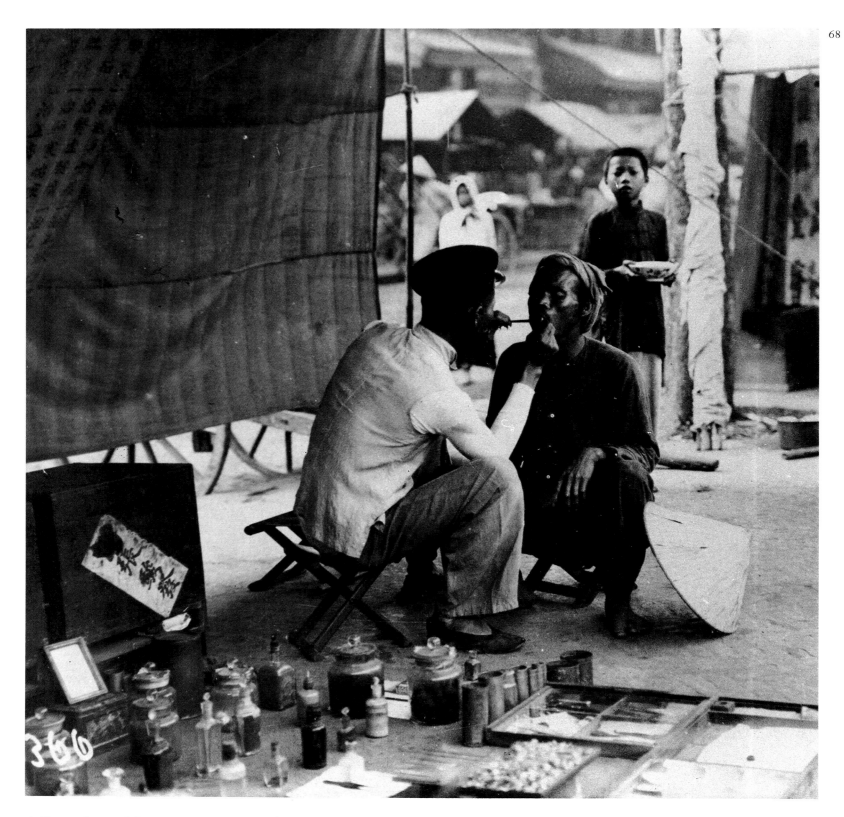

A Chinese dentist of the 1930s examines a patient's teeth in a Saigon street stall. Kulturhistorische Sammlung des Bundesverbandes der Deutschen Zahnärzte, Cologne.

Dental Care Today

During most of its history, China has suffered from a shortage of trained dental practitioners. Street-corner "specialists" were for years to be found in every city and town. These itinerants attracted clients by beating a drum and other acts of showmanship. Today the government is making strenuous efforts to discourage them and has made great strides in increasing the number of dentists in the country; yet there is still a woeful shortage of properly qualified dentists—currently, one university-trained specialist for about 150,000 people. During the Cultural Revolution of 1966–69, formal professional education was discouraged and the number of trained dentists fell drastically. Filling the gap, especially in the vast rural areas, are specially trained technicians known as "barefoot dentists." These young people are trained to offer many kinds of dental care: simple fillings, extractions, and treatment of gingival ailments. Having completed six months of formal training, they are essentially first-line dental corpsmen. In the communes they have at their disposal dispensaries with simple but functional equipment and supplies, including anesthetics but seldom any X-ray facilities. The care they provide helps to keep the populace in a reasonably good state of dental health, although extractions, rather than reconstructions, are routine. However, in emergencies patients can be referred to larger specialized dental facilities at the county seat or provincial capital.

The first modern dental school in China was established in 1918 at the West China Union University, a missionary school run by the United Board of Christian Colleges. Originally a department in the faculty of medicine, the dental school was reorganized after a year as a separate faculty.

The Chiang Kai-shek government in 1935 named a committee of education in dentistry, and the result was the establishment of a dental technicians' school at the National Center University in Shanghai, where in 1938 a six-year course was inaugurated.

Other centers of dental education were set up in 1942 at the National Defense Medical College and the Chunking Dental Demonstration Center. Later, Nanking and Shanghai opened dental schools, and in 1947 Peking University included a dental department in its medical college.

Chinese dentists in the modern tradition receive their training in a formal university setting to which each student is admitted after ten years of preliminary education. Four years of dental school are followed by a two-year internship at the school clinic. Upon graduation, the new dentist is assigned to a post wherever the government chooses. There is no private practice in China.

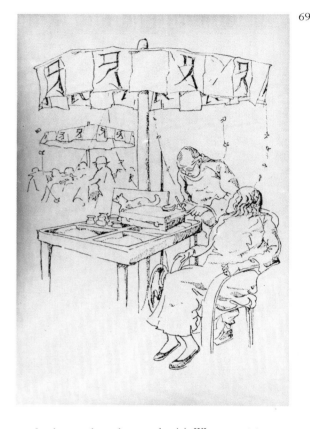

In this modern drawing by M. Wong, an itinerant Shanghai dentist has set up shop at an outdoor fair. He uses a foot-treadle drill to fashion a dental prosthesis for his patient, who curiously eyes his work.

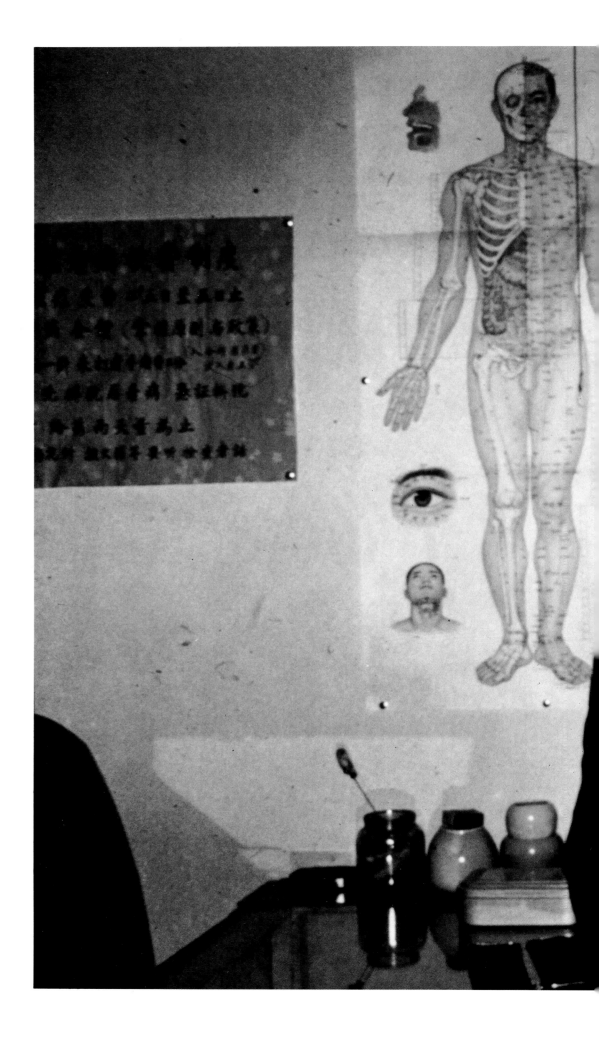

In an apartment-house clinic, a modern Chinese acupuncture specialist stands in front of large charts that show the points on the human body to be pierced by his needles in treatment. The chart on the left deals with the mouth and its adjacent structures.

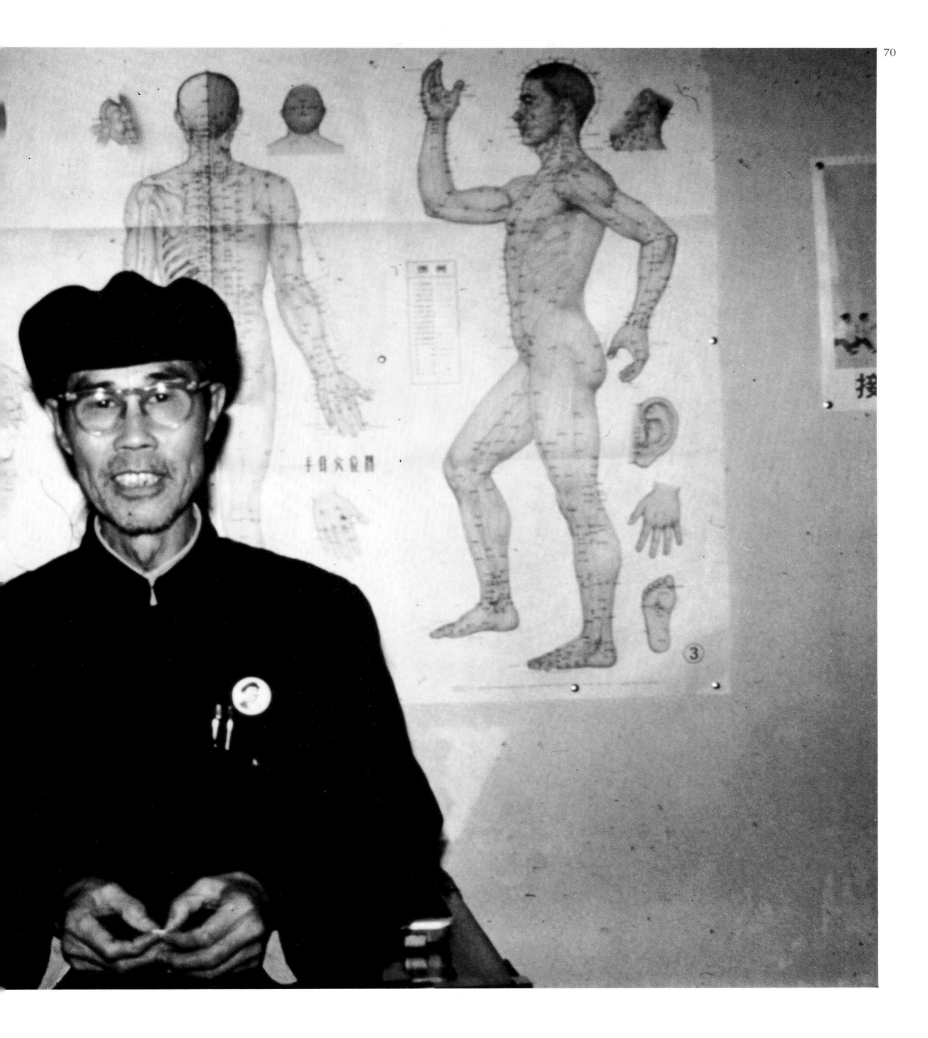

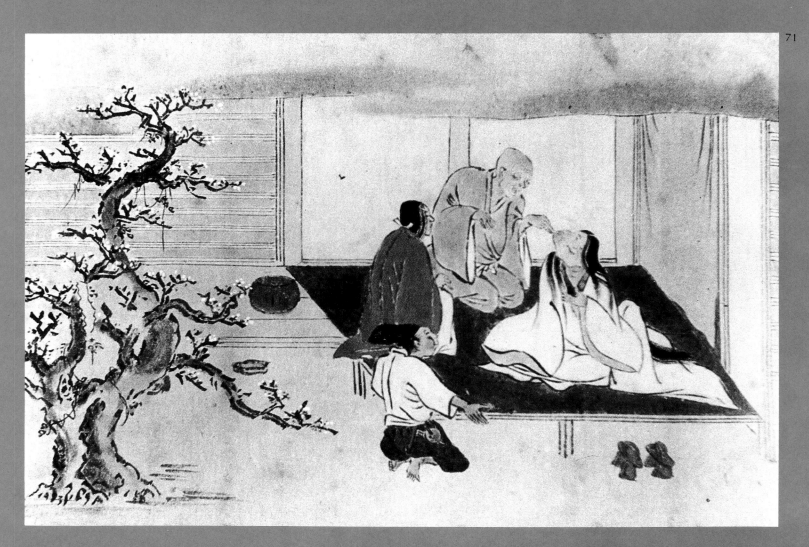

This lively sketch of a twelfth-century dentist examining a patient, who probably suffers from a
maxillary tumor, illustrates the *Yamai-no-soshi* (*Collection of Disease Pictures*) by Mitsungagy Gosa.

Japan

Since civilization spread from China to Korea and later to Japan, both China and Korea exercised a marked influence on the development of the healing arts of their neighbor to the east. In A.D. 414 the Japanese emperor Ingyo appealed to the Koreans for a qualified doctor, and King Shiragi sent a physician named Kimbu to serve at the Japanese court. Another Korean, Tokurai, emigrated to Japan in A.D. 459, became a naturalized citizen, and was designated *naniwa kusushi*, or physician.

Late in the sixth century came a development in the medical arts in Japan, for Buddhist missionary-priests brought with them a number of venerable Chinese medical texts. We also know that the toothbrush—then a tufted twig—was introduced to Japan by Buddhist priests, who were required by the dictates of their religion to brush their teeth and scrape their tongues every morning before prayer.

Centralized government was established in Japan about 650, and by the end of the century a formal legal code was adopted to deal with all aspects of civil and criminal law. This code, the *Taiho Ritsuryo*, consisted of seventeen volumes, eleven of which were concerned with civil matters. One of these, *Ishitsuryo*, is the earliest Japanese book of law to deal with medical practice. With the idea that medical treatment is the responsibility of the government as a premise, it provided that officers should be named to oversee medical and pharmaceutical practice.

The government, in addition, supervised all medical education, and students were trained at government expense. The course of study was divided into areas that reflected the four recognized medical specialties: internal medicine, surgery, pediatrics, and oto-ophthalmo-stomatology. Toward the end of the Heian era, during the 1100s, dentistry was recognized as a specialty separate from otology and ophthalmology.

With the establishment of the Heian government in Kyoto in the year 794, commercial and cultural exchange with China, which had begun early in the Christian Era, began actively to flourish. In the tenth century Yasuyori Tambano, descendant of a Chinese emperor, emigrated to Japan and became not merely a citizen but the most acclaimed medical practitioner of his time. It was under the supervision of this foreign doctor, the father of Japanese medicine, that *Ishinho*, the oldest existing Japanese medical book, was produced. This treatise, of about 980, dealt at length with the entire spectrum of disease; treatment of disorders of the teeth, lips, and mouth occupies eighteen pages of the fifth volume.

Fuyuyori Tambano, a descendant of the father of Japanese medicine, achieved fame during the Kamakura era (1185–1333) for skillfully extracting the carious teeth of Emperor Hanazono. It is Fuyuyori's son, Kaneyasu, however, who is remembered today as the first Japanese dentist, since he was the first practitioner officially appointed to the court, and because his descendants served in that capacity for many generations. The Tambano family kept its techniques secret, transmitting them only to members of the clan from generation to generation. Ultimately, however, they were gathered together in book form, and *Chikayasu's Dental Secrets*, issued in 1531, remains a well-known treatise.

About 1185 control of the country fell into the hands of the Minamoto family. Although the emperor continued to reign, the office of *shogun* (Generalissimo) was established, and those who held it were the effective rulers of Japan. During the Tokugawa shogunate, in the early 1600s, Gentai Kaneyasu served as dentist to Hidetawa, the second *shogun*. Other *shoguns*, and emperors too, followed suit, commanding well-known dentists to serve at their courts. These dental specialists were regarded as the professional equals of medical doctors. The outlying provinces were controlled by feudal lords known as *daimyos*, and these, too, had their own dentists to treat them and their retinues.

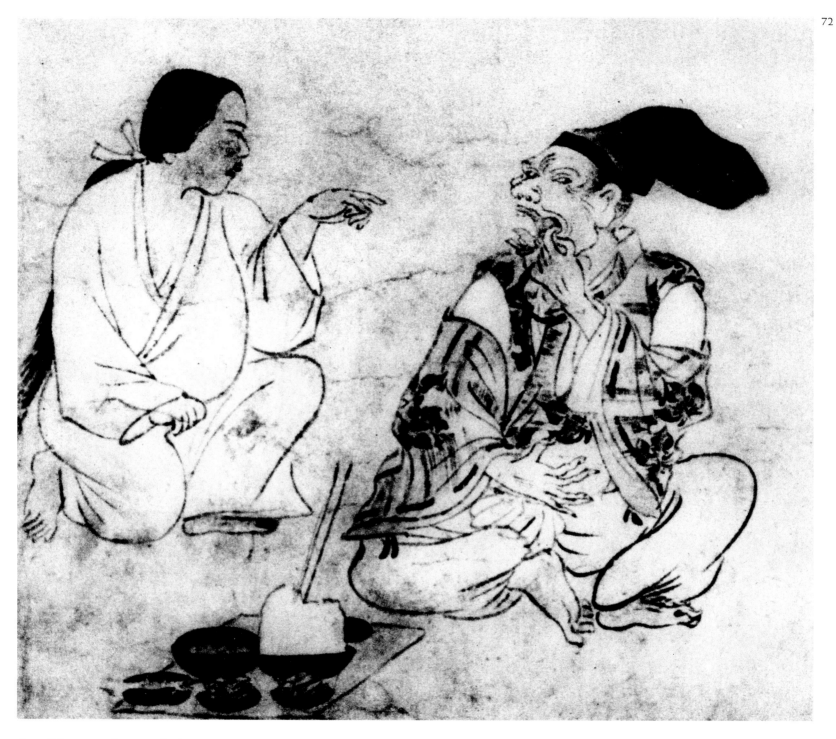

A twelfth-century Japanese husband complains to his wife during dinner that he has trouble chewing hard food because his teeth are loose. Evidently he suffers from severe periodontal disease. From Mitsungagy Gosa, *Yamai-no-soshi* (*Collection of Disease Pictures*).

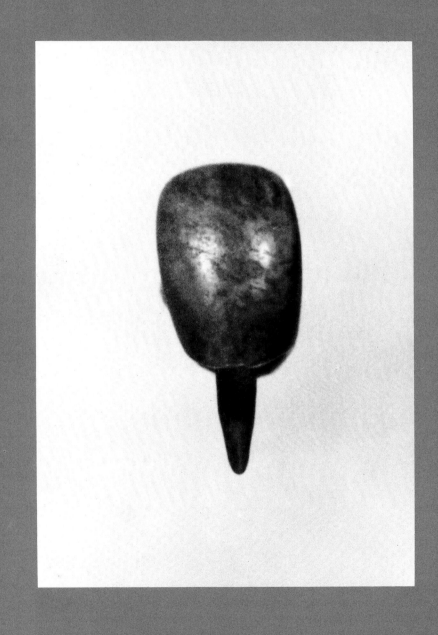

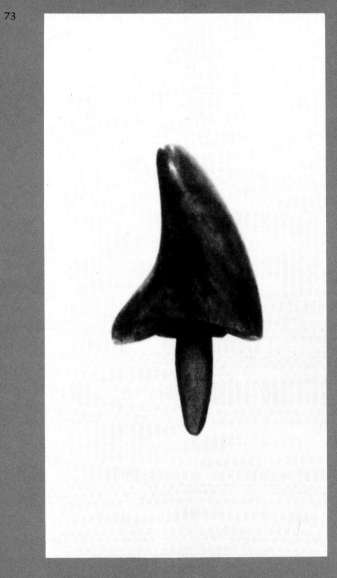

This wooden dental prosthesis of the Tokugawa era was designed to function like the modern dowel crown. The pin was inserted into the root canal of a non-vital tooth, whose natural crown was missing.

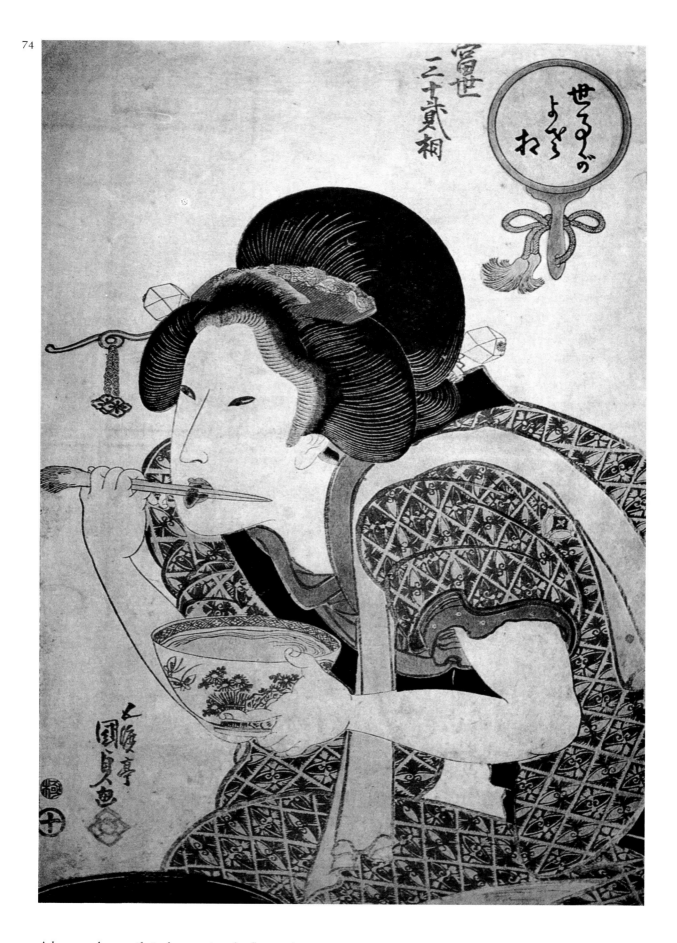

74

A Japanese housewife is shown using the flattened side of a toothbrush to scrape her tongue in this colored woodblock print by an artist of the Tokugawa period (1603–1867). In her hand she holds a bowl of water with which she will rinse her mouth.

The Tokugawa (Edo) Shogunate (1603–1867)

Dental treatment from the 1600s to the mid-1800s varied in nature and was provided by a variety of practitioners. Relief of toothache was sought in acupuncture, moxibustion, and cautery with a hot iron, and by the use of charms and incantations. When all these failed, extraction was resorted to.

Dental practitioners set up offices in the major cities and through extensive advertising and extravagant claims attracted a primarily middle-class clientele. Some specialized in extraction, others did mostly prosthetics. The common people were treated by quacks and charlatans who operated in the street, luring patients by dazzling feats of acrobatics, swordplay, and top-spinning tricks. In the mid-1600s in the city of Edo (the first name for Tokyo) 5,600 of these charlatans were plying their trade!

A school of Chinese medicine was established in Kanda, in Fukuoka prefecture, in 1765. In a few years it fell under the direct control of the shogunate and became known as the Medical Science School. Thereafter, various clans in the outlying parts of the country founded medical schools within their own domains, and the Wakayama, Yamaguchi, and Takanabe clans established independent courses in dentistry to educate specialists.

A major milestone in furthering education in the Western style was the publication in 1774 of *Katai shinsho*, a translation of a German anatomical text. It introduced modern medical science in a systematic format into university curriculums and had a profound influence on the development of scientific professional education.

A number of dental practices of the Tokugawa period are portrayed in *ukiyo-e*, "pictures of the floating world." Immensely popular in bourgeois circles, these colored wood-block prints depict beautiful women of the amusement quarters, famous actors, and scenes of everyday life. One of the most striking of these customs to Western eyes was the blackening of teeth by married women and courtesans as an enhancement of their beauty. When in the 1850s Commodore Matthew Perry arrived in Japan, which for centuries had been closed to the West, he was taken aback by this custom. "When the young women smiled bashfully and opened their ruby red lips," he wrote, "black teeth, lined up frighteningly in diseased gums, appeared unexpectedly." Indeed, so struck was he by their appearance that he called the strange country Black-toothed Japan.

The custom, rooted in antiquity, had gradually become proof of the married status of women. Before a new bride entered her husband's home, she visited the establishments of seven relatives to receive dye and then underwent what was called "the first blackening." Its significance is expressed in the adage, "As the color black never changes, neither does the intimate bond between a husband and wife." Blackened teeth were evidence that a wife had sworn eternal fidelity to her spouse. The dye, derived primarily from ferric tannate, was applied by women not well-to-do with a brush made of a crushed twig. The rich used brushes made from the feathers of a pheasant or mandarin duck. The dye was reapplied periodically as the color wore off. By the 1700s the custom had been adopted by prostitutes. Before a novice entertained her very first customer, she collected tooth dye from seven experienced courtesans and then blackened her teeth with it.

During the Tokugawa era, toothbrushes were customarily made from willow twigs beaten to separate the fibers. The length of the twig was cut thin and flat so that it might be used as a tongue-scraper. Women's toothbrushes were made softer than men's in order to preserve the black dye on their teeth. A polishing agent, a specially prepared earth mixed with salt and scented with musk, was applied to the teeth with a twig-brush whose end had been moistened with water.

Toothpicks, essentially similar to those used today, were crafted by hand and sold, along with the brushes and tooth powders (commercially prepared tooth powder was on the market as early as 1634), in special shops. Beautiful models and showgirls enticed customers into these establishments, which had become numerous by the beginning of the nineteenth century: more than two hundred lined the streets leading to an important Edo temple!

When Buddhism was introduced into Japan in the sixth century, new arts and techniques arrived as well. By the eighth century the Japanese had mastered the art of carving wooden Buddhas, and it is possible that the earliest wooden dentures were made at that time. Certainly by the beginning of the Tokugawa era the technical aspects of denture manufacture had been perfected.

In his classic work of 1728 the great Western dentist Pierre Fauchard describes two complete upper dentures of his devising that depended solely upon atmospheric pressure for their retention. The full significance of his great discovery apparently eluded him, for he continued to advocate the use of springs in denture construction. But the Japanese were constructing complete upper and lower dentures that were retained by adhesion and atmospheric pressure alone more than two hundred years earlier. And of equal interest is the fact that these dentures were made of wood! More than 120 complete wooden dentures have been found, dating from about the early 1500s to the mid-1800s.

The early Japanese denture was carved from a single piece of wood, usually of a sweet-smelling species such as box, cherry, or apricot. An impression of the patient's edentulous jaw was taken in beeswax and a model was made, also usually of wood. The denture was carved to conform roughly to this model. Then the inside of the patient's mouth was painted with vermilion pigment or india ink and, by recording high spots, the inside of the denture was carved to match the inside of the mouth. (This procedure is not unlike the later Western method of shaping ivory denture bases to the mouth.) The base was extended well into the mucobuccal fold to enhance retention, and even the impression of the irregular ridges of the hard palate were carved into the surface of the denture.

The false teeth themselves were made of marble chips or animal bones carved to shape, and natural human teeth were used as well. Instead of posterior teeth, copper or iron nails were driven into the wood base to increase chewing efficiency. Should the client require it, teeth and borders were painted black to indicate that the wearer was a married woman, and then the entire denture was covered with lacquer, which would resist the action of saliva.

The oldest extant Japanese upper denture belonged to a Buddhist priestess, Nakaoka Tei, familiarly known as Hotoke-hime, or Lady of the Buddha, who founded the Ganjo-ji Temple at Wakayama about 1500. Among her personal effects, which are treasured in her temple, are a mirror, an inkstone, a fan, a bell, some relic bones, and the denture (fig. 76), which the priestess is said to have made herself. Traces of iron oxide indicate that at one time it was painted black. It seems probable that wooden dentures were common at that time in urban centers, for in the sixteenth century Wakayama was a remote, rural area.

The Opening of Japan to the West

Portuguese Christians flocked to Japan in the 1500s and made a substantial number of converts. The Dutch too penetrated what had hitherto been a closed area and established a flourishing trade. In the beginning, these foreigners were accepted or tolerated by the Japanese. In time, however, internal political problems created an atmosphere of animosity toward the foreigners, especially the missionaries, and anti-Christian edicts were promulgated.

When the first Tokugawa *shoguns* were beset by internal rebellion, they feared that the Europeans might lend support to the rebels. They summarily ordered the expulsion of foreign missionaries as well as of all Spaniards and Portuguese, while other aliens—principally Dutch and Chinese—were confined to Nagasaki, where a very limited foreign trade was permitted. In addition, all Japanese were forbidden to travel abroad. Thus, by 1640, Japan was virtually isolated from the outside world. Young people thirsting for Western knowledge made their way surreptitiously to Nagasaki, where they faced the formidable task not only of obtaining banned foreign books but of learning Dutch and then coining appropriate Japanese terms for foreign concepts. In 1832 Philip von Siebold, a German

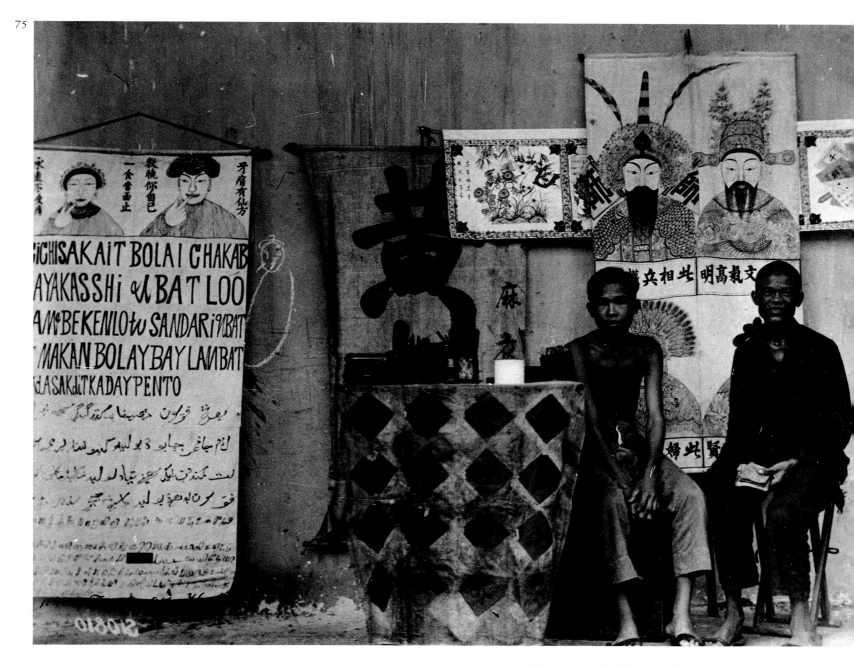

These youthful Malaysian dentists rendered treatment in the street about 1930. Kulturhistorische Sammlung des Bundesverbandes der Deutschen Zahnärzte, Cologne.

physician in Dutch employ, arrived in Nagasaki and began a series of lectures on clinical medicine. The *shoguns*, tacitly conceding the value of Western medicine, closed their eyes to his illegal activity, and thus scientific knowledge began to spread in Kyushu.

With the opening of Japan to Western trade by Commodore Perry in 1854, isolation came to an end. The Japanese turned from translating Dutch works to the study of British and American treatises. Foreign influence became pronounced and resulted in the adoption of Western techniques in medicine and dentistry.

In 1860 an American dentist, W. C. Eastlake, arrived in Yokohama and opened an office, thus becoming the first foreign dentist in Japan. He was followed in the early days of the Meiji era (1868–1912) by a number of colleagues, who introduced American practice with its emphasis on advanced prosthetics. These men had a profound influence upon Japanese dentistry, which today must be rated very high indeed. In 1875 formal examination for licensure was instituted, and in the following year Dr. Einosuke Obata became the first licensed *shika*, or dentist, in Japan.

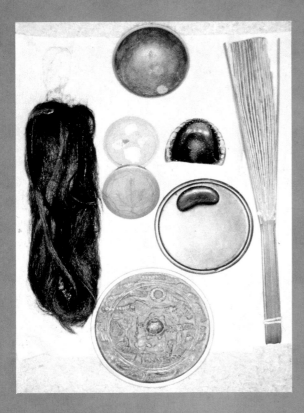

Nakaoka Tei was priestess at the Buddhist temple at Wakayama in southern Honshu until her death in 1538. The painting shown at right is believed to be her self-portrait. If so, Nakaoka Tei was manually proficient, for the full upper denture seen opposite is believed to have been carved of boxwood by the priestess herself. With her other personal effects, shown at left—a lock of hair, an inkstone, a fan, a bell, a mirror, and some relic bones—the denture, painted black at one time, is still preserved at the temple.

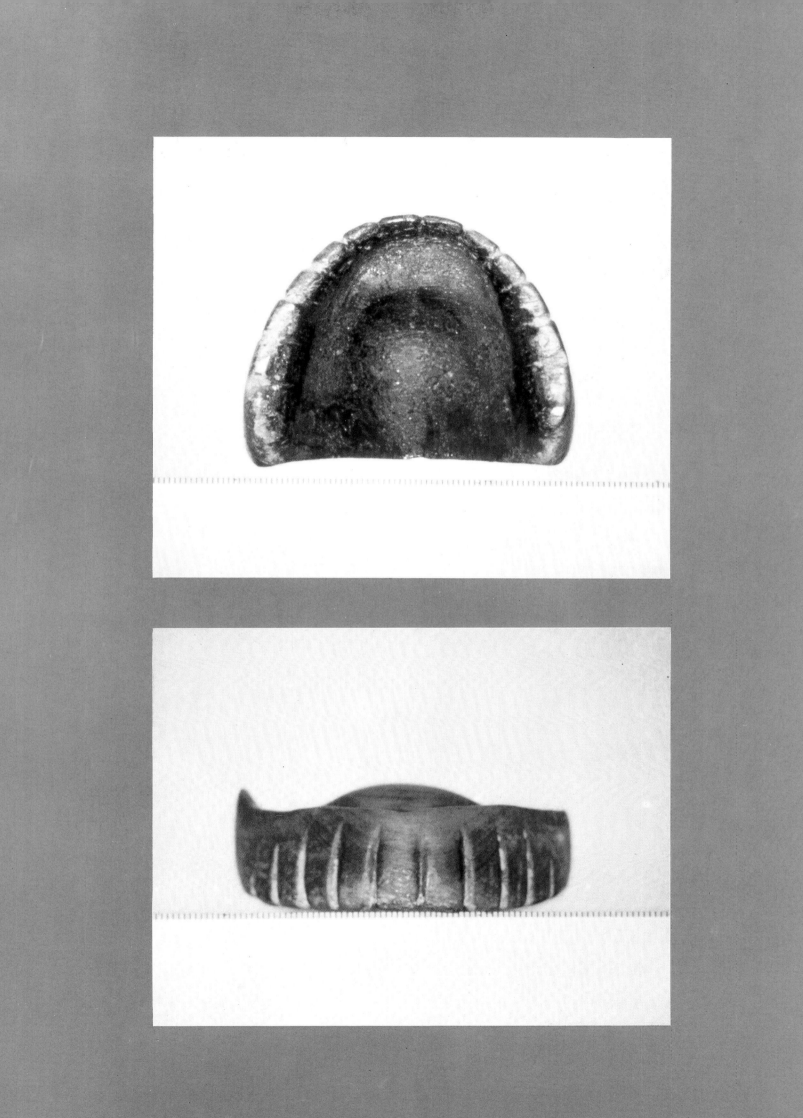

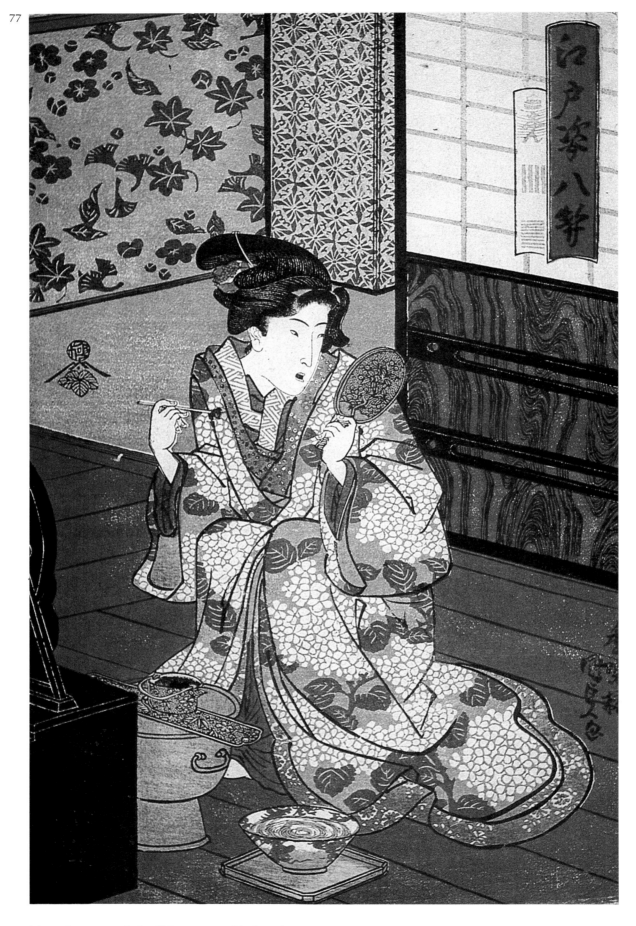

Married women of the Tokugawa era blackened their teeth as a token of conjugal fidelity, and—partly in imitation, partly as a beauty measure—prostitutes adopted the practice. In this colored woodblock print of about 1800, a courtesan dips a twig brush into a bowl of black pigment.

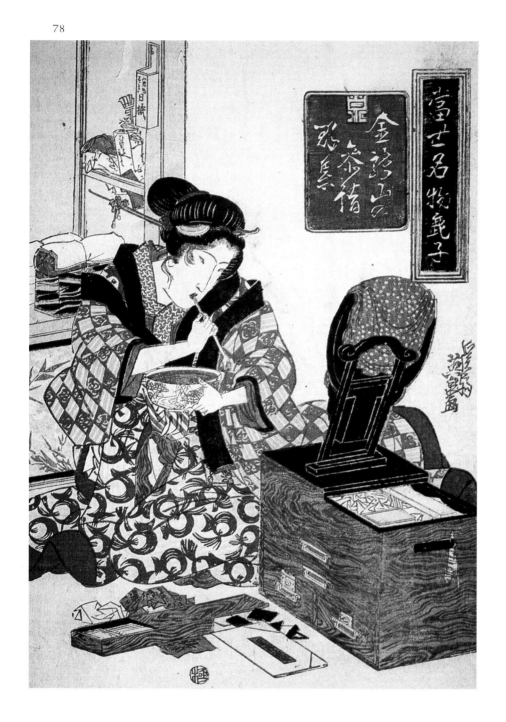

Gazing into her mirror, an open box of tooth powder before her, a Japanese woman of about 1830 brushes her teeth with the end of a beaten twig.

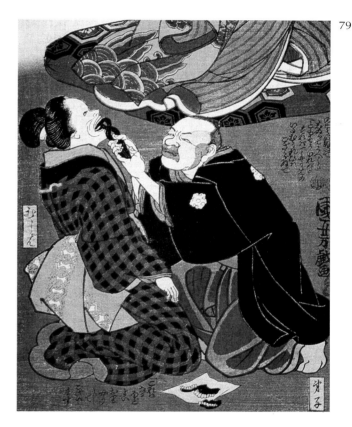

79

Facing each other as they kneel for the operation in Japanese style, a dentist extracts a patient's front tooth in this colored woodblock print of about 1800. Several wooden dentures lie on a piece of rice paper beside them.

The fifteenth-century *Epistle of Othea* by Christine de Pisan contains this illustration of a medieval physician examining a bottle of urine while the patient's servant waits for a diagnosis. Uroscopy, or the diagnostic study of urine, was very highly regarded throughout the Middle Ages. It simplified the treatment of illness, since the physician did not need to examine his patient but only to study a urine sample. Bibliothèque Royale, Brussels (Ms. 9392, fol. 42).

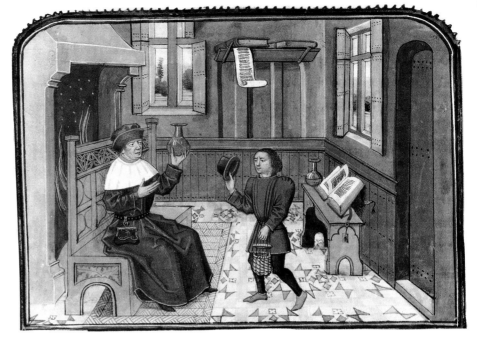

Until the fourteenth century, anatomical dissections of the human body were rarely performed at the European universities. In this woodcut illustration from Bartholomeus Angelicus, *La propriétaire des choses* (Paris, 1510), we see a group of medical men standing around a dissected corpse in attitudes of wonder and amazement. Houghton Library, Harvard University, Cambridge (Ms. Typ. 515.10.194).

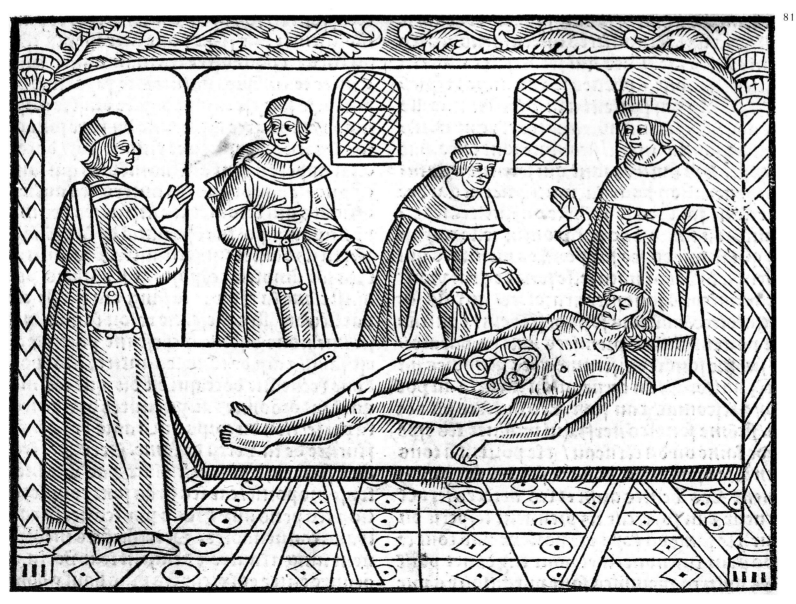

VII

THE LATE MIDDLE AGES IN WESTERN EUROPE: THIRTEENTH TO SIXTEENTH CENTURIES

"Except for some advance in anatomy and surgery at certain southern schools, like Bologna and Montpellier, the medieval universities made no contributions to medical knowledge, for no subject was less adapted to their prevailing method of verbal and syllogistic dogmatism" (C. H. Haskins, *The Rise of Universities*, 1957). During the thirteenth and fourteenth centuries, the medical curriculum continued to be based on the writings of the ancient Roman and Greek authors translated into rude Latin. Some attention was also paid to the writings of Muslim doctors, whose works had also been translated but in most cases attributed to one or another contemporary European scholar. There was no clinical teaching of any kind and, until the fourteenth century, no dissection. Eventually, following the example of the University of Bologna, whose school of law undertook dissections as a means of securing legal evidence, medical faculties in a number of cities adopted the practice, but it was never considered a central part of the curriculum.

When the medieval student had completed his medical studies satisfactorily, as evidenced by his mastery of the Greek and Latin classics, he was awarded a cane with a gold knob and allowed out into the world to earn his living. Needless to say, the medicine he practiced was of the most primitive kind, based largely on venerable superstitions and pseudo-scientific postulates. For example, diagnosis based solely on study of the patient's urine, or uroscopy, became so popular that observation of the patient was not considered necessary. The physician assiduously studied a sample of urine and then rendered an opinion and prescribed a course of treatment.

That ancient scapegoat the mythical toothworm was still blamed for toothache, whose intermittent pains were explained as being due to the worm's fitful movements. Elaborate liquid prescriptions were applied as drops on an aching tooth to conquer the worm. Following the methods of the Arabic writers, specialists applied harsh acids like aquafortis, taking care to shield the rest of the mouth from damage. One innovative method of protection was to build a small cofferdam of wax around a carious tooth before filling it with caustic liquid. Today we know that any relief that did ensue resulted from the destruction of the nerves in the dental pulp, though our ancestors attributed it to the death of the toothworm.

Generally, however, dentists attacked the toothworm by fumigation with henbane or leek seeds. These were mixed with sheep tallow to form little balls. The patient would stand or kneel near a brazier and hold a funnel with the large opening over the fire and the small end directed toward the tooth. Then the seed balls were dropped on the fire. The burning vapors that entered the tooth were supposed to drive out the worm.

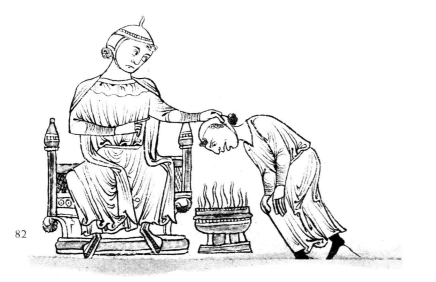

82

A patient bends over a brazier containing burning henbane seeds, the fumes of which were believed to cure toothache by driving out a "worm" consuming the tooth. The illustration is from a thirteenth-century gloss on Roger of Salerno's *Practica chirurgia*. Three other illustrations from Roger's influential work are shown in figure 89. Trinity College Library, Cambridge (Ms. 0.1.20).

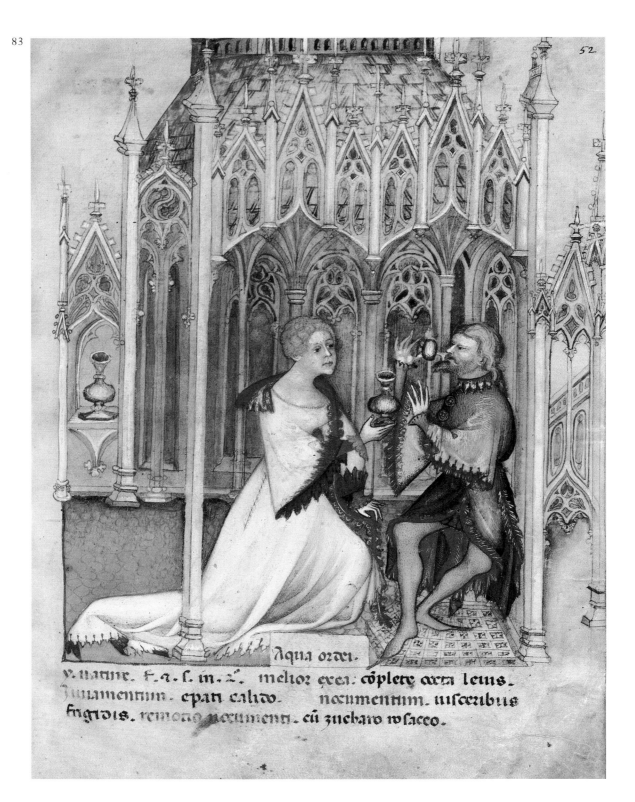

Aqua ordei.

In the early Middle Ages great reliance was placed on the supposed curative value of common plants. This miniature from *Tacuinum sanitatis*, a medico-pharmacological treatise of 1405, based on a tenth-century Arabic work, shows a patient being offered *aqua ordei* (barley water, which was classified as "cold and dry") to relieve a coldness of the intestines. Bibliothèque Nationale, Paris (Ms. Nal. 1673, fol. 52).

84

The author of one thirteenth-century medical manuscript (Bodleian Library, Oxford, Ms. Ashmole 1462) offered advice on relieving pain in certain areas of the body by cauterizing others. In the lower half of this illustration he shows the hot cautery points for the treatment of toothache ("ad dentium dolorem"). It is interesting, but probably not significant, that these points also appear on the Chinese acupuncture specialist's chart for oral structures (figure 70).

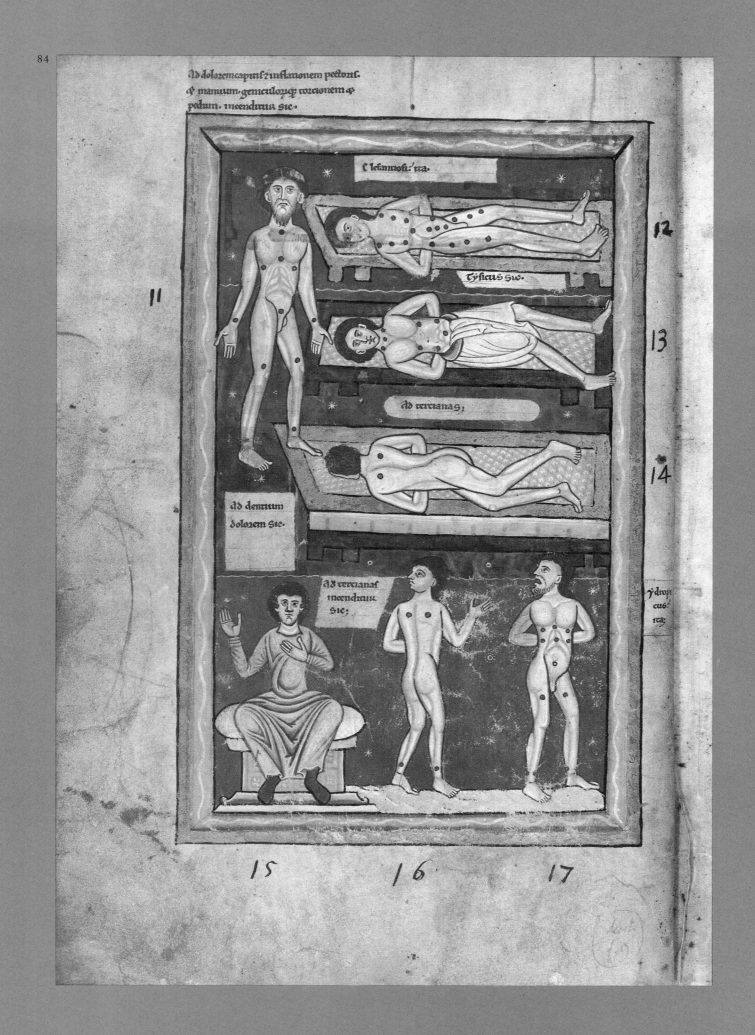

est iouis barba uncia una · tape semen uncia una · flar
tos titios uncia una · eupatori uncia una · ueto radicem
hec est capsella uncia una · erpeti uncia una · trifoli se
men quod mulieres in capite utuntur uncia una · a
morn uncia una · serpulli sicci uncia una · centaine
uncia una · aristolocie uncia una · rute agrestis uncia
una · Erute semen uncia una · lacam radicem hec est si
psana siue armodia semen uncia una · pruca semen un
cia una · hec omnia contunduntur in uno in puluere
leuissimu et ita cum melle attico teres bene commis
ces et sic condi ligent abis in buri reco2 nea utize quo
moto uoluens · uel ante lucem dabis in magnitudine
ab chiane hec si usus fueris usq ad diem definitionis
tue saluus eris ·

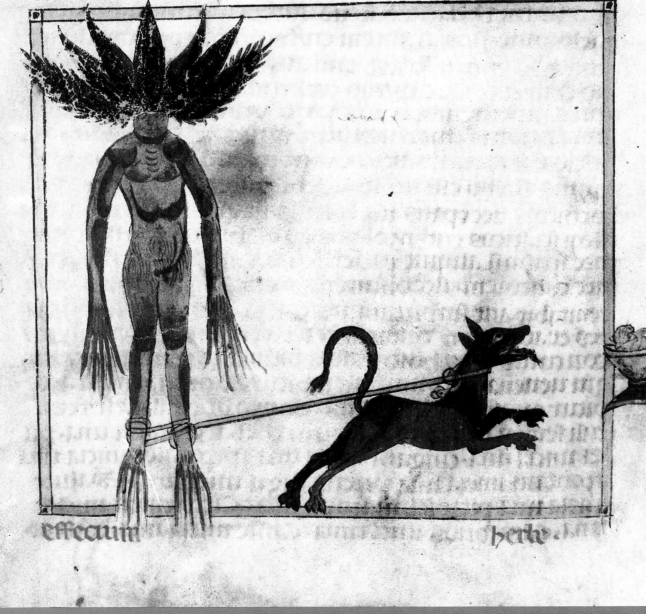

effectum   herbe

Herbal Medicine and Folk Remedies

Not yet free from the ignorance and superstition characteristic of the earlier Middle Ages, Western doctors still depended on folk medicine and especially on botanicals, which were prepared and administered in a multitude of ways and introduced into the body through every possible orifice. One of the most widely relied upon medicinal concoctions was theriac, a universal antidote dating back to the court of Mithridates, king of Pontus (ruled 120–63 B.C.), who sought to protect himself from poisoners. He is said to have achieved this by feeding ducks with a variety of toxic substances and ingesting their blood. The search for polyvalent drugs of this nature continued until the eighteenth century A.D. A popular theriac of the 1600s contained 230 ingredients, including ants, worms, and dried vipers!

Because its root resembles a human body, *Mandragora officinalis*, or mandrake plant, was highly valued as a curative. Used by the ancient Babylonians and Egyptians as a narcotic, it was recommended in the first century by Celsus, who boiled it and used the liquid to treat toothache; and its importance in the pharmacopoeia grew still greater in the later Middle Ages. The mandrake's anthropomorphous shape gave rise to many legends. A manuscript widely copied and circulated in the late Middle Ages gives these instructions for securing the plant:

> A man should not [dig up the root] because it would endanger his life.
> Therefore, the top part of the plant is tied to a black dog, and the animal has to be driven until the mandrake is lifted out of the earth. At this moment the plant will utter a terrible shriek and the dog will fall dead on the spot. To survive, the root-gatherer must plug his ears beforehand.

By the end of the Middle Ages, a genuine mandrake cult existed in Europe and the plant was eagerly collected.

Many other nonsensical beliefs were propagated and perpetuated. Pervasive was the idea that the liquor left after boiling little green frogs would loosen the teeth and make them fall out. Hieronymus Brunschwig, a German surgeon of the Renaissance—quoting Rhazes—said unhesitatingly that if a cow grazing in a field accidentally took a little green frog into her mouth, all of her teeth would fall out in an instant. Garlic crushed and carried on the thumbnail of the hand on the same side as the toothache was believed to cure that affliction, as was the juice of pellitory, ivy, chicory, and rose petals dropped into the ear or nostril on the side of the offending tooth. And in an attempt to improve upon a tried-and-true remedy for odontalgia—cautery with hot needles—dentists disregarded the tooth itself, plunging the needle instead into one of several sites on the body that they believed to be directly connected to the aching tooth. Or the needle might be plunged into the earlobe on the same side of the head. Later another school of thought claimed that to be effective the needle must be inserted into the earlobe on the *opposite* side of the head—and the two factions, the "same siders" and the "opposite siders," maintained a fierce rivalry.

85

Because of a fancied resemblance to the human body, the mandrake plant was credited with many magical attributes during the Middle Ages; moreover, it was believed to utter such a hideous shriek when uprooted from the earth that any human being nearby would fall down dead. In this illustration from Antonius Musa's thirteenth-century *De herba vettonica*, the usual method of harvesting the plant is shown. A dog tied to a rope attached to the plant pulls it out out of the earth, while his master presumably whistles for him from a safe distance. The mandrake (*Mandragora officinalis*) does indeed contain a narcotic that acts as a painkiller. Wellcome Institute Library, London.

si collū disiungitur fit uirtū inuucturā colli. eu
nisi mediuc ato suciurit morit desacili. 7 sus
focatur infirm. cu festinat sic ē subueniens.

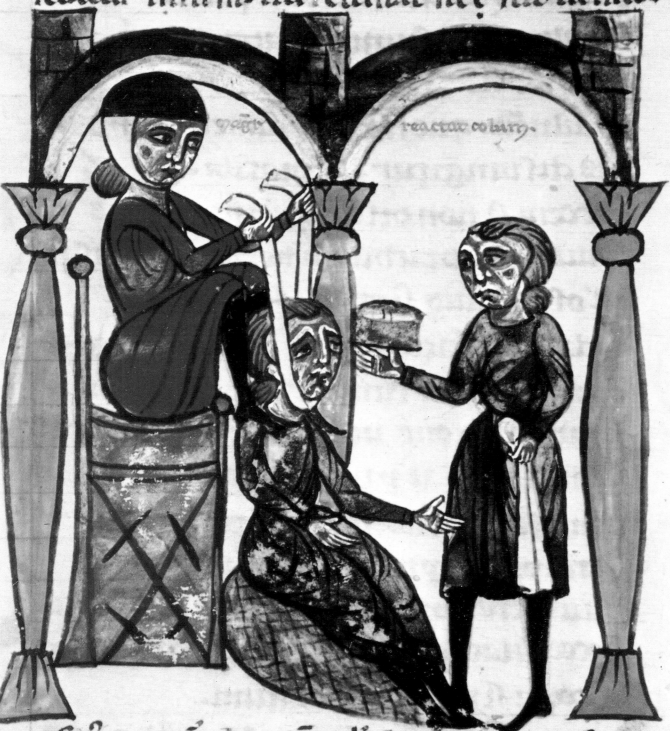

magist   reactuoc colurg.

ofsi apiut. 7 lignū ul' amo tile ut osap
tum teneit inoit mittit cuirt postea ep si
uiuenit ē7 de nouo disiūctio sit. sic atipia
tur perpillos l simutitate capitis 7 eleuetū
subito. 7 fasciolus subuminou bul' ponatū

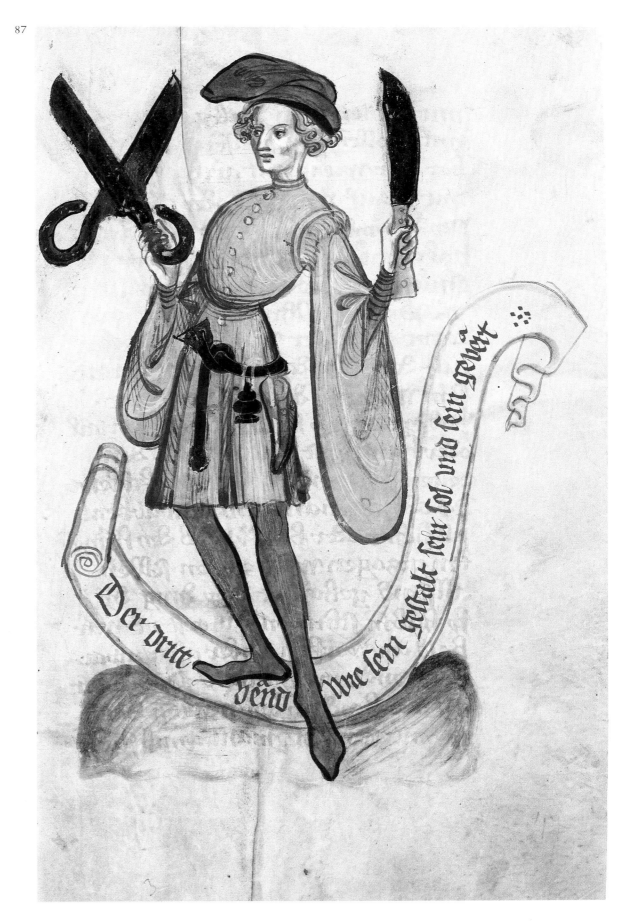

Der dritt bend Wie sein gestalt sein sol und sein gewert

86

A female practitioner places a bandage under the jaw of a patient, possibly to stabilize a fracture or a reduced dislocation. From a fourteenth-century gloss on Roland of Parma's *Chirurgia*. Biblioteca Casanatense, Rome (Ms. 1382, fol. 9).

Decorating a page of Jacobus de Cessolis, *Schazabelbuch*, of about 1408, a colorful barber-surgeon flaunts the tools of his trade: a shears and a knife. Houghton Library, Harvard University, Cambridge (Ms. Typ. 45).

In this detail of *Superbia*, a satirical engraving by
Pieter van der Heyden in the style of Brueghel, a
medieval barber investigates the mouth of a customer, who holds a basin beneath his chin. Metropolitan Museum of Art, New York. Harris Brisbane
Dick Fund, 1976.

88

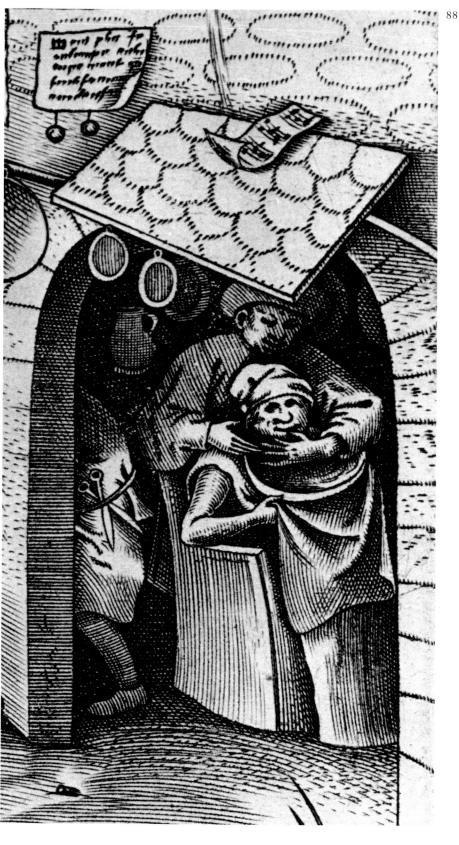

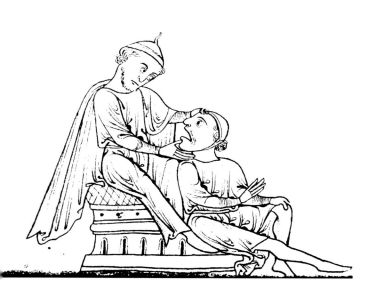

89

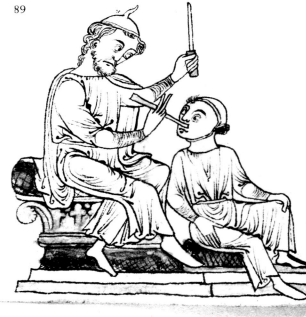

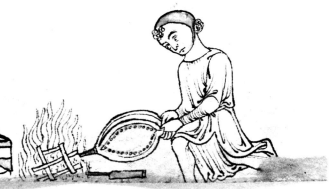

The Rise of Surgery

Since the early days of the Church, medical treatment had for the most part been the province of the monks. The Edict of Tours of 1163 wrought a major change, as we have already observed. Since monks were forbidden to perform any more operations, this duty fell to the barbers who had previously assisted the monks in their surgical ministrations. Barbers had been frequent callers at the monasteries, especially after 1092, when beards were banned, shaving the monks and cutting their hair in the tonsure prescribed for each particular order—hence their name, *barbi-tonsoribus*. The barbers soon widened the scope of their activities, performing many types of surgery, such as couching cataracts, cutting for bladder stones, lancing abscesses, letting blood, and extracting teeth. In Germany the barber was often the keeper of a bathhouse (*balneator*), who, in addition to cupping and bleeding, also gave enemas and extracted teeth. He proved his competence in examination by the way he sharpened his knives and razors and prepared his salves and plasters.

How professional surgeons rose from the barbershops of medieval Europe can be deduced from what happened in France. There the guild of barbers was organized in 1210, in Paris. As some of its members claimed more knowledge than others, eventually a division occurred between surgeons (or "surgeons of the long robe") and lay barbers (also called barber-surgeons, or "surgeons of the short robe"). Various royal decrees in the fourteenth century forbade members of the latter group from practicing surgery without first being examined by the former. Several operations were performed by both groups—bleeding, for example, and the extraction of teeth. In time, however, bleeding, cupping, giving enemas, leeching, and extracting teeth became nearly the exclusive province of the barbers.

The earliest surgeons to gain prominence in their field wrote extensively of their work, and their treatises served as guides for successive generations of practitioners. The first of these were Roger of Salerno and Roland of Parma, who lived in the late twelfth century and early thirteenth century, respectively. Their works were copied repeatedly in succeeding years, and glosses and commentaries on them give us an interesting picture of dental treatment in that early time. Expressing the opinion of specialists since the days of Hippocrates, they advised against tooth extraction except as a last resort because of its danger, recommending instead fumigation and cautery. In their treatises we find discussion of the treatment of mandibular fractures and dislocations, letting blood from a vein under the tongue, and the all-too-familiar "remedies" for toothache, including insertion of raven manure into a carious tooth!

In England John of Gaddesden, working in the early 1300s, authored a curious book, *Rosa anglica*, in which he reiterated most of the folk remedies popular at the time. He believed that the brains of a hare rubbed on the gums would not only facilitate teething but make teeth grow in the mouths of those who had lost them! And although he too considered extractions a last resort, he must have performed them, for he says, "Take an iron, wide at the front and sharply cutting on the inside and force the tooth down, and it will thus fall out." What kind of instrument he used is unclear; probably it was a forerunner of the pelican.

In Italy the Church's interdiction against the practice of surgery by the clergy was occasionally violated. A prominent example was Teodorico Borgognoni (Theodoric of Cervia, 1205–1296), who ultimately became a bishop. He was the first to make note of the copious salivation of patients treated with mercury for syphilis.

Similar to John of Gaddesden's *Rosa anglica* was *Lilium medicinae*, by Bernard de Gordon, an English physician settled in Montpellier. Written about 1285, *Lilium*

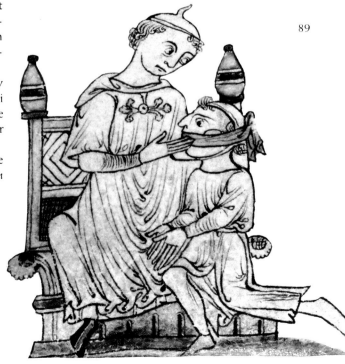

These three illustrations from a thirteenth-century French gloss on Roger of Salerno's *Practica chirurgia* show, from left to right, a doctor examining a patient, cauterizing his aching tooth with a hot iron, and bandaging his sore mouth. Trinity College, Cambridge (Ms. 0.1.20).

89

facto i sublunato regis z abstinē
cia aq̄ z oim cibioz frioz z
i oigestibiliuz. Et sic cib̄ cū
panis bñ coctus z bñ ferme
tatus caro arietis castrāy
al. coluina. pullina. poia
na z isilia hys rubeiz sit m
nuz. aar isbia i ootoz aio
materz.

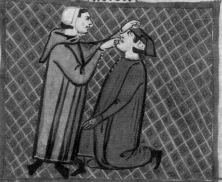

Pleniq̄ Do nap
ta ccūr sup ca z cu
fluitas quc̄ra,
q̄bur hoīmib. q̄ uul go
dr napta. Et ē spi ma
gnū carnosū z molle.
ut plimū sic figus z nō est
i eo oloz nz caloz nz pulsa
tō z foztasse er ea ē q̄ nigra
ē atco. ut super cēs alias sup
fluitates cozpis. Et ia moi
que dū septoz z oriī. ip̄i q̄ hē

bat naptaz i humo suo Et
ē uioisse euz putabaz cū ha
bere pulluinar i humo Bñ
oetecto collo uioi egisse. Et
p̄sidēta eḡne fuit z siluit me
uiz ut nō tagēt sz remaneit
ē comino suo timui p̄ mag
tuoiuez ei z moris mei sp̄ē
p̄siluiz tiicisionib muiq̄ oaiz
ū por aliq̄ piculuz er iciisio
nib cuēie. Vir aut in̄epto
p̄siilio meo accessir ao q̄idā
cyirurgie in notuz z iiaoir eui
z popr me liliiuir. et riur n
naptaz. Vu lcbs z aplius poū
ter. Vuguī hē er raio rit gēt
b) **C**Et mod curatois et
ē ur ierdaz z ercorieiz er oī p
te cuz facilitate z ecilatur.
Vui ioc eauti cei p optiē p̄
sagus flurir q̄ mltosiciens
post icisionē accerē p̄iueuir
Jntō. n. n̄ fiar cautiçatio
mozbi reoir. **C**Si u̅ napta
fuir nimis q̄ sic raoicas cui
ciisio ueciā ē. Vn̄ iciioc ēcame
oietarz cū i cauticā iesi ou
uir. Et q̄n raoir eius ē sbtil
ualoe z pene sic testiculus
tē nō oz ercoziare ip̄m, sz ia
ois ear tē raoicē z cautiça.

Teodorico Borgognoni (also known as Theodoric of Cervia, or of Lucca), an illustrious surgeon, authored his important *Cyrurgia* (*Surgery*) between 1267 and 1275, the same years he served as bishop of Cervia. This illustration from an early fifteenth-century edition shows a dentist examining a patient. Bibliotheek der Rijksuniversiteit, Leiden (Ms. Vossius Latinus 3, fol. 117).

Folio 54, verso, of Aldo Brandino da Siena's *Le régime du corps*, a fifteenth-century treatise on hygiene, shows a man rubbing his teeth with liquid from one or more of the bottles arranged on a table before him. Pierpont Morgan Library, New York (Ms. 165, fol. 54).

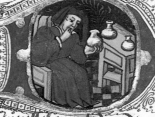

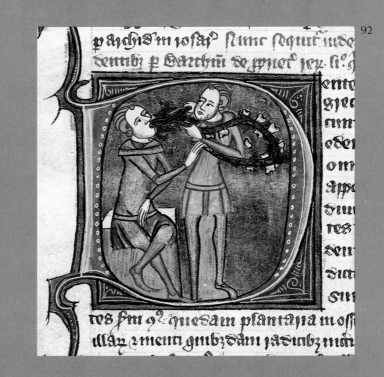

The initial letter *D* from Jacobus the Englishman's *Omne bonum*, a fifteenth-century English manuscript written in Latin, is enlivened by the sketch of a dentist extracting the tooth of a patient. British Museum, London (Royal Ms. 6 E VI).

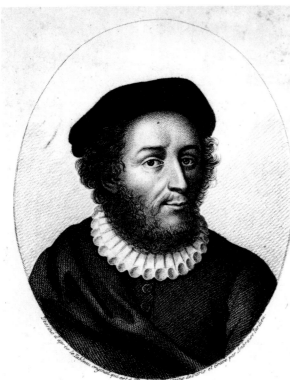

GUY DE CHAULIAC
(Médecin – Anatomiste),
Docteur de la Faculté de Montpellier,
Médecin des Papes Clément VI, Innocent VI
et Urbain V.

Guy de Chauliac was the most influential author on surgery in the fourteenth century. As A. Tardieu's engraved print indicates, de Chauliac was a member of the faculty of the great French hospital at Montpellier and personal physician to three popes. Wellcome Institute Library, London.

medicinae must have been widely known, for a number of manuscript copies of it exist today. Although de Gordon's writing was extremely literate, he introduced little that was new. Among his numerous comments on dentistry is the popular observation that there are internal and external causes for tooth ailments. Among the external ones de Gordon listed are eating hot foods immediately after cold ones; cracking hard foods with the teeth; neglect of oral care; and too vigorous rubbing of the gums. His internal causes included humors that flowed down to the teeth from the head and vomiting up stomach acids. He astutely warned surgeons against the injudicious use of opiates and urged caution in extraction, advocating first loosening the tooth with corrosive agents enclosed in a wax cofferdam.

Guy de Chauliac

Far and away the most important personage in the field of surgery during the fourteenth and fifteenth centuries was Guy de Chauliac (c. 1300–1368). He studied medicine at Toulouse and Bologna but preferred surgery, receiving his training from Henri de Mondeville, surgeon to Philip the Fair and professor of anatomy at the Holy Ghost Hospital in Montpellier (fig. 93).

In 1343 de Chauliac wrote his great work *Inventorium...Chirurgicalis Medicinae*, which soon became the principal surgical work of his time, and which in 1592 was translated into the vernacular French (*Grande Chirurgie*) for the benefit of practicing surgeons. It was also translated into Provençal, Italian, English, Dutch, and Hebrew, and published in about 130 editions. The importance of de Chauliac's work in his own day, before the advent of printing, must have been very great, for there are extant today about thirty-five manuscript copies of his magnum opus.

In *Inventorium...chirurgicalis medicinae* de Chauliac discussed the anatomy of the teeth and their eruption, citing "evidence" that adults occasionally erupt an additional set of teeth. He also listed the maladies to which the teeth are subject: pain; corrosion; congelation; "setting on edge"; and looseness. Their cures he divided into two categories: "universal" and "particular." The universal category of treatment consisted of adherence to rules of hygiene; the use of purgatives; letting blood from a cephalic vein or veins under the tongue; cupping; friction; scarification; and the cure of disorders of the head. His hygienic rules were sound and for the most part hold true today:

1. Avoid food that putrifies readily.
2. Avoid food or drink that is either too hot or too cold and especially avoid swallowing extremely cold food after extremely hot food, and vice versa.
3. Do not bite into things that are too hard.
4. Avoid foods that stick to the teeth, such as figs and confections made with honey.
5. Avoid certain foods known to be bad for the teeth [his example was leeks].
6. Clean the teeth gently with a mixture of honey and burnt salt to which some vinegar has been added.

When de Chauliac speaks of "particular" treatment, he repeats many of the remedies suggested by the Arabic writers. In addition, he recommends washing carious teeth with decoctions of wine and mint, pepper, or other agents, and afterward filling the cavities with either gallnut powder, mastic, myrrh, camphor, or one of a host of other substances. He advised the use of astringents and other agents to tighten loosened teeth, suggesting that if they fell out they might be replaced with human teeth or teeth fashioned from the bone of cattle and held in place by ligatures of gold wire. De Chauliac was extremely brief in his discussion of dental prosthetics. He mentioned the materials used in his time to fill teeth but gave no indication as to how they were applied or in what proportions they were mixed. While on the subject of extraction, he described the double-lever pelican and its method of use. However, whether he himself used it or merely watched the barber-surgeons use it is not clear.

Whereas Albucasis had declaimed strongly against the barbers because they had the temerity to undertake operations on the teeth for which they were ill-prepared, de Chauliac was of a very different opinion. He maintained that operations on the teeth were "proper to the barbers and *dentatores*," though they should be performed under the supervision of doctors, and advised the physicians who supervised the barbers to acquaint themselves with the techniques of the *dentatores* so that they might be in a position to give proper advice. This is the very first time that the term *dentatores*, signifying a specific group of practitioners, appears in the literature. The inventory of instruments de Chauliac lists as their necessary equipment makes it clear that the *dentatores* were not just barbers who occasionally extracted teeth. The list includes razors, iron scrapers, straight and bent spatulas, single- and double-armed levers, forceps, probes, lancets, scalpels, cannulas, and drills. These up-to-date practitioners clearly offered a complete range of dental services.

Though much of his writing is based on superstition and unfounded convention, de Chauliac was wiser than many of his contemporaries. Considering the assertions by his colleagues that teeth could be removed by applying unguents of frog fat and similar decoctions without recourse to forceps, he remarks, "These remedies promise much but deliver little."

One other important fact emerges from de Chauliac's treatise. Surgeons at that time were apparently using drugs to prevent their patients from feeling pain during operations. Among the stupefacients they used were opium, hyoscyamine, mandrake root, ivy, and hemlock. De Chauliac describes how they were administered. A new sponge was soaked "in these juices and left to dry in the sun; and when [surgeons] have need of it they put the sponge into warm water and then hold it under the nostrils of the patient until he goes to sleep. Then they perform the operation." It appears that the narcosis achieved was truly intense since de Chauliac describes how a surgeon could awaken his patient by holding another sponge, soaked in vinegar, to his nostrils, or by dropping the juice of rue or fennel into his ears.

De Chauliac's Successors

De Chauliac's influence was great and perdurable—not only because of his writings but also because he trained a number of students, perhaps the most distinguished of whom was Pietro d'Argelata (died 1423). A professor at Bologna, d'Argelata wrote his own *Cirurgia*, published in Venice in 1480, a treatise in six volumes in which diseases and treatment of the teeth occupy a large part. Though he introduced little that was new and repeated much of what de Chauliac had said without attributing it to him, d'Argelata helped to lay the basis of dental practice. He and the surgeons who came after him added, each in small measure, to the growth of this branch of healing.

Giovanni Arcolani (or Arculanus), who died in 1460, followed d'Argelata as professor at Bologna from 1422 to 1427. He too authored a treatise—*Cirurgia practica*, published in Venice in 1483—in which he dealt extensively with dentistry and, as a result, he is also considered one of the pioneers in the field.

Arcolani repeated many of de Chauliac's sound general admonitions and dealt extensively with dental anatomy as well as with all manner of dental problems and their treatment. Yet it is for two quite different reasons that he holds a position of importance for historians of dentistry. First, to elucidate his remarks on tooth extraction, he illustrated the instruments most commonly used for that operation, including the pelican, by his time a tried-and-true dental aid and destined to remain so until modern times. Still more significant is a passage on

Prima pars practice in chirurgia.

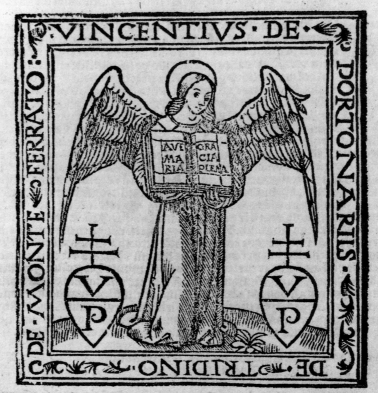

VINCENTIVS · DE · PORTONARIIS · DE · TRIDINO · DE · MONTE · FERRATO

AVE MA RIA · GRA CIA PLENA

Practica in arte chirurgica copiosa Joannis de vigo Iulij.ij. Pon.Mar. Continēs nouē libros ifra scriptos.

Primus:	De anathomia chirurgo necessaria.
Secundus:	De apostematibus in vniuersali et particulari.
Tertius:	De vulneribus in vniuersali et particulari.
Quartus:	De vlceribus in vniuersali et particulari.
Quintus:	De morbo gallico:et dislocatione iuncturarum
Sertus:	De fractura et dislocatione ossium.
Septimus:	De natura simplicium et posse eorum.
Octauus:	De natura compositorum:et est antidotarium.
Nonus:	De quibusdam additionibus totum complentibus.

Cum gratia et priuilegio.

carious teeth, where at the end of a long paragraph on fillings he mentions gold leaf—the first documentation of the use of gold for filling diseased teeth. We deduce that the practice was well established by Arcolani's time since he does not single it out for special mention, and we therefore have a convincing piece of evidence that operative dentistry had developed mightily by the end of the Middle Ages.

In the authoritative surgical treatise of the sixteenth and seventeenth centuries, *Practica copiosa in arte chirurgica* (1514), by Giovanni da Vigo (1460–1525), we find more specific discussion of the way carious teeth were filled with gold. "Corrosion occurs in the great teeth through rottenness with sharp and evil moisture which grows and bites them. You may remove the corrosion with trephines, files, and other convenient instruments, filling the cavities afterward with leaves of gold." It is very likely, though not certain, that da Vigo himself carried out this procedure (by his day about a hundred years old), for very frequently he states that he himself has tried and personally "proved" one or another remedy or treatment. He may even have filled the teeth of his princely patron, Pope Julius II, who brought him to Rome as his personal physician after ascending the papal throne in 1503 (a noteworthy move, for the surgeon da Vigo thereby achieved the same status as a medical doctor).

Although this leading surgeon of his day was probably himself skilled in tooth extraction, he nevertheless urged his readers to go to the barber-surgeons in order to learn their methods and thus improve their own dexterity: "When all remedies fail . . . we must come to handy operation, to draw out the teeth, whereunto an expert man is requisite, wherefore the surgeons do remit this cure to the barbers and vagabond tooth-drawers. Howbeit, it is good to have seen and to mark the working of such."

In his open-mindedness and curiosity, and in many other ways, da Vigo was ahead of his times. For outside the great medical universities and the sophisticated metropolises, dentistry remained backward and inadequate. As late as 1500 a renowned German surgeon, Christopher Wirtzung, was recommending that a condition he described as "a swelling and falling down of the palate"—which was probably an infection of the soft palate or a peritonsillar abscess—be treated by smearing the palate with a paste made of *album graecum,*

> that is, a white dog's turd (of a dog that eats nought but bones). If the patient has long hair, then let a strong man take hold of it and pull it upward violently, until one may perceive that the skin is severed or parted from the skull; then also doth the palate ascend, because it is fastened to the skin; it has been found by experience that it has helped immediately, and has preserved the patient from choking.

Da Vigo, who enjoyed a close friendship with Giovanni Anthracino, the most eminent member of the Roman medical faculty, and who moved in the sophisticated circles that included Michelangelo, Raphael, and Bramante, was never guilty of such excesses, though he clung to the theory of the cardinal humors, blaming abscesses of the jaws on an excess of humors in the head, much as had Galen thirteen hundred years earlier.

Da Vigo recognized how important healthy teeth are to human psychological and physiological well-being: "The teeth serve for comeliness, for chewing meat, and for pronunciation, and therefore they must be cured with all diligence." He vigorously advocated good oral hygiene, prescribing numerous concoctions composed of plantain, pomegranate, wild olive, and other materials "wherewith the gums are to be rubbed." He also specified in detail how tartar should be scraped from the teeth. Like de Chauliac, d'Argelata, and Arcolani, he must be remembered as one of the pioneers of the late Middle Ages in the advancement of surgery, which eventually resulted in the birth of the modern profession of dentistry. Because of their example, dentistry in Europe would never again lose significant ground to the forces of superstition and intellectual stagnation. It would now be possible to "begin where older knowledge left off—where it had reached the limits of its understanding."

94

Born in 1460, the close contemporary of Leonardo and Macchiavelli, Giovanni da Vigo belongs chronologically to the Renaissance, but because his vocation lagged behind other arts, he stands only at the threshold of the modern age in medicine. During his lifetime, and in part because of his efforts, surgery rose rapidly in repute. He himself developed better methods of ligating arteries and veins, and his *Practica copiosa in arte chirurgica*, which contained extensive dental writings, remained *the* important treatise on surgery during the next two centuries. Illustrated here is the title page of the edition issued in Leiden in 1518, which served also as a short table of contents, outlining what the reader would find within. National Library of Medicine, Bethesda.

BARTHOLOMAEI

EVSTACHII

SANCTOSEVERINATIS

LIBELLVS DE

DENTIBVS.

Cum priuilegijs.

VENETIIS,

M D LXIII.

The first major book on dental anatomy, *Libellus de dentibus*, published in 1563, was Eustachius's great contribution to dentistry. Illustrated here is the title page. The ornament includes the ancient medical symbol of twined snakes.

VIII
THE RENAISSANCE

The most important achievements of the Renaissance were two: the rediscovery and absorption of the thought and art of the Romans and Greeks and the rebirth of the spirit of Classical inquiry, which made it possible to free science from theology and superstition. During the fifteenth century a number of events predisposed Europeans to what Jacob Burckhardt called the "discovery of the world and of man," which separates the Middle Ages from the Renaissance. The invention of printing with movable type and the invention of engraving were of tremendous importance for the development and diffusion of knowledge. The discovery of America and the opening up of the rest of the world to exploration revealed new aspects of nature. The capture of Constantinople by the Turks in 1453 forced many Byzantine scholars to flee to the West, and they brought with them knowledge of the ideas of Plato and Hippocrates, which did much in time to unseat the Galenists, who clung to beliefs not based on facts or observation and stubbornly ignored new techniques and medications.

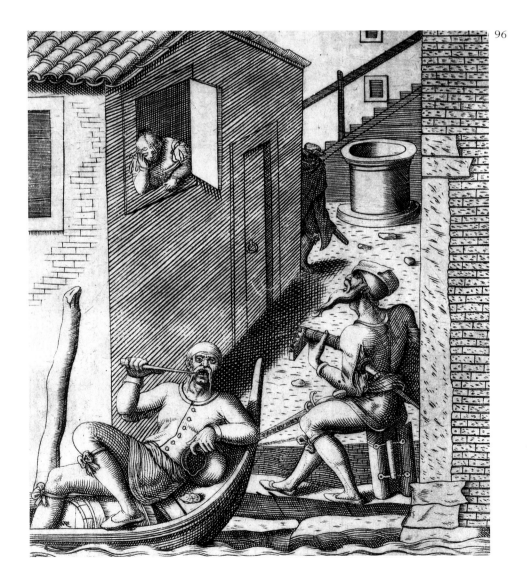

96

This illustration from *Naspo Bizaro* by Alessandro Caravia (1565) shows that oral hygiene of a sort was practiced in Venice in the sixteenth century. A gondolier, who has just finished a meal, cleans his teeth with an oversized pick while his passenger serenades his inamorata. Houghton Library, Harvard University, Cambridge (Ms. Typ. 525. 65. 260).

Advances in Anatomical Knowledge

At the basis of progress in medicine during the fifteenth and sixteenth centuries was the renaissance of anatomy. Artists manifested a new interest in the human body, and many studied it in order to improve the accuracy of their renderings. Leonardo da Vinci (1452–1519), however, studied anatomy for anatomy's sake, conducting the most painstaking dissections and studying and sketching almost every part of the body, internal and external, leading the eighteenth-century English anatomist William Hunter to call him the greatest anatomist of his epoch. Leonardo studied the skull in great detail (fig. 97), depicting the maxillary antrum some 150 years before Nathanael Highmore. He described the teeth carefully, and for the first time made a distinction between molars and premolars. Probably with an eye to his painting he delineated the effect loss of teeth has upon the physiognomy.

Da Vinci's influence upon medical science was ultimately pervasive because in his painstaking dissections (with no accurate nomenclature to guide him) he broke from a slavish subservience to Galen and broadened the acceptance of free inquiry. However, as Charles Singer and E. Ashworth Underwood have pointed out (*A Short History of Medicine*, 1962), although Leonardo's work remained in manuscript until fairly recently, we must not assume that his ideas were without effect on his contemporaries. Certainly, within a few years of his death, the questions he had raised about the heart and the blood vessels were attracting widespread attention.

These studies of the human skull made by Leonardo da Vinci about 1489 show the maxillary antrum some two hundred years before Nathanael Highmore described it. Lost for three hundred years, Leonardo's superb anatomical drawings now in Windsor Castle had little direct influence on his contemporaries, yet in spirit they herald the fifteenth-century renaissance in anatomy and, consequently, in surgery. Royal Library, Windsor Castle. Copyright reserved to HM the Queen.

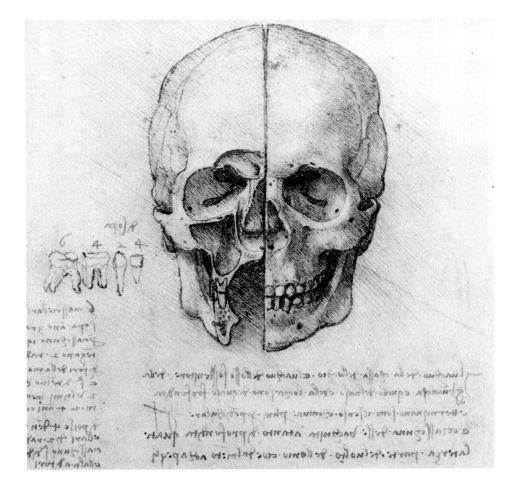

DE DENTIBVS, QVI ETIAM
ossium numero ascribuntur.   Caput XI.

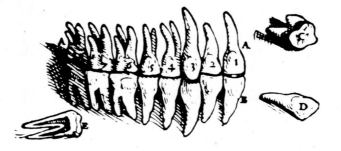

PRAESENTIS VNDECIMI CAPITIS FIGVRAE,
ac ipsius characterum Index.

HAC figura tam superioris maxillæ, quàm inferioris dentes, in altero latere exprimun tur. quum enim utriusque lateris par sit ratio, abundè est alterius lateris dentes ex maxillis eru tos delineasse. Si uerò dentes maxillis adhuc infixos contemplari uisum sit, superioris Capitis. figuræ inferiorem commonstrant seriem, quemadmodum tertia & quinta sexti Capitis figuræ superiorem. ubi & quarta eius Capitis figura alueolos promptè ostendit, quibus dentes insigun tur. Quandoquidem ex caluaria, quam illa figura expressimus, studio superioris maxillæ den tes euulsimus.

AA *Dextri lateris octo superiores dentes.*
BB *Dextri lateris dentes octo inferiores.*
1,2 *Duo dextri lateris incisorij.*   3 *Dens caninus dexter.*
4,5,6 *Quinque molares dextri. Hunc numerum & inferiori & superiori dentium classi accommo*
7,8 *dare integrum est. Nomina autem dentium, cum uarijs reliquorum ossium nomenclaturis, ex hu ius libri calce sumenda ueniũt: quòd in eum locum nomina, quæcunque mihi hactenus occurrere, duxerim reijcienda.*
C *Basis notatur molaris dentis.*   D *Acies dentis incisorij.*
E *Media molaris dentis pars hic delineatur, sinum in dentibus conspicuum ostensura.*

This page of Vesalius's *De humani corporis fabrica* deals with the teeth. Illustration E, a bicuspid tooth seen in section, shows the pulp canals. Elsewhere in his book the great anatomist discusses the development of the primary teeth and articulation of the jaws.

Vesalius

Andreas Vesalius (1514–1564) made anatomy what it remains today, a living, working science (fig. 99). Born in Brussels, of German parentage, he studied under Jacques duBois (Jacobus Sylvius), a Galenist who was to become his bitterest critic.

In 1534 Vesalius joined the faculty of the University of Padua, a city not under papal control where dissecting was not forbidden, and among his duties as public prosecutor were autopsies. In 1539 he was given the task of editing a new edition of Galen, and while engaged in this he discovered many errors and also outright falsehoods that were being perpetuated by the Galenists. He concluded, as he subsequently stated, "Galen never dissected a human body lately dead."

Vesalius was the author of one of the great works in anatomy of all time, *De humani corporis fabrica*. The illustrations were probably made by a pupil of Titian under the direct supervision of Vesalius himself, and the book was published in 1543 in Basel. Because, as Fielding H. Garrison has explained (*An Introduction to the History of Medicine*, 1929), it disposed of Galen's osteology and muscular anatomy and recreated the whole gross anatomy of the human body, it had an immense effect upon Vesalius's contemporaries and marked a break with the past and an overthrowing of Galenical tradition. Unfortunately, its author's challenge to established authority was followed by persecution, and in anger he left Padua to become physician to Emperor Charles V. On a pilgrimage to the Holy Land he was shipwrecked on a remote island, and there he died of an obscure disease at the age of fifty. His influence, however, long survived him.

Only a small portion of *De humani corporis fabrica* deals with the dental structures, but here too the author broke with Galen in maintaining that teeth are not bones; he did, however, share Galen's belief that teeth continue to grow throughout a person's lifetime, mistaking for growth the extrusion that occurs when an opposing tooth is missing.

Vesalius's Successors

The first important pupil of Vesalius was Matteo Realdo Colombo (1516?–1559), who freely borrowed from his master and others in compiling *De re anatomica*, which was published in 1559, the year of his death. Nevertheless, Colombo made some important discoveries: while dissecting fetuses he found the follicles of teeth, and thus was able to refute the widely held belief that the primary teeth form from the milk the child ingests. However, he perpetuated Vesalius's incorrect notion that permanent teeth form from the roots of the deciduous ones.

A clear demonstration of how teeth form was the achievement of another outstanding anatomist, Gabriello Fallopio (Fallopius, 1523–1562). Clearly describing the dental follicle, he proved that a permanent tooth develops independent of a primary one. And in the course of his study of many bodies of children, he disproved the idea that the mandible consists of two bones. "In all the corpses of children who have not passed their first year which I have dissected, I always found the mandible to consist of two bony parts connected in the middle by a cartilaginous mass." But with those who had died after the age of seven, he said, he found it undivided. He observed the similarity between the growth of a tooth follicle and the development of a bird's feather, laying the groundwork for the embryological study of tooth development and, what is more important, disproving the idea held since Galen's time that teeth are bones.

Among Fallopio's discoveries that proved of importance to dentistry were the trigeminal, auditory, and glossopharyngeal nerves, as well as the *chorda tympani* and the semicircular canals.

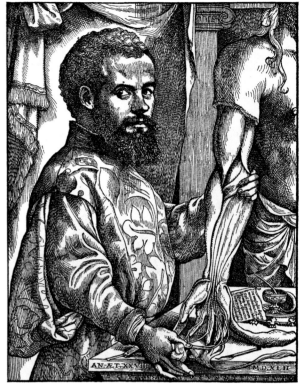

Andreas Vesalius's monumental *De humani corporis fabrica* (1543) revolutionized the study and teaching of medicine. In this illustration from the great anatomical treatise the author is portrayed at the age of twenty-eight, in the year before its publication.

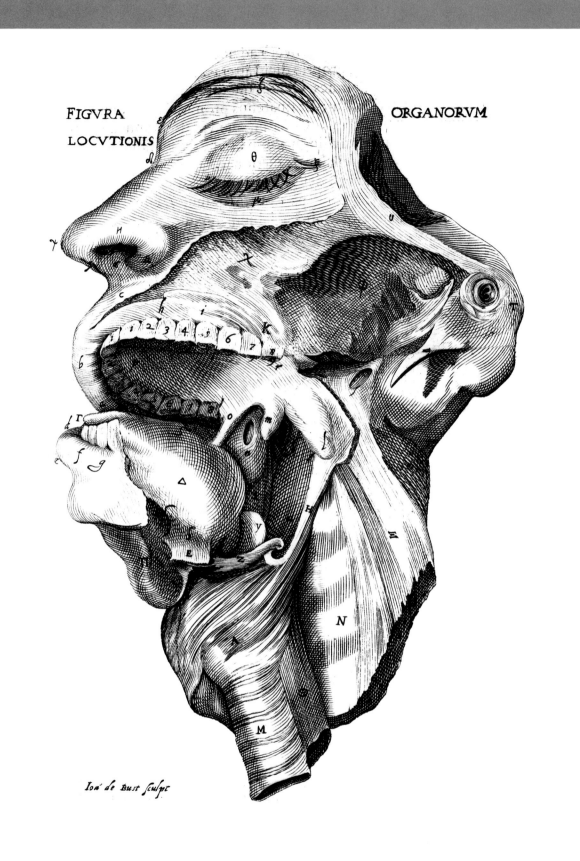

Hieronymus Fabricius ab Aquapendente (1537–1619) was professor of anatomy and surgery at Padua for forty years. One of the giants in anatomy, he is also considered the founder of embryology. This detailed illustration from his *De locutione* (1604) shows the organs of speech. Wellcome Institute Library, London.

Eustachius

The first dental anatomist, also a pupil of Vesalius, was Bartolommeo Eustachio, called Eustachius (died 1574). He made many contributions to the field, among them the description of the Eustachian tube, the abducens nerve, and the muscles of the throat and neck. His greatest achievement was to prepare for publication in 1563 *Libellus de dentibus (Pamphlet on the Teeth)*, the first book devoted to the anatomy and histology of the teeth. Divided into thirty chapters, it gathered together all current knowledge of dental morphology, histology, and physiology, containing descriptions of the formation of the teeth, their blood supply, and their pulp chambers, as well as the way in which they grow. He described in detail the function of each tooth, showing how its shape contributed to its usefulness in performing its task. He observed that teeth are not equally hard in all animals, and noted that even the most powerful dogs become cowards upon loss of their teeth.

Eustachius remained the principal authority on his subject until the eighteenth century. Nevertheless, he remained a staunch supporter of Galen to the end of his life. He defended Galen on one occasion against the accusation that he knew nothing of the existence of dental pulp with the trustful assertion that such a conscientious observer of nature's creatures as Galen must have known of it!

In 1552, while he was professor at the Collegia della Sapienza in Rome, Eustachius completed his *Tabulae anatomicae*, a set of superb plates drawn by himself, which lay unpublished in the papal library for 162 years. Finally printed in 1714, with notes by G. B. Morgagni, they are among the first anatomical studies engraved on copper, and although they lack the artistic beauty of Vesalius's work, they are more accurate and sharp (fig. 101).

Eleven years before his *Libellus de dentibus* was published, Eustachius prepared a set of drawings of parts of the human body; however, these anatomical studies, very beautifully engraved on copper, were not published until the early eighteenth century. In this plate from the 1714 edition of *Tabulae anatomicae*, Eustachius shows the upper and lower incisor, canine, premolar, and molar teeth.

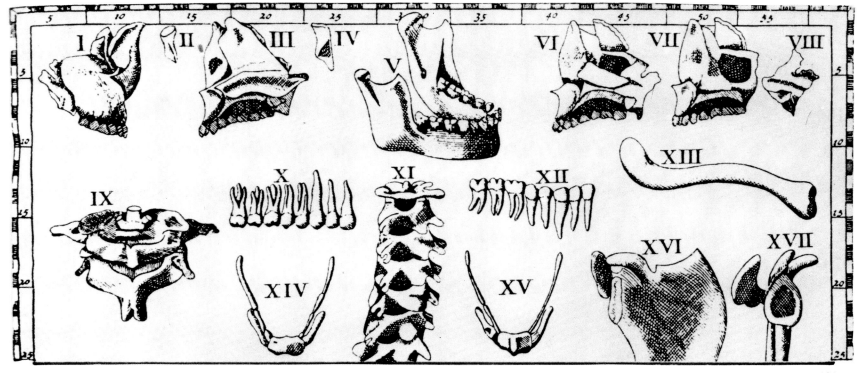

101

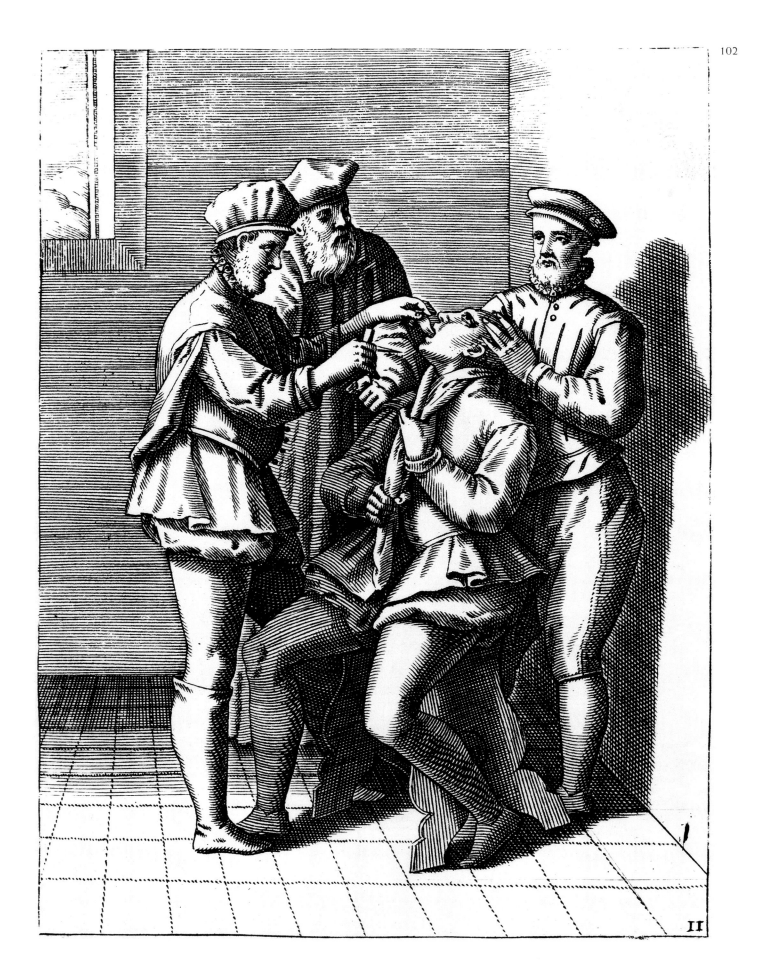

Advances in Pharmacology: Paracelsus

Far ahead of his time was Theophrastus Bombastus von Hohenheim, known as Paracelsus (1493–1541). In the same way that Vesalius laid the groundwork for scientific anatomy, so did Paracelsus pioneer rational pharmacotherapeutics. Son of a Swiss physician, he had a keen, retentive mind, and his incurable wanderlust sent him traveling all over Europe collecting information from people of every walk of life: barbers, executioners, gypsies, midwives, and fortune-tellers.

Appointed professor of medicine at Basel in 1527, he began his tenure there by publicly burning the works of Galen and Avicenna, and lecturing in his native German, instead of Latin, on findings based on his own experiences. He discounted Galenism and the theory of the cardinal humors, substituting rational therapeutics based on his theory that diseases are specific in nature and can be cured by specific remedies. He countered alchemy with chemistry and decried uroscopy, which was still extremely popular, as well as the study of the heavens as an aid to diagnosis and treatment. He stressed that it was nature that healed wounds, not officious meddling. He greatly enlarged the pharmaceutical arsenal with valuable drugs, many of which had been newly introduced from the Americas (quinine and ipecacuanha are two examples still in use today, and from caoutchouc is made gutta-percha, used even today for root-canal fillings).

Though his influence today is greatly diminished, Paracelsus remains for us a prime example of the Renaissance mind, probing and examining, casting aside whatever ran counter to observable truths despite the sanctity that enveloped many irrational beliefs of the ancients.

Letting blood from under a patient's tongue to cure maladies of the head and mouth caused by an imbalance of humors is very ancient. By the late Middle Ages, the treatment had become the province of the barber-surgeons. In this illustration of 1584 from *Discorsi intorno al sanguinar i corpi humani* by Paolo Magni, a practitioner is about to bleed his patient with a lancing pin, an instrument still in use as late as the eighteenth century. Wellcome Institute Library, London.

Many services were performed by barbers, as this sixteenth-century satirical engraving indicates. Under the same roof one could have one's wounds treated, blood let, teeth pulled, and hair cut. Bibliothèque Nationale, Paris (Ms. RF 1 rés., fol. 66).

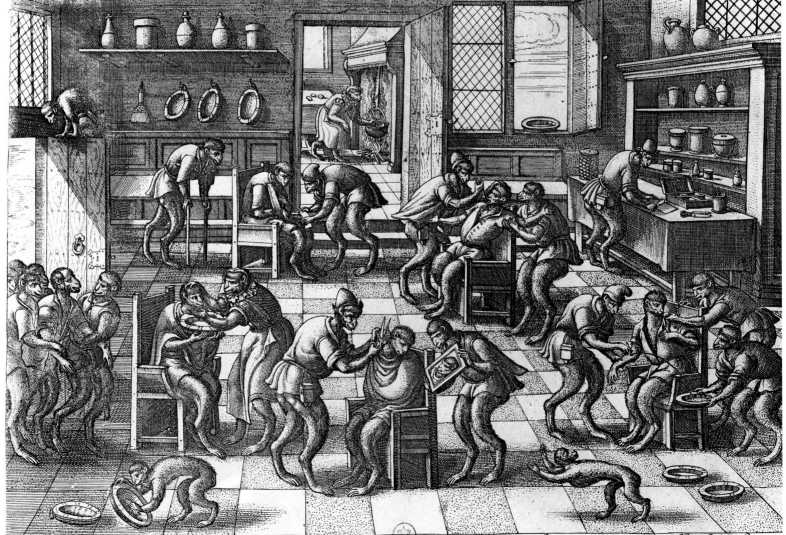

Et capita hirſutis tradunt ſpolianda capillis,
6.   Membraq; Tonſori ſaucia curet, agunt.

Chez le Barbier ſe tondre veꝛ phlebotomer ſont,
Arracher dent, curer, lors que naurez ils ſont.

Mey laet, mey trext dey tant, ey mey ſcheevt hiev dey baevt,
Maev thie dat dey baevbier ghee̅y gvoot ghelt ey gaevt.

Advances in Surgery

In Chapter Four we chose the example of France to show how the profession of surgery rose out of the multifaceted trade of barbering during the late Middle Ages. Slightly later, the same process took place in England, and in the Tudor period we have documentation of the establishment of a group of true dental specialists within the guild of barber-surgeons.

A guild of master surgeons was organized in England in 1368, and in 1462 a Mystery (Company) of the Barbers of London became incorporated. Though many members of both associations were doubtless reputable and skilled, there were hordes of incompetents as well because of an absence of professionally enforced standards. (William Clowes, the greatest surgeon of the Tudor period, inveighed against the unskilled practitioners of his own time, characterizing them as "no better than runagates or vagabonds ... shameless in countenance, lewd in disposition, brutish in judgment and understanding ... tinkers, tooth-drawers, peddlers, ostlers, carters, porters, horse-gelders, horse-leeches, idiots, apple-squires, broom-men, bawds, witches, conjurers, soothsayers, sow-gelders, rogues, and rat-catchers!"—a pretty assortment, and doubtless the situation had been no better a century earlier.) The ranks of the surgeons were also swelled after 1535 by the many monks with an elementary knowledge of medicine and surgery who had been forced out of the monasteries closed by Henry VIII.

Competition between the surgeons and the barbers reached a high pitch in the early fifteenth century, with acrimony and hard feelings on both sides. Peace was eventually brought about by Henry VIII, who prevailed upon the two groups to form a Royal Commonalty of Barber-Surgeons. The occasion of his granting a royal charter to the group is commemorated in a famous painting by Hans Holbein (fig. 107). Among the practitioners depicted are ten whose names we know. Four were surgeons, four were barbers, and two were "outsiders," who had not belonged to either company. The charter of the company delineated the bounds within which each group would operate: the surgeons would henceforth give no haircuts or shaves and the barbers would refrain from practicing surgery. The only fields left open to both were tooth extraction, cupping, leeching, and bloodletting. But the Royal Commonalty of Barber-Surgeons also included in its ranks practitioners who limited their activities to removing teeth, for the minutes book for 1551 notes that "John Brysket, tooth-drawer, hath been admitted for a brother into this house." We may conclude that there was by the mid-sixteenth century in England a group of people practicing some dentistry who enjoyed a special status and privileges conferred upon them by virtue of their membership in the guild.

The rise in the skill of European surgeons during the fifteenth and sixteenth centuries is in part attributable to the great advances that were being made in anatomy, and in part to the demands placed upon them by the continual warfare and carnage of the period. Scarcely a year passed in which warfare between the kingdoms of Europe and between the kings and the Holy Roman Emperor was not raging, and after the introduction of gunpowder in the fourteenth century, the wounds inflicted during an engagement tended to increase in number and in gravity. Many practitioners advanced to the forefront of the medical profession, accepted as the equals of the medical doctors in the highest circles. Giovanni da Vigo, who, as we have seen, became the personal physician of Pope Julius II, had received his training as battle-surgeon to the pope, then Cardinal Giulano della Rovere; William Clowes, later surgeon to Queen Elizabeth, came to London's St. Bartholomew's hospital in 1581 after a distinguished military and naval career. In fact, the first salaried professionals at St. Bartholomew's (appointed in 1549) were surgeons; the first physicians joined the staff only in 1568.

The first important treatise on military surgery is *Buch der Wund-Artzney* (*Book of Wound Surgery*) by Hieronymus Brunschwig (c. 1450–1533), published in Strasbourg in 1497. Brunschwig introduced a number of innovative techniques, such as tying off a blood vessel with a ligature and suturing a wound to bring the edges

Walter Hermann Ryff published *Gross Chirurgey* (*Great Surgery*) in 1545, and it appeared in several later editions, including one of 1559, in which these drawings of scalers appear. Ryff's illustrations were both detailed and accurate. It is a shame that the book on dentistry he proposed to write (the last sentence on this page announces forthcoming pamphlets on the eyes and teeth) was never published.

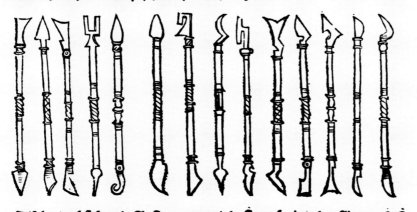

Teutſchen Chirurgei. XXXVIII

güt den mund fein gemach vnnd ſeuberlich damit auffzuſchtauben/mit allein dem Patienten luffe vnd labung zugeben/ſonder jm auch vnderweilen mit bequemer artznei zuhelffen ꝛc.

So wir nun des munds gedencken / kommen vns auch die zän für / welche mit jrem ſcharpffen vnleidlichen ſchmertzē trefflich vil Inſtrument durch die notturfſte erfunden haben.

Vnd ſeind alle diſe Inſtrumentlin ſo hernach verzeychnet ſtehn/ nicht anders geordnet/dann allein die zän damit zuſeubern / reinigen/ vnnd ſchaben/ Werden von den alten Dentrificia genant welche diſer zeit bei den Walhen/ die ſich leibliches ſchmuckens vil mehr wann wir Teutſchen gebrauchen/ noch im brauch/die zän damit friſch vnd ſauber zubehalten.

Diſe hernachfolgende Inſtrument/ wie du ſie nach einander fürgemalt ſiheſt/ Als nemlich Entenſchnabel/Pellican/Zänzangen/Vberwürff/Geyßfüßlin vnd dergleichen/wie ſie genant werden mögen/ ſeind mancherley art vnd geſtalt geformiert/ nach dem ſie ein jeder Meyſter nach ſeiner hand weyß zubrauchen vnnd regieren. Deren hab ich dir die aller gemeyneſten vnnd gebreuchlichſten fürreiſſen oder malen laſſen. Wie ſie aber zugebrauchen ſeind/ ſampt der gantzen zänartznei/ findeſt du hernach in folgender Chirurgei weitern bericht in einem beſondern Capitel/in dem letſten Theyl. Wiewol wir auch kurtz verſchinener zeit ein beſonder Büchlin haben außgehn laſſen/ darinnen alle fehl vnd gebrechen der augen vnnd zän gnügſamlichen beſchriben vnd angezeygt werden.

together. Of greater interest to us, however, are his illustrations of instruments and operations, for these give us a fine idea of the kind of surgery practiced in his day.

Brunschwig offered no advice on the repair and replacement of teeth, though he discussed wounds of the mouth and surrounding tissues. He devised a clever support for the chin in cases of jaw fracture: a leather cup fastened by straps across the top of the head. He noted that when the fragments of the mandible were displaced, the patient's teeth were to be brought into articulation and wired together. He also dealt with dislocations of the mandible, electing to treat them with supportive bandages.

A surgeon of dubious moral character who was expelled from numerous cities, Walter Hermann Ryff (1500–1562) is nevertheless important because he wrote a surgical treatise, *Gross Chirurgey oder Vollkommene Wundtartzeney* (issued in 1545 and in 1559), with wonderful illustrations of dental instruments (fig. 104). Although no part of the text concerns dentistry, Ryff included these pictures in his book, as he states, because he intended to deal with dental afflictions in a later volume, which his death unfortunately prevented him from completing.

Ambroise Paré (1517?–1590), the preeminent surgeon of his era, shown here at about the age of seventy, had an extensive dental practice and wrote at length on dental treatment. National Library of Medicine, Bethesda.

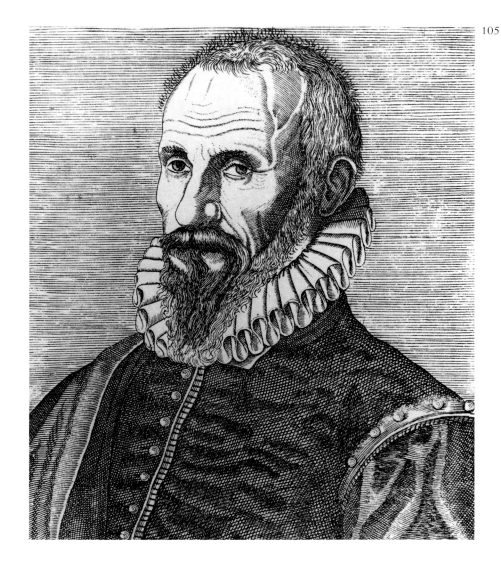

Ambroise Paré

In a century notable for advances in surgery, one name stands above all the rest, that of Ambroise Paré, who has often been called the father of surgery (fig. 105). He was born in Laval in northwest France about 1517, the son of a cabinetmaker. His sister Catherine married Gaspard Martin, a barber-surgeon of Paris, and his brother, Jean, also became a barber-surgeon, in Brittany. Ambroise Paré received his early training as a barber's apprentice, possibly in the shop of his brother.

In 1532, when he was fifteen, Paré was bound over to a barber-surgeon of Paris as an apprentice and in time secured appointment as "companion surgeon," or wound-dresser, at the Hôtel-Dieu hospital. At a later date Paré reported that he studied surgery for nine or ten years and then was employed at the hospital for three, and during his residency there he passed the examination that admitted him to the rank of master barber-surgeon.

Seeking wider scope for his talents, in 1537 he became a military surgeon. His operating skills brought him to the attention of the commander of the French forces in Piedmont, who appointed him military surgeon with the title Master Barber-Surgeon.

Soon after, Paré made a momentous discovery. It was then the established practice to cauterize gunshot wounds with boiling oil. After a particularly bloody battle, the supply of oil ran out and Paré merely dressed the wounds of his remaining patients with an unguent of egg whites, oil of roses, and turpentine. To his surprise, the next morning he found that the soldiers whose wounds had been treated with boiling oil were in grievous pain and had high fever, while the others were much more comfortable. "Then I resolved within myself," he said years later, "never so cruelly to burn poor, wounded men."

Later in his career, Paré entered a long period of service as a surgeon to a succession of French kings, and during this period he greatly enlarged the scope of his work and began publishing books on surgery, obstetrics, anatomy, and the plague and other diseases. Since he had had no classical education, his books were written in vernacular French instead of Latin.

At that time in France, surgeons were still divided into two groups: "surgeons of the long robe," the Confraternity of St. Côme, and "surgeons of the short robe," the barber-surgeons (whom the former considered altogether inferior). Both groups were looked down upon by the physicians. Paré, especially at the height of his fame, incurred the wrath of the medical faculty of Paris University, not only because he had attacked the profession's more dubious remedies but because, as an upstart barber-surgeon, he had dared to encroach on their domain. This drew from Paré the reply: "Dare you teach me surgery, you who have never come out of your study? Surgery is learned by the eye and by the hands. You, *mon petit maître*, know nothing else but how to chatter in a chair." (His *Complete Works*, published in 1575, enraged not only the physicians, who had been alarmed by Paré's treatises as well as by da Vigo's and Galen's in translation, but also the surgeons of St. Côme, who unsuccessfully sought to have its publication banned by an act of parliament.)

Paré also had an extensive dental practice, and his books contain much information on the subject. He discussed dental anatomy, although not with the exactness of Eustachius or even Vesalius. His practical methods of treatment were, for the most part, rational and sound. He suggested stabilizing jaw fractures with ligatures of gold wire. Caries he treated by cauterization with acid, although he made no mention of filling the cavity. Broken teeth, or those that stood above the occlusal plane and were causing problems, he filed down with special instruments that are shown in his books (fig. 108). He replanted teeth that had been accidentally avulsed, binding them to firm teeth with wires. Paré also dealt extensively with problems of teething, offering the gratuitous advice that in difficult cases the child's gums might be rubbed with the roasted brain of a hare!

He designed several instruments for extracting teeth (fig. 108)—one to push the gum away from a tooth prior to its removal; others to pry out roots; and several varieties of pelicans (fig. 109), one of which he called a *daviet*.

Paré cautioned against the use of excessive force in extracting teeth.

> The extraction of a tooth should not be carried out with too much violence, as one risks producing luxation of the jaw or concussion of the brain or eyes, or even bringing away a portion of the jaw together with the tooth (the author himself has observed this in several cases), not to speak of other serious accidents which may supervene as, for example, fever, apostema [abscess], abundant hemorrhage and even death.

Paré devised artificial teeth and published drawings of them. In this illustration from *Dix livres de la chirurgie* (1563), we see bridges of different lengths. The ivory teeth, inserted in a base made probably of gold, were bound to adjacent natural teeth with gold wire. New York Academy of Medicine, Rare Book Room, New York.

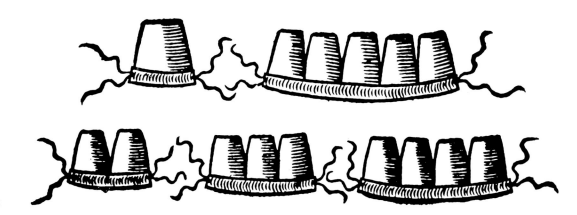

106

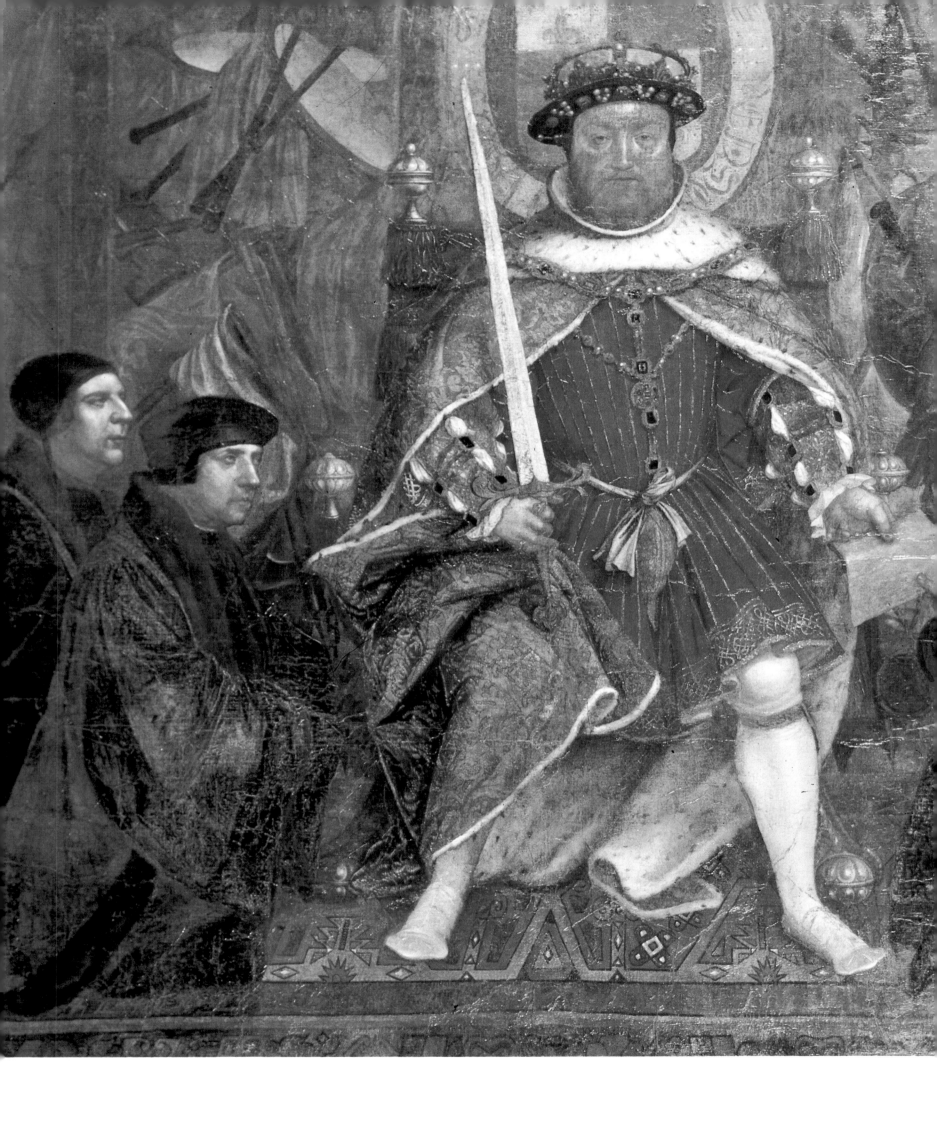

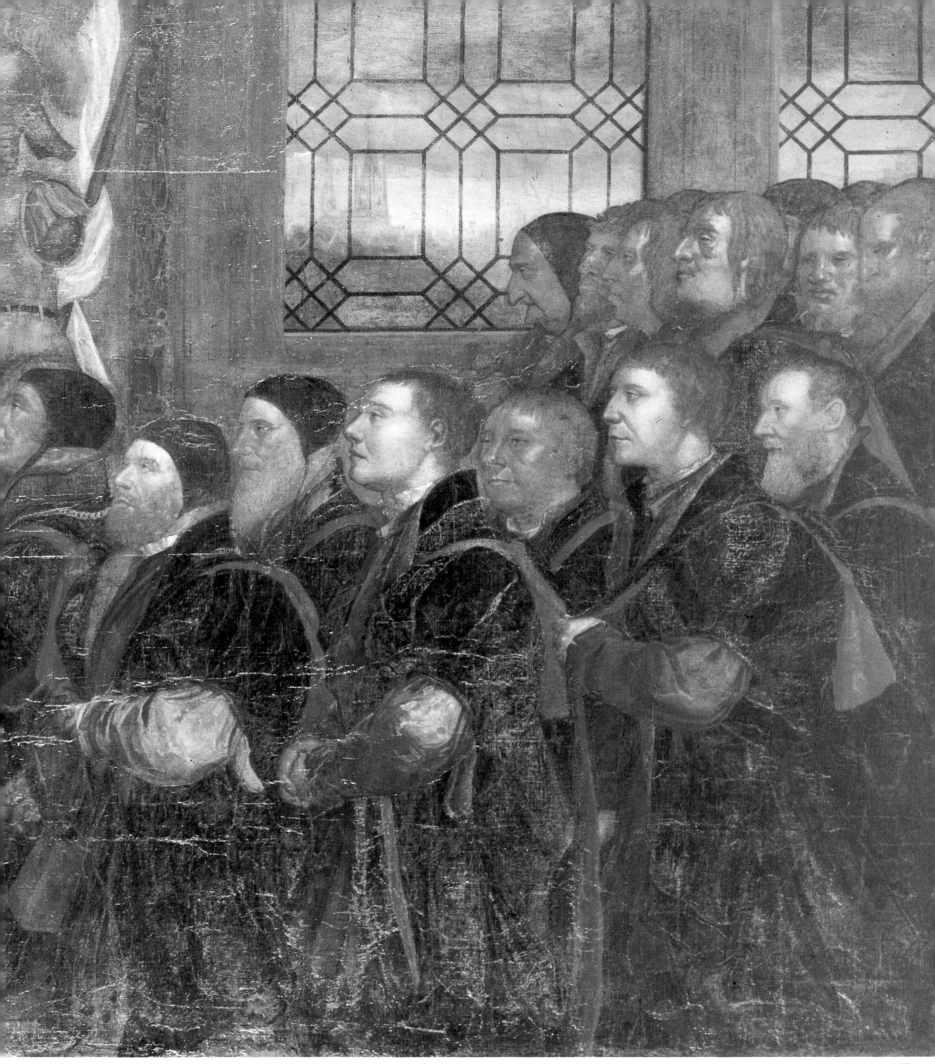

In 1540 Henry VIII of England granted a charter to the Royal Commonalty of Barber-Surgeons. In a painting executed in the same year by Hans Holbein, the king is shown handing the royal document to Thomas Vicary, a surgeon. The new charter circumscribed the areas in which surgeons and barbers could practice. The extraction of teeth was permitted to both groups. Royal College of Surgeons of England, London.

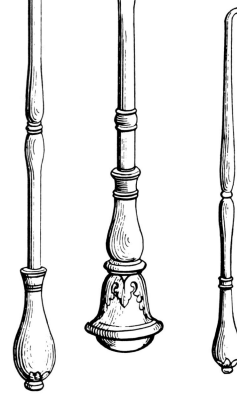

These illustrations from Ambroise Paré's *Complete Works* (1575) show, on the left, two lancets used to loosen the gums around teeth to be extracted and a "poussoir," used to pry out tooth roots. On the right are files for smoothing out the fractured edges of teeth.

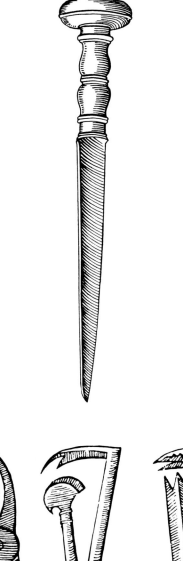

In his *Dix livres de la chirurgie*, Ambroise Paré included this drawing of two kinds of pelicans and, at left, an extraction forceps.

After an extraction it was necessary, Paré said, to let the wound bleed freely to eliminate "morbid humors." Then the alveolus should be pressed firmly on both sides with the fingers to reposition the bone that had been disturbed.

Paré described a method of restoring missing teeth, probably limited to the anterior ones, for, as he said, when the front teeth are lost, often as a result of a blow, the result is not only disfiguring but also causes speech defects. After waiting until the gums had healed, he substituted for the lost teeth artificial ones made out of bone or ivory, tying the bridge to the neighboring teeth with gold wire (fig. 106).

One of his great contributions to prosthetic dentistry was the palatal obturator. Although the physician Amatus Lusitanus had described an obturator in 1560, it was Paré's *Ten Books of Surgery*, first published in 1563, that brought it to public attention (fig. 110). The need for an obturator was very much greater in those times than at the present because of the epidemic of syphilis. Because no effective treatment was known, the new disease frequently progressed to perforation of the hard palate. Paré's simple and effective device consisted of a curved sheet of gold large enough to cover the hole and shaped so as to conform to the roof of the mouth. On the convex surface was soldered a small clip into which a sponge could be fitted. This was introduced into the nasal cavity, where it absorbed secretions and swelled up, keeping the gold plate in place. Admittedly not the most esthetic or sanitary device, it nevertheless effectively closed the opening, allowing the patient to eat, drink, and speak more normally. Later Paré devised a similar appliance which, instead of a sponge, had an ovoid knob that could be inserted through the palatal hole and then, by means of a special forceps, rotated to make it securely engage.

In sum, Paré's importance lies in his awareness that the surgeon needs a solid grounding in anatomy as well as practical experience. He did much to elevate his profession from a despised handicraft to a major branch of the healing art, one that in his time was far in advance of the others!

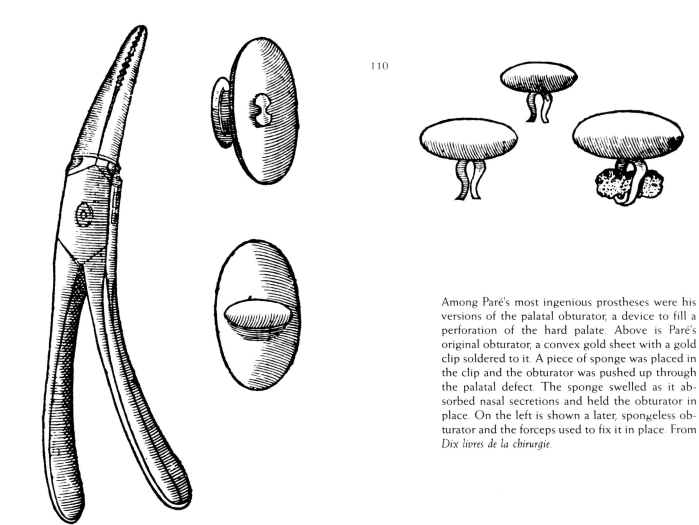

110

Among Paré's most ingenious prostheses were his versions of the palatal obturator, a device to fill a perforation of the hard palate. Above is Paré's original obturator, a convex gold sheet with a gold clip soldered to it. A piece of sponge was placed in the clip and the obturator was pushed up through the palatal defect. The sponge swelled as it absorbed nasal secretions and held the obturator in place. On the left is shown a later, spongeless obturator and the forceps used to fix it in place. From *Dix livres de la chirurgie*.

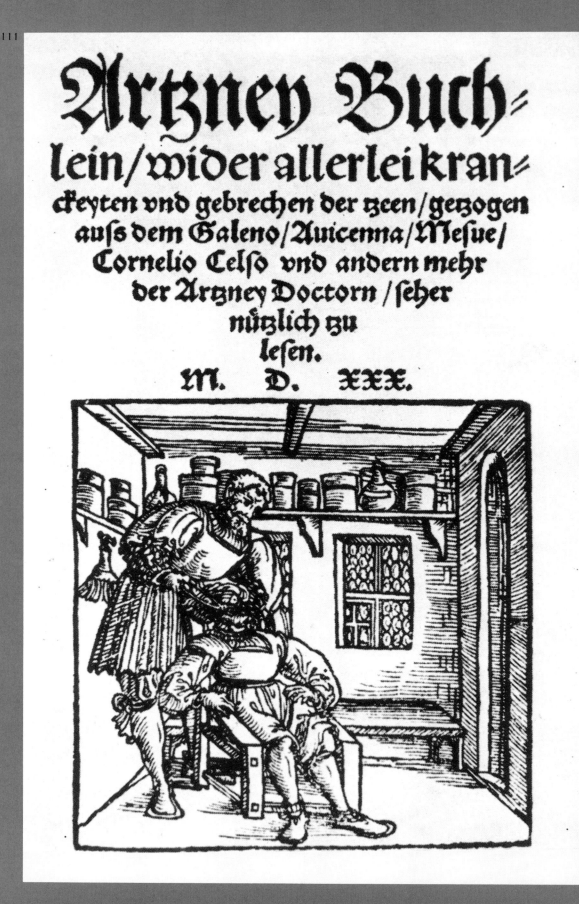

Artzney Buch=
lein/wider allerlei kran=
ckeyten vnd gebrechen der zeen/gezogen
auß dem Galeno/Auicenna/Mesue/
Cornelio Celso vnd andern mehr
der Artzney Doctorn /sehr
nützlich zu
lesen.
M. D. XXX.

The first book devoted to dentistry was written in vernacular German. Entitled *Artzney Buchlein (Little Book on Medicine)*, it addressed the barbers and surgeons who treated afflictions of the mouth. Illustrated is the title page, which states that the contents will make "very profitable reading."

The Anatomie.

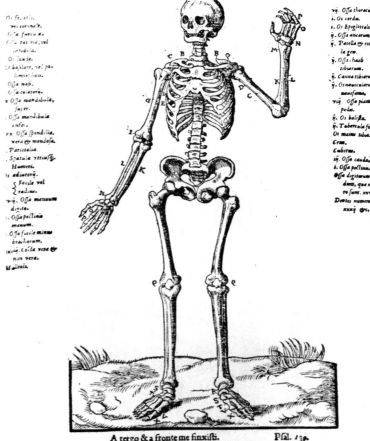

A tergo & a fronte me finxisti. Psal. 139.

William Bullein's *Bulwarke of Defence Against All Sicknesse*, a Tudor health manual, was published in 1579 in London. This illustration is one Bullein copied from Vesalius.

Dental Literature

The year 1530 saw the publication, in Leipzig, of the first book devoted entirely to dentistry; moreover, it was written in German instead of Latin, addressing itself to the barbers and surgeons who treated the mouth, rather than to the university-trained physicians, who ignored all diseases of the teeth.

Artzney Buchlein wider allerlei Krankeyten und Gebrechen der Tzeen (Little Medicinal Book for All Kinds of Diseases and Infirmities of the Teeth) was based on the writings of Galen, Pliny, Celsus, Avicenna, and other classicists and Arabic writers, much of the material coming by way of Giovanni da Vigo. The book is short—only forty-four pages—but it had an immediate success, for during the ensuing forty-five years more than fifteen editions were released. It covered such subjects as drilling carious teeth and filling them with gold (here following da Vigo's advice), oral hygiene, fumigation of the teeth with henbane seeds to discourage toothworms, and extractions, which, the author made clear, should be performed by a surgeon rather than a physician.

Who wrote the *Artzney Buchlein* will probably forever remain a mystery. We believe it may have been written by an educated German surgeon who avoided using his own name because dentistry was considered such a lowly profession. It may, however, have been put together by an enterprising printer who recognized a marketable commodity. The fact remains that the publication of this rude little book marked the beginning of professional dental literature.

About fourteen years later, the disreputable surgeon Walter Ryff, whom we have already met, published the first monograph for the layman on dentistry. Perhaps inspired by the popular success of the *Artzney Buchlein*, Ryff wrote his small pamphlet of sixty-one pages, *Useful Instruction on the Way to Keep Healthy, to Strengthen and Reinvigorate the Eyes and the Sight, With further instruction on the way of keeping the mouth fresh, the teeth clean, and the gums firm*, for the ordinary person, not the professional, encouraging the practice of oral hygiene and simple dental care. The first part of the book deals with the eyes, the second with the teeth proper, and the third with the primary dentition. Since it was intended for the instruction of the lay person, it includes no discussion of filling or pulling teeth.

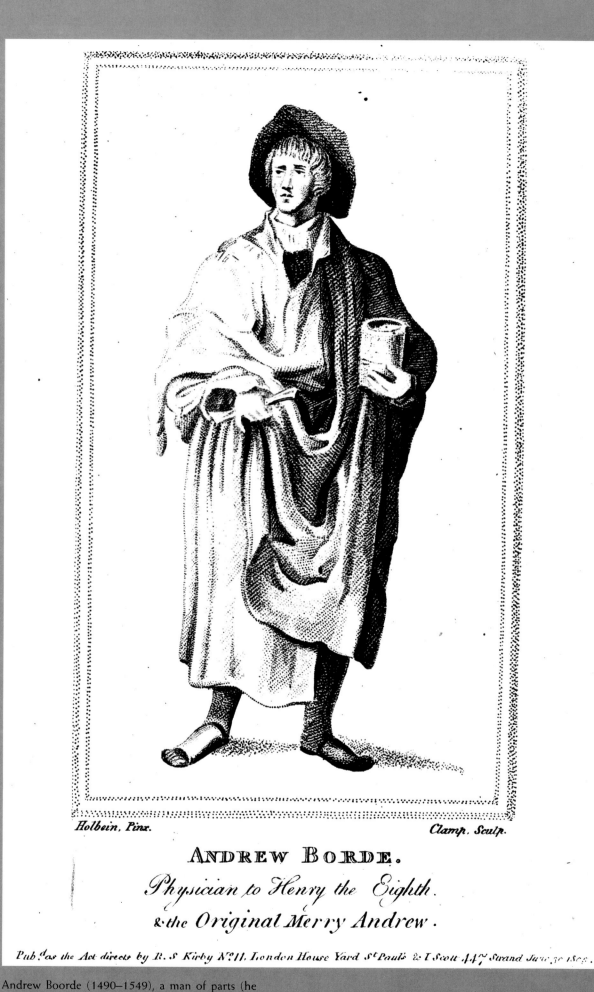

Holbein, Pinx.   Clamp. Sculp.

ANDREW BORDE.

Physician to Henry the Eighth.

& the Original Merry Andrew.

Pub.ᵈ as the Act directs by R. S Kirby Nº 11. London House Yard St Pauls & I Scott 447 Strand June 30 1805.

Andrew Boorde (1490–1549), a man of parts (he was priest, physician, and ambassador), wrote *Breviarie of Helthe*, which was published in 1547. Most of the recommended remedies are worthless, but this early English medical treatise gives a good idea of the kind of dental treatment rendered in sixteenth-century England. Engraving by Clary, after Holbein. Wellcome Institute Library, London.

Dentistry and Oral Hygiene: The British Isles

Although during the fifteenth and sixteenth centuries the practice of dentistry in the British Isles was somewhat old-fashioned by comparison with dentistry on the Continent, the people of England, Scotland, and Wales cared for their teeth and had them attended to in very much the same way their European contemporaries did and, for that matter, very much the same way their grandfathers had. In the case of Tudor England we have an excellent record of what went on, for many treatises by physicians and surgeons of the time have come down to us.

In 1547 the priest-physician Andrew Boorde (fig. 113), who was also political emissary of the Church of England to the courts of Europe, published *Breviarie of Helthe*, one of the earliest English medical books. He shows much interest in dental treatment, though his understanding of pathology was in large part founded on his belief in the cardinal humors. What we today recognize as a swelling of the submandibular salivary gland as a result of the blockage of its duct Boorde calls an "impostume," or abscess. "This infirmity," he asserts, "doth come of too much humidity flowing to the place where the impostume is. A remedy: first purge the matter with pills of cochee [?] and use a gargarice [gargle], and if need be exhaust two ounces of blood out of a vein under the tongue." Like this one, most of his recommendations are worthless by our standards. A strong believer in fumigation to drive out the toothworm, Boorde advised his patients to inhale the fumes of burning henbane seeds while bending over a dish of water. The worms would supposedly fall into the water, "and then you may take [them] out . . . and kill them on your nail."

Though Boorde probably saved few teeth, he did at least believe in trying to do so—something many doctors of the day did not—and his compassion for suffering shines through: "A tooth is a sensible bone, the which being in living man's head hath feeling, and so hath no other bone in man's body; and therefore the toothache is an extreme pain." His patients must have suffered grievously from toothache, for the diet of the upper and middle classes, at least, was extremely rich in sugar. In *Romeo and Juliet*, Mercutio remarks that ladies' lips are plagued with blisters "because their breaths with sweetmeats tainted are." Entrees were topped by a mixture that included half a pound of sugar and a saucer of rosewater; and cakes, jams, and jellies were favorite foods (L. E. Pearson, *Elizabethans at Home*, 1957).

Philip Barrough, one of the most renowned medical doctors of his day, like Boorde believed in the effectiveness of letting blood. In *The Methode of Physicke*, of 1583, he reiterates again and again that dental ills are "a corruption of humors" and advises that by studying the color of ulcers in the mouth one can determine which "humor" is at fault. Thus, a yellow ulcer indicates an excess of bile in the system, a white one too much phlegm, and so forth.

William Bullein, a cleric and physician, was the most prolific writer on topics concerning the health of the public during the Tudor period. His *Bulwarke of Defence Against All Sicknesse, Soarenesse and Wounds That Doe Dayly Assaulte Mankind*, published in London in 1579, is a compendium of the medical practice of the day and offers sound advice on health, general hygiene, and the use of herbs in treating disease. Moreover, it includes a section on the surgical treatment of wounds and tumors illustrated with pictures copied from Vesalius. Most interesting is the picture he gives us of the medical men of his day, including the pharmacists and herbalists.

114–16 (pages 138–39, 141)

These three portraits of Queen Elizabeth of England reflect the changes in her appearance from youth to old age. As gradually she lost her teeth, her face contracted, particularly in the area of the upper lip, heightening the impression of senescence. In the portrait by Gheeraerts, she is still probably only in her fifties.

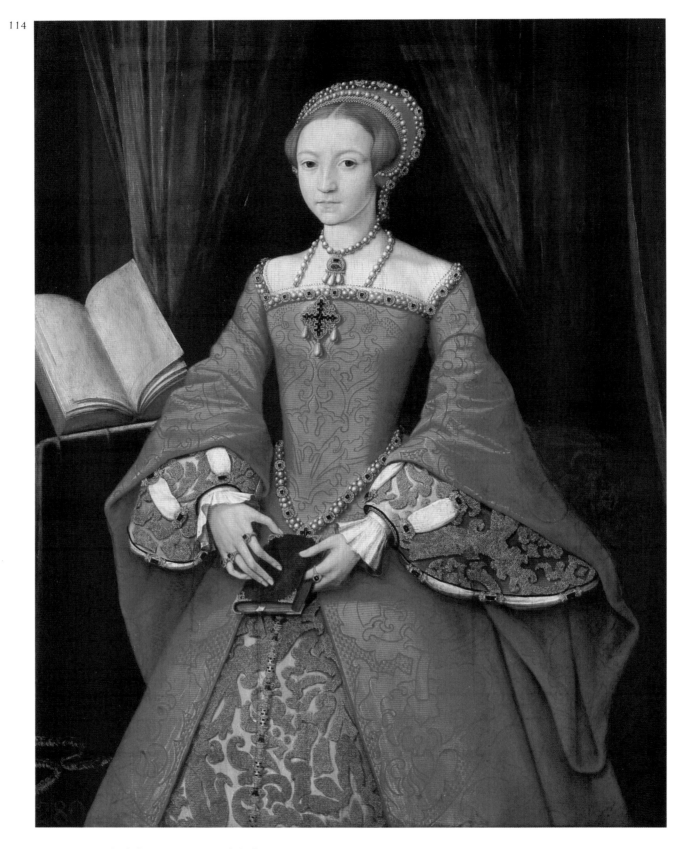

Anonymous. *Elizabeth I as Princess*. Royal Collection,
by permission of the Lord Chamberlain, London.

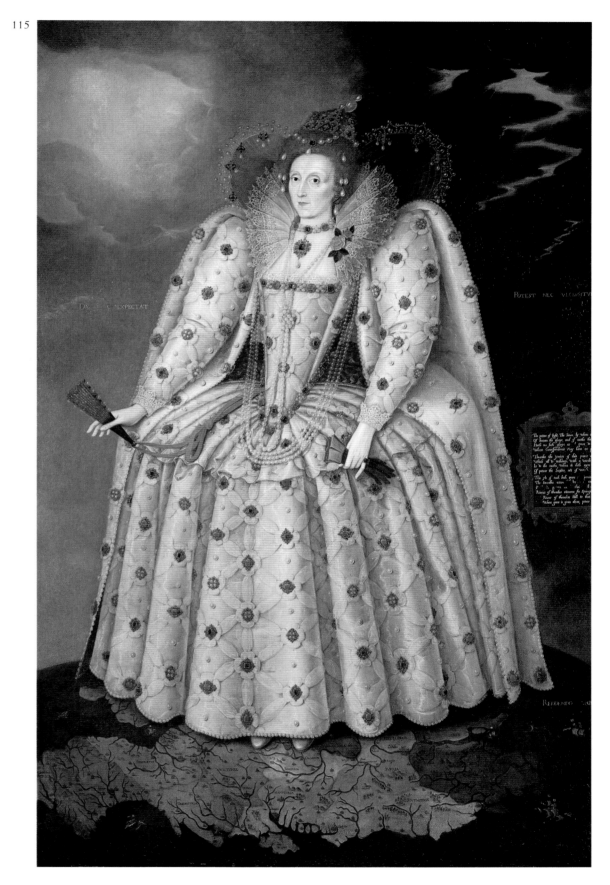

Marcus Gheeraerts the Younger. *Elizabeth the First.*
c. 1592. Collection National Portrait Gallery, London.

James IV, who ruled Scotland from 1488 to 1513, was adept in medicine and surgery, treating the members of his court for ulcers, letting blood, and touching for the king's evil, or scrofula.

In 1503 the king called a barber in to extract one of his teeth and apparently learned from him the technique. Thereafter, he offered simple dental care to his courtiers and his servants, extracting teeth and cauterizing aching ones. A note of 1507 in the royal archives indicates that the king paid two shillings for "an iron to burn sore teeth." The records also show that James bought numerous dental instruments for his armamentarium, including forceps, elevators, and tooth files. A foresighted monarch, he was responsible for the incorporation of the barbers and surgeons of Edinburgh, granting them his royal charter in 1506, thirty-four years before Henry VIII took a similar step in England.

James's niece Elizabeth I of England apparently suffered all her life from severe toothache. Even her teething was not easy, for her governess wrote that "my Lady has great pain with her great teeth, and they come very slowly forth, and cause me to suffer her Grace to have her will more than I would." As a grown woman we know that at all times she carried at her belt a small bag filled with sweets. These may indeed have been responsible for the rapid destruction of her teeth, though she may have sucked them to mask the fetid breath that comes from carious teeth.

Over the years Elizabeth endured repeated bouts of toothache that were often so severe as to necessitate her cancelling official audiences. After she ascended to the throne, foreign envoys regularly reported to their governments on the state of the queen's health, and in 1567 the Spanish ambassador wrote to Madrid that the queen had suffered from toothache and fever for forty hours, which greatly weakened her.

On October 17, 1578, the earl of Leicester wrote Lord Burghley that "the Queen has been marvelous ill for many days with a pain in her cheek." By December her condition had become so serious that her surgeon was called for. Although he is not named, he may have been William Clowes or perhaps Thomas Balthrop, who had served her father, Henry VIII. Elizabeth, however, feared extraction so much that the bishop of London, "a man of high courage," offered to have one of his own teeth extracted to show the queen that she had little to fear. This was done—the bishop sacrificed a tooth—and it was later (1701) recorded that, "accordingly . . . she was . . . encouraged to submit to the operation itself."

When her contemporaries described her, they often mentioned Elizabeth's unsightly teeth, which they called either "black" or "yellow." As she aged, Elizabeth's face was affected by the loss of her teeth, and by 1594, a woman of sixty-one, she had very little left of her youth except her straight back and her beautiful hands. She still dressed as a young girl in spite of her wrinkled face, false hair, and missing teeth" (Marchette Chute, *Shakespeare of London*, 1950). Three years later the French ambassador described her with candor: "As for her face, it is, and appears to be, very aged. It is long and thin, and her teeth are very yellow and unequal, compared with what they were formerly, so they say, and on the left side less than on the right. Many of them are missing so that one cannot understand her easily when she speaks quickly."

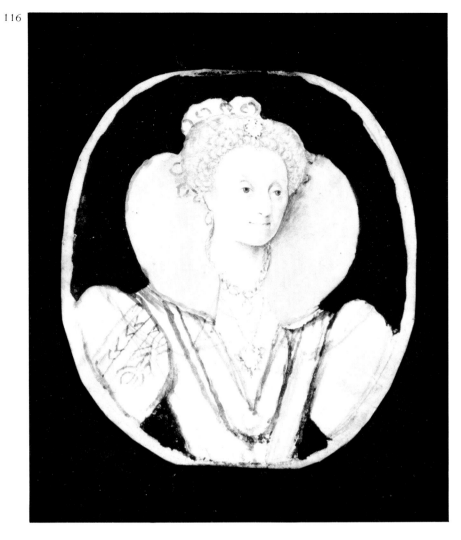

Anonymous. *Queen Elizabeth as an Old Woman.* Victoria and Albert Museum, London.

Oral Hygiene

During the 1500s the English placed little emphasis on personal cleanliness. Queen Elizabeth herself is reported to have taken a bath once a month "whether she required it or not." Soap was in short supply and was very expensive since it had to be imported. Nevertheless, the need for cleansing the mouth was frequently stressed in writings of the time, and a variety of dentifrices were described. One writer, however, advised that clean water was all that one needed:

> *Keep white thy teeth, and wash thy mouth*
> *With water pure and cleane,*
> *And in that washing, mannerly,*
> *Observe and keep a meane.*

The toothbrush was apparently not in common use, although some cleaned their teeth by rubbing them with a cloth-wrapped finger, but using a toothpick was fashionable among the nobility and gentry, who imported them from France, Spain, and Portugal; they are itemized in the royal list of import duties along with ear picks. Elizabeth in 1570 received a gift of six gold toothpicks as well as "tooth cloths" edged in silver and black. Indeed, these toilet articles were used as ornaments as well. At one time James IV of Scotland purchased two gold toothpicks with a chain, for the custom was to wear the picks suspended around the neck. His son, James V, in 1541 ordered from the royal goldsmith "ane pennare of silver to keip pyke teeth in"—a little silver case for toothpicks.

Shakespeare alludes to toothpicks many times in his plays, and a contemporary writer on etiquette in 1577 advised,

> *Pick not thy teeth with thy knyfe*
> *Nor with thy fyngers ende,*
> *But take a stick, or some cleane thynge,*
> *Then doe you not offende.*

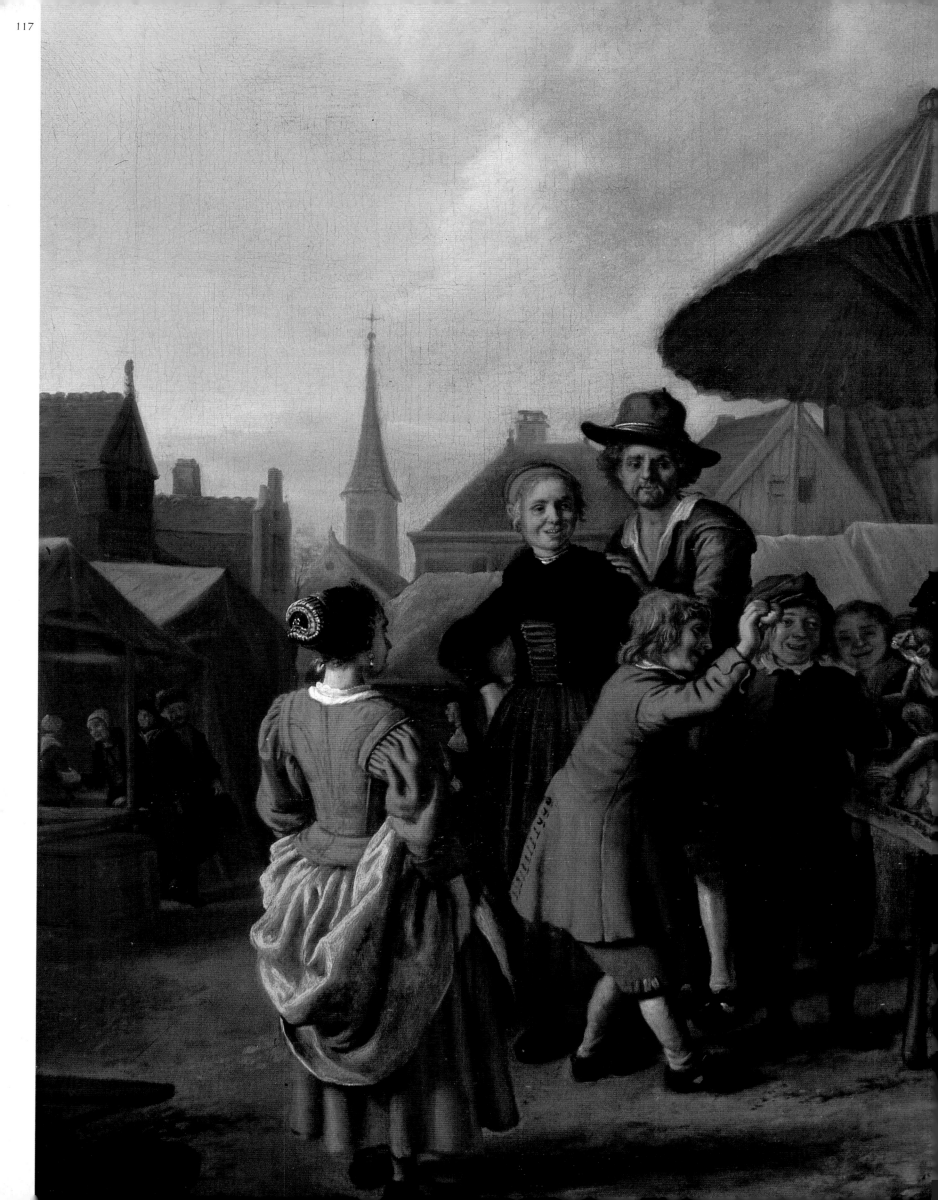

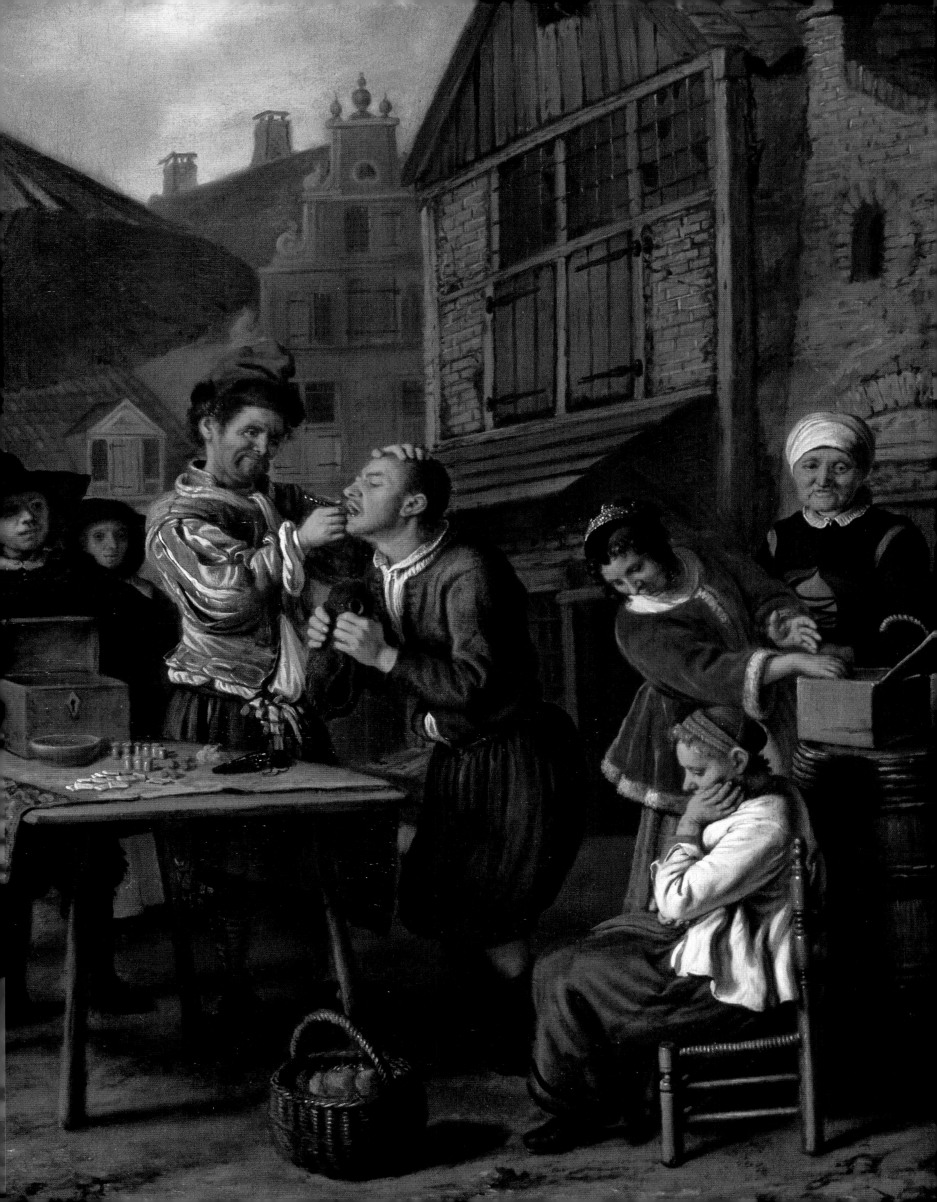

The dentist depicted in this painting by the Dutch artist Jan Victors (1620–1676) was prosperous, if his gorgeous jacket and handsome red velvet hat are as new as they look. The girl awaiting her turn in the foreground is anxious-faced, but the spectators and even the patient in the chair look relatively cheerful. Kulturhistorische Sammlung des Bundesverbandes der Deutschen Zahnärzte, Cologne.

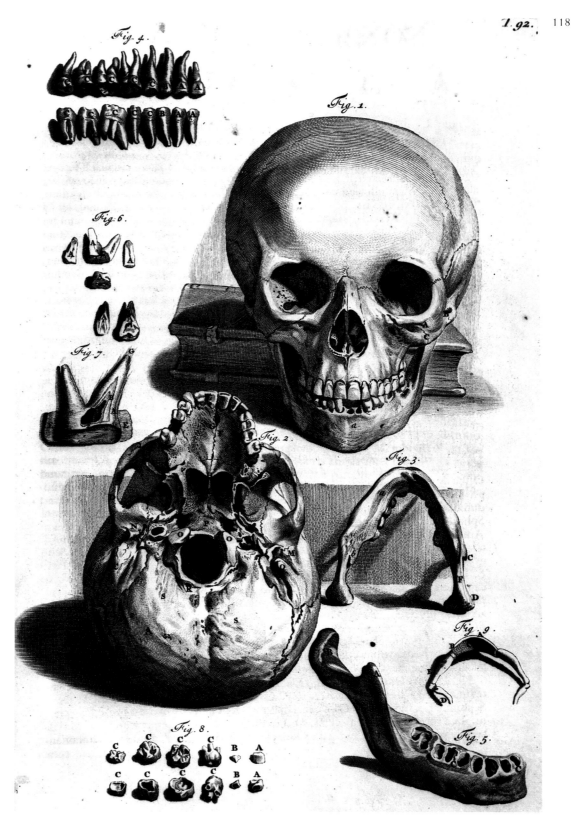

During the seventeenth century, scientists began to ask *how* rather than *why* things happen. This engraving of the human skull and dentition from Govert Bidloo's *Anatomia* (1685) displays the kind of precise, detailed observation of natural phenomena that was imposed by the rephrasing of the question. Edward G. Miner Library, University of Rochester, School of Medicine and Dentistry.

IX
THE SEVENTEENTH CENTURY IN EUROPE

During the seventeenth century great discoveries in the fundamental sciences were made, discoveries that would form the basis of modern medicine, but medical practice still languished in superstition and ignorance.

Scientific Discoveries

Of paramount importance was the English physician and anatomist William Harvey's discovery of the circulation of the blood. By demonstrating his findings, which were published in 1628, Harvey effectively established the science of physiology.

During the 1600s extensive anatomical studies, based on the work of Vesalius, led to a more complete understanding of the functioning of the human organism, though unfortunately little of this knowledge was translated into practical therapy. The introduction of the copper plate made it possible to render anatomical structures in remarkable detail. One of the finest books of this period, the *Anatomia* of the Dutch physician Govert Bidloo, published in Amsterdam in 1685, became the standard by which other works in the field were judged.

Progress in anatomy led to the growth of two other sciences: comparative anatomy and histology. Outstanding in the former field was Edward Tyson, who was graduated from the University of Cambridge in 1678 and who published elaborate monographs on the anatomical structures of the lower animals. It was Harvey's demonstration of the circular course of blood flow that led Marcello Malpighi (1628–1694) to investigate the link between arteries and veins, culminating in his discovery of the capillaries in 1666. Malpighi's studies of other minute structures justify his being designated the founder of histology.

The invention of the microscope in the seventeenth century opened a new world for scientific study. The great early microscopist Anton van Leeuwenhoek (1682-1723) advanced knowledge immeasurably. Leeuwenhoek, who was not a university-trained scientist but a draper, nonetheless earned for himself a place of honor as a Fellow of the Royal Society of England, for during his long lifetime he sent 375 scientific papers to that august body and 27 to the French Académie des Sciences.

Among Leewenhoek's findings of importance to dentistry were the tubules in the dentin and the microorganisms, including bacteria, that he found in the *materia alba* adhering to the teeth. When the president of the Royal Society sent him several worms that, he was told, had been taken from a carious tooth, Leeuwenhoek effectively disproved that they were toothworms by proving microscopically that they were identical to the maggots that infest overripe cheese. He postulated that the maggots had entered the carious lesion when the owner of the tooth ate the cheese, for, as he said, he had extracted maggots from the damaged teeth of his own wife after she had partaken of infested cheese.

The painstaking and minute zoological studies of the Dutch scientist Jan Swammerdam (1637–1680) led him ultimately to the study of the function of the blood itself as well as of the lungs and to the establishment of a solid foundation for the study of physiology. Using the microscope, the English philosopher Robert Hooke (1635–1703) discovered that parts of plants are cellular, paving the way for the advance of cell theory in the nineteenth century.

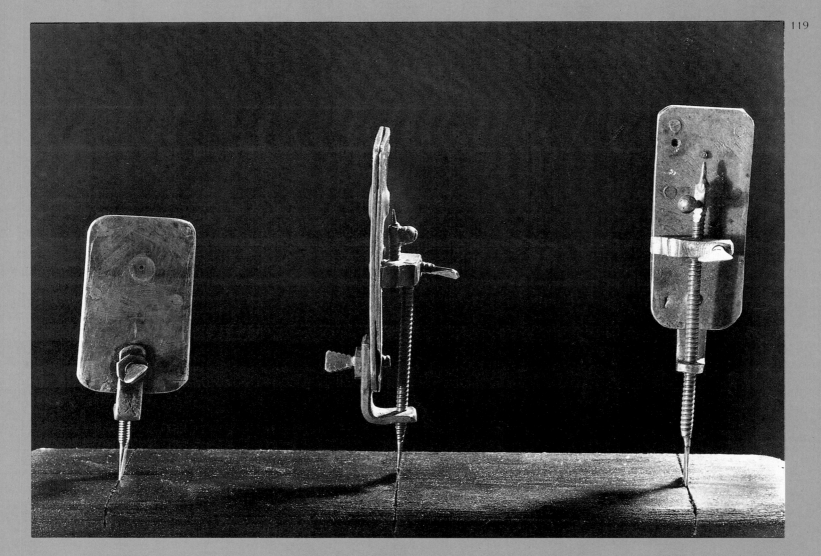

With these microscopes of his own invention, Anton van Leeuwenhoek saw for the first time in history both the microorganisms that infest the *materia alba* adhering to human teeth and the dentinal tubules in sections of teeth he ground thin. Rijksmuseum voor de Geschiedenis der Naturwetenschappen, Leiden.

Medical Practice

The Physicians

The physician of the seventeenth century was virtually unaware of the intellectual ferment in the sciences. Even the great clinician Thomas Sydenham (1624–1689), who classified diseases by their symptoms as well as their responses to modes of treatment—thereby laying the basis for the future science of pathology—saw little of practical value in the recent discoveries in science and medicine. Training in the medical schools on the Continent and in England was still based on the Classical and Arabic writers, and anatomy was inadequately taught. Uroscopy was at the zenith of its popularity. Astrology was fervently believed in, and alchemy provided the medical community with an unending flow of "magical potions" and amulets such as the bezoar stone, an inorganic mass found in the stomachs of ruminant animals that was highly prized for its supposed curative properties. The great twentieth-century medical historian Fielding H. Garrison summed up the caliber of doctoring four hundred years ago in these words, "By the seventeenth century, the physician had become a sterile pedant and coxcomb, red-heeled, long-robed, big-wigged, square-bonneted, pompous and disdainful in manner, making a vain parade of his Latin and, instead of studying and caring for his patients, tried to overawe them by long tirades of technical drivel, which only concealed his ignorance of what he supposed to be their diseases."

The *materia medica* of the period gives a good indication of the state of medicine. The first edition of the *London Pharmacopoeia*, published in 1618, mentions compounds made of worms, dried vipers, foxes' lungs, and oil of ants. Succeeding editions swelled the medicine chest with "blood, fat, bile, viscera, bones, marrow, claws, teeth, hoofs, horns, sexual organs, eggs and the excreta of animals of all sorts; beeglue, cock's comb, cuttlefish, fur, feathers, hair, isinglass, human perspiration, saliva of a fasting man, human placenta, raw silk, spider webs, sponge, seashell, cast-off snake skin, scorpions, swallow's nests, wood-lice . . . and a bone from the skull of an executed criminal."

The absolute nadir of rational pharmacotherapeutics was reached when in 1696 Christian Franz Paul, a German court physician, brought out his book *Heilsame Dreck Apotheke (Healing Excrement Pharmacy)*. It listed innumerable disgusting materials, many of which were recommended for dental problems, such as a paste of honey and dog excrement for sores on the gums and mouse or raven droppings used to make a carious tooth fall out. It was reissued in five editions until 1734.

The Surgeons

Looked down upon though they were by the physicians; it was the surgeons who made the greater strides, building upon the work of Paré and other pioneers. They still received much of their training in the military, and an idea of their rank can be gained by the realization that in many armies they were expected to shave the officers in addition to performing surgery. Many barber-surgeons began to improve themselves by study, especially since there were now books directed specifically to them—for example, Tiberio Malfi's *Il barbiere* (1626)—which covered bloodletting, would dressing, extractions, and other simple oral surgical procedures.

The leading German surgeon of the period was Wilhelm Fabry of Hilden (1560–1624), who clung to the views of the ancients yet was a bold and innovative operator and the inventor of many new instruments. He wrote *Observationes et curationes (Observations and Counsels)*, a compilation of case histories gleaned from his practice. We read that he used wooden mouth props wired to the teeth to separate and immobilize the jaws after a tumor had been removed by cauterization and corrosive agents. Another case indicates that Fabry also removed tumors by ligating them with a thread and then excising them with a knife. He also re-

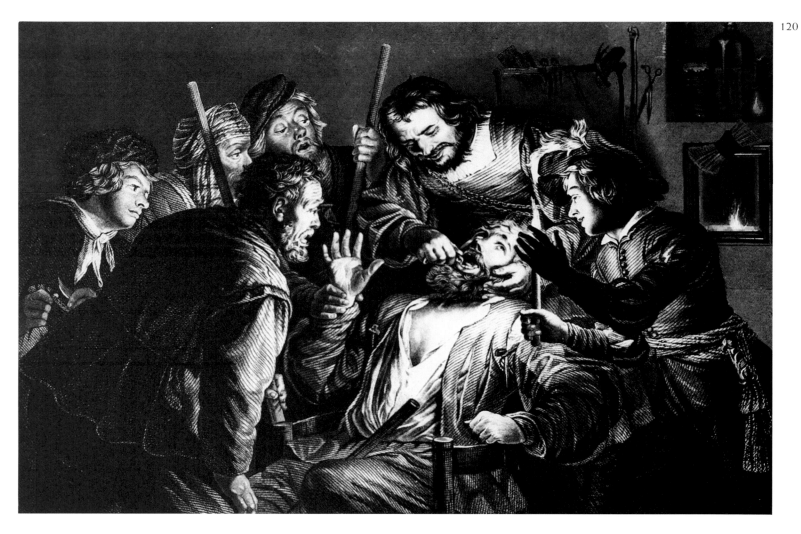

A dentist using a forceps extracts a lower anterior tooth by candlelight. That he was a barber-surgeon can be deduced from the instruments in the background: razors, scissors, and shaving brushes. Etching after the painting *Der Zahnarzt* of 1622 by Gerard von Honthorst.

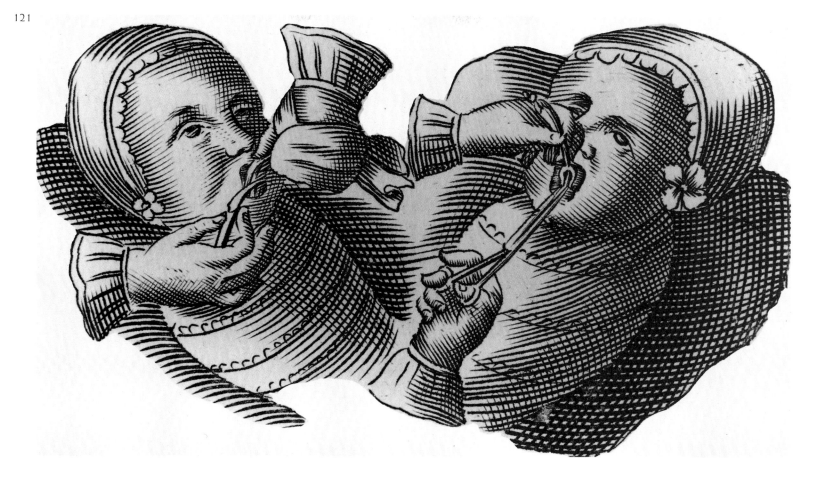

cords the case of a woman who had for years suffered from headaches, whom he cured by removing four decayed maxillary teeth.

In England, Richard Wiseman (1622–1676), surgeon to Charles II, raised his profession to equality with medicine. His *Several Chirurgical Treatises* (1672) deals with amputation in cases of gunshot wounds and relief of gonorrheal stricture by urethotomy and gives a good account of the king's evil (scrofula). He dealt with dental problems as well. The 1676 edition of his book details a case "of a person of about fifty years of age, of a strong constitution, [who] by cracking of an apricot-stone, caused a great pain amongst the great teeth of his upper jaw. From that time that part of the gum swelled and one tooth grew loose and after some time a fungus thrust the tooth out." Wiseman decided to treat the "fungus" by cauterization, and, to the surprise of other medical attendants who despaired of saving the tooth, the tooth held "seven years or thereabouts." In another case of tumor, Wiseman "placed the patient in a clear light then pulled out the teeth that lay loose and, as it were, buried in the fungus."

There is an extensive discussion of the surgical treatment of dental problems in the work of Johannes Scultetus (Johann Schultheiss) of Ulm, Germany, whose book *Armamentarium chirurgicum* first appeared in 1655 and was later reprinted in several languages, including English (entitled *The Chyrurgeon's Store-House*, it was published in 1674). Scultetus, an ardent follower of Galen, relied on the Roman doctor's methods to prepare his patients for operation. Thus, in the case of a woman who had a cyst of the maxilla, he initiated treatment with bleedings, purgings, sweatings, and the application of various drawing ointments to remove the excess "moist humors." This done, he placed the lady in her bed, tying her hands to her side, and incised the cyst. There "flowed out a thick yellow matter like honey, and the tumor subsided." Sculteus followed the operation with vigorous treatment of the cystic cavity for a period of two months and apparently achieved healing.

This illustration from the French edition (1712) of *Armamentarium chirurgicum* by Johannes Scultetus shows two methods of treating a short lingual frenum by surgical incision. National Library of Medicine, Bethesda.

In 1686 an event occurred that was to have a profound effect on the social and professional status of surgeons. Louis XIV of France, who suffered from an anal fistula that had resisted every ointment, tincture, and dose the royal physician could devise, turned in desperation to the royal surgeon, C. F. Félix, who operated with complete success. In gratitude the king made him a nobleman, gave him a country estate and a fee of 15,000 louis d'or, three times the honorarium received by the royal physician! This incident gave the surgeons of France a considerable boost in prestige, and the profession continued to rise in public esteem during the next century.

Since 1533 in France, surgeons of the long robe had been educated at the Collège de St. Côme rather than the medical school of Paris University, whose faculty despised them. The surgeons, however, imitated the manners of the physicians, putting on airs and substituting three ointment boxes for the traditional three barber's basins on their guild banner—which behavior drew down upon them the ire of the jealous physicians, whose chief, Guy Patin, the dean of the Paris faculty, branded them "booted lackeys...a race of evil, extravagant coxcombs who wear mustaches and flourish razors." In turn, the surgeons looked down upon the barbers. In 1655, however, the surgeons were obliged to swallow their pride and form a union with the barber-surgeons. The former benefited from the practical experience of the latter, the barbers from association with their colleagues of higher status. And in 1660 both groups came under the supervision of the king's surgeon, who as we have seen was shortly to become a person as important and influential as any physician.

The Dentists

During the seventeenth century most barbers continued to offer a range of services to their clients, but many advertised themselves as being skilled in extractions, and a variety of names were given them, including *Zahnbrecher* (literally, "tooth-breaker") in Germany; *cavadenti* in Italy; and *arracheur des dents* (literally, "snatcher of teeth") in France. In England the dentists styled themselves "operators for the teeth."

The humblest practitioners pursued their vocation wherever they could attract clients. One of the most common was the marketplace in village or town, where they would set up tables or chairs under umbrellas or else put up platforms. Sometimes they advertised themselves by flying brightly colored banners with pictures of sufferers successfully treated, or by hiring drummers, musicians, jugglers, and even sleight-of-hand artists to draw a crowd. Successful professionals maintained their own shops, where, on the evidence of a large number of contemporary genre paintings, more than mere extraction was performed. These early dentist-barbers also lanced abscesses, filed and smoothed fractured teeth, and performed many other simple dental operations, including scaling and cleaning the teeth. Cintio d'Amato, whose *New and Useful Practices of All Kinds for Diligent Barbers* was published in Italy in 1632, emphasized the importance of these measures.

> It happens in general that owing to vapors that rise from the stomach, a certain deposit is formed on the teeth, which may be perceived by rubbing them with a rough cloth on waking. One ought, therefore, to rub and clean them every morning, for, if one is not aware of this, or considers it of little account, the teeth become discolored and covered with a thick tartar, which often causes them to decay and to fall out. It is then necessary that the diligent barber should remove the said tartar with the instruments designed for this purpose.

The overwhelming majority of the wandering practitioners were inept and poorly trained at best and at worst unblushing quacks who promised to rid teeth of worms (and at the same time the bowels of their worms, too) and to cure head-

This page from the 1712 French edition of Johannes Scultetus's *Armamentarium chirurgicum* depicts operations in and around the mouth. Figure I illustrates a method of repairing a cleft lip; figures V and VI deal with hot cautery; in figure VII extraction by means of a dental forceps is depicted; and figure VIII shows a method of opening the mouth in cases of trismus.

TABLE. XXXV

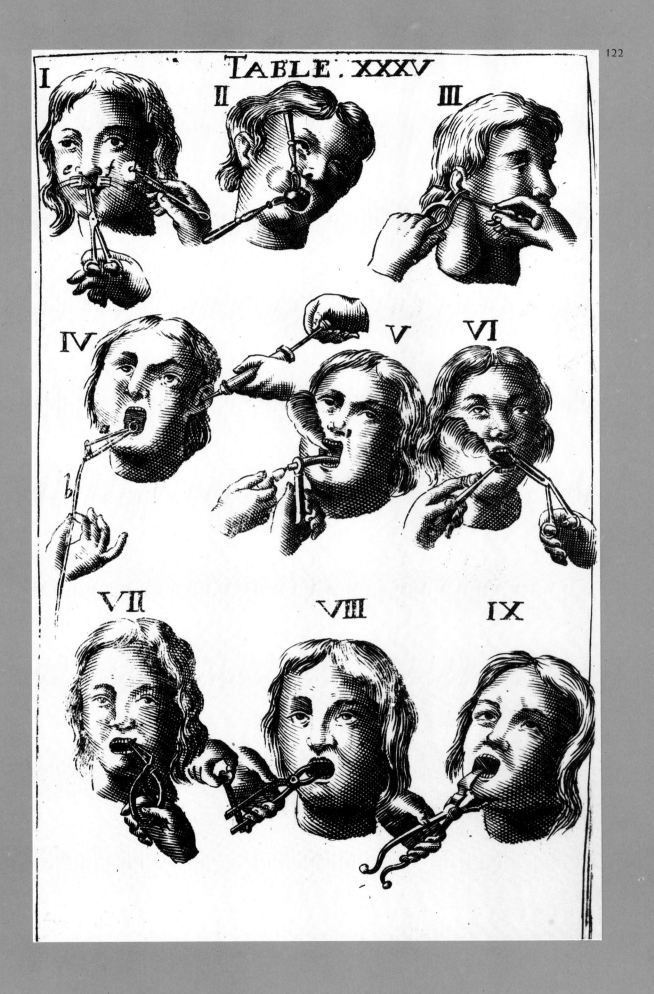

aches by removing stones from the head or an unusually large tooth from the mouth. It was an age of extravagant claims—in dentistry as in other fields. One Professor Jacobaens of the University of Copenhagen claimed that after scraping about in a carious cavity he saw a worm, which when extracted and put in water swam energetically about! Another physician, Philip Salmuth, maintained that by applying rancid oil he was able to drive out toothworms as big as earthworms! Some methods of treatment, though doubtless offered in good faith, were so excessive and scattershot one wonders why the patient did not turn on his torturer and murder him with his own instruments. Lazare Rivière, a seventeenth-century professor of medicine at Montpellier, was nothing if not thorough in treating toothache, as the following description quoted in Vincenzo Guerini's *History of Dentistry* (1909) indicates.

> Where the pain was occasioned by hot humors, the treatment began by bleeding in the arm. The following day an aperient was administered. Afterward, if the pain still persisted, the sufferer was cupped in the region of the scapula or spine; blisters were created behind the ears or the nape of the neck; resinous plasters were placed at the temples. In addition to this, various remedies were introduced into the ears, various operations were performed on the aching part itself. And this was followed by extracting the offending tooth.

We have evidence, however, that some real advances were made in prosthetic dentistry in the 1600s. In 1953 a farmer's wife in Vaison-la-Romaine, in Provence, found a small object of bone that was recognized by the curator of the Natural History Museum in Avignon as being a dental bridge (fig. 124). This was studied by experts, who have dated it to the middle of the seventeenth century. Made of one piece of bone carved to simulate three anterior teeth, it was fixed in the mouth by silver posts that were cemented into the canals of the tooth roots on either side of the missing tooth. (The teeth on either side may have been badly carious, suggesting to the operator that he cut them off at the gum line.) This prosthesis is obviously in advance of Paré's device of a century earlier, by which he ligated pontics to the adjacent teeth with gold wire, but it is of obviously cruder construction than the prosthesis Fauchard would devise in the next century. In 1964, again not far from Avignon, there was found an adult skull that showed gross periodontal destruction, with many teeth missing and the remainder having lost most of their bony support. In the anterior region, however, three natural teeth were ligated together with gold wire, effectively stabilized and apparently usable until the death of their owner. This skull is firmly dated to the middle of the seventeenth century (fig. 125).

But on the whole, dentistry made little progress during the seventeenth century. Evidence of this is found in the first book on dentistry published in English. Entitled *The Operator for the Teeth* and authored by a self-styled "professor," Charles Allen, who was in all probability a barber-surgeon, it first appeared in 1685 and was reissued twice. In his book Allen deals superficially with the preservation of the teeth, suggesting filling cavities with materials as to whose composition, unfortunately, he leaves us in the dark. He describes extractions and illustrates several instruments, including what he called a "polican." Allen gives us little that is new. Dentistry had to wait until the next century to become a true science.

123

A traveling dentist has set up shop in the Dutch village depicted here by Jan Steen (1629–1679), and his ministrations provoke both consternation and amusement in the spectators. Mauritshuis, The Hague.

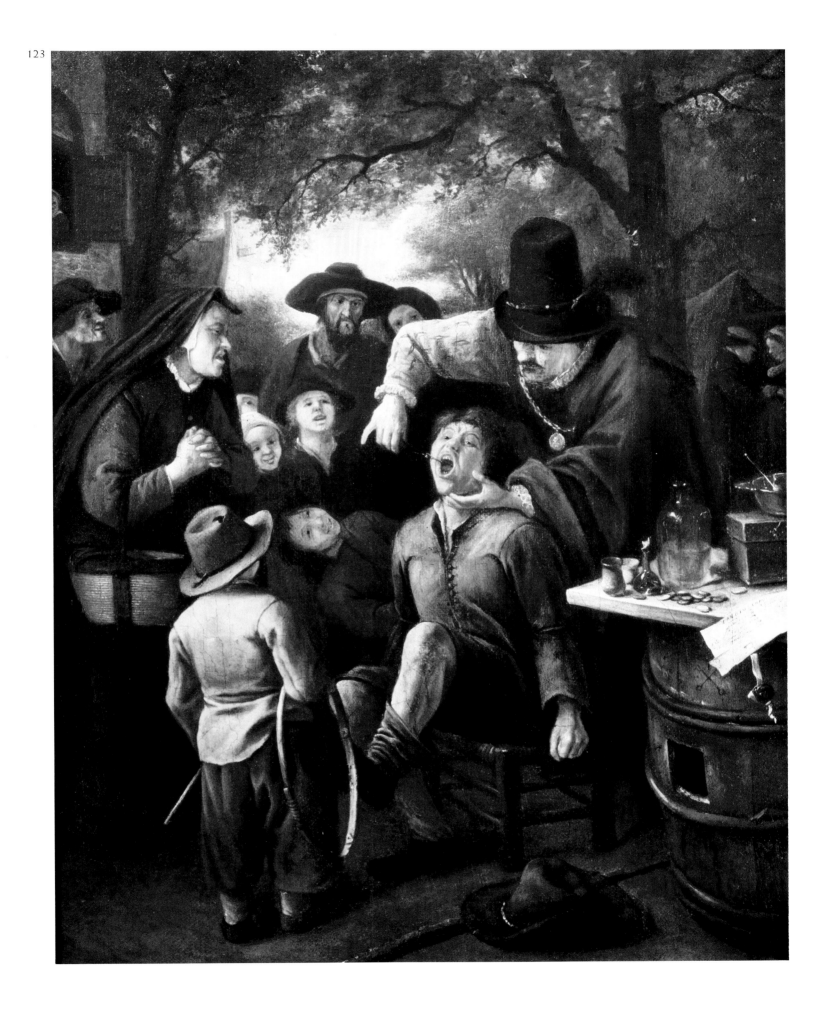

124

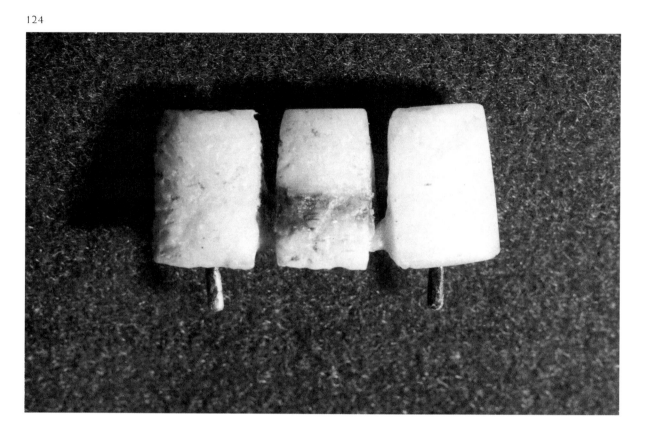

The construction of the silver posts in this French dental bridge found at Vaison-la-Romaine dates the prosthesis to the middle of the seventeenth century. The posts were cemented into the root canals of the teeth on either side of the missing tooth.

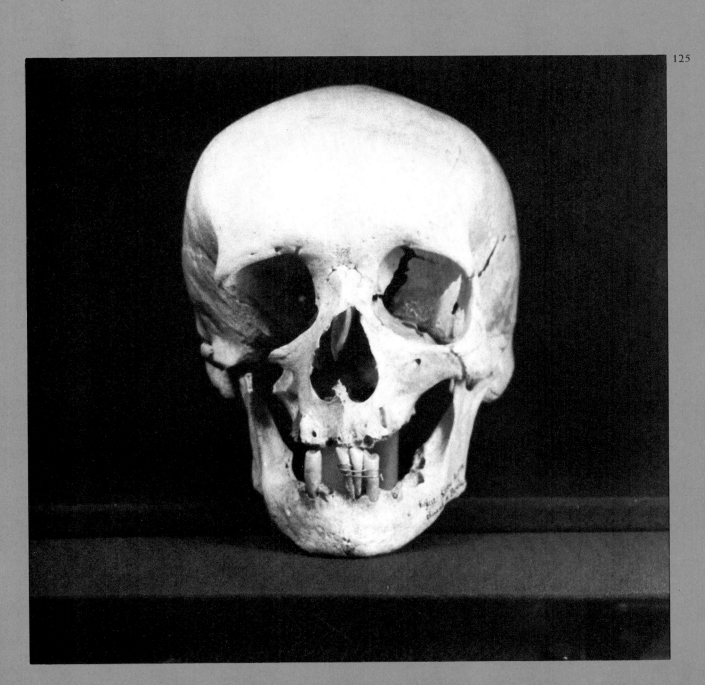

Three lower teeth of this mid-seventeenth-century skull from Avignon have been ligated together with gold wire in an effort to stabilize them. Advanced periodontal disease weakened their bony support and caused the loss of many posterior teeth as well.

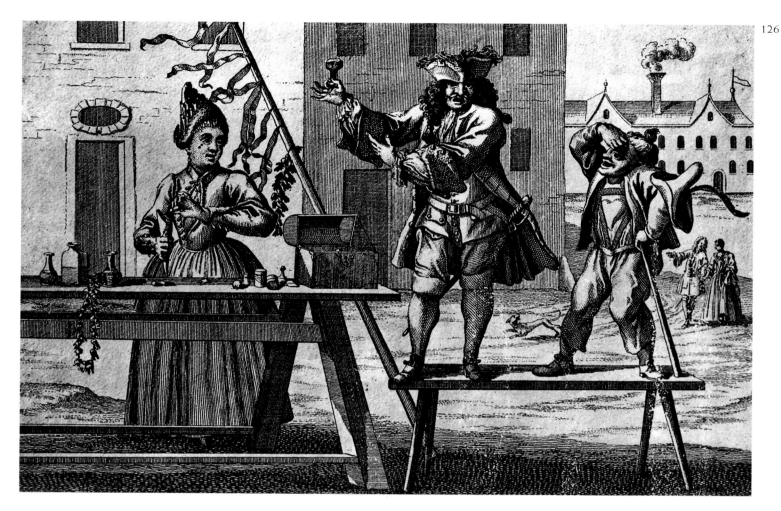

A German charlatan of about 1700 exhibits a huge tooth, which he pretends to have removed from the mouth of the patient beside him. His female assistant is preparing a medicinal powder, for in addition to toothache he claims to cure dizziness, cough, the complications of pregnancy, urinary gravel, and kidney stones. Over the edge of the table hangs a chain of extracted teeth. The Francis A. Countway Library, Harvard Medical Library/Boston Medical Library, Rare Book Collection, Boston.

The subject of this mid-eighteenth-century print entitled *Sans Douleur (No Pain)* is a peripatetic French charlatan-dentist. He displays a tooth he has just extracted, while his trained monkey mimics him in the background. Lithograph by Engelman after Roehn. Cabinet des Estampes, Bibliothèque Nationale, Paris.

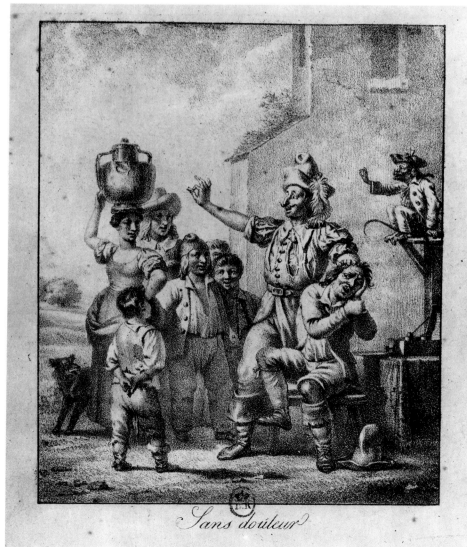

Sans douleur

X
THE EIGHTEENTH CENTURY IN EUROPE

The eighteenth century ushered in profound changes in the practice of dentistry, the impetus for which came from the scientific discoveries of the preceding century. Dentistry ultimately became an independent scientific discipline—not overnight, however, but after much painstaking experimentation and dedicated effort on the part of several generations of practitioners.

By the beginning of the century, France had become the most civilized and cultured country in Europe, and surgery was one of the many fields in which this superiority was reflected (medicine, however, still languished far behind). By about 1725 the surgeons of the Collège de St. Côme had publicly demonstrated their independence from the physicians, and they themselves lobbied for legislation to regulate the practice of surgery.

In 1699 the French parliament passed a law stipulating that dental practitioners (*experts pour les dents*), along with such other specialists as oculists and bonesetters, had to be examined by a committee of surgeons before being allowed to practice in Paris and its environs. In other countries, too, a sincere attempt was made about this time to protect the people by regulation from harmful mistreatment by quacks. Fourteen years before France, as Professor Walter Hoffmann-Axthelm has rightfully pointed out, the German state of Brandenburg-Prussia passed an edict regulating the practice of the Collegium Medicum in Berlin and "what physicians as well as apothecaries and surgeons are to observe." All those who wished to practice dentistry were obliged to appear before a government commission in order to receive a license. "When oculists, operators, lithotomists, hernia-operators, tooth-drawers, etc., wish to advertise themselves and wish publicly to practice and offer for sale their art and science, then they should be inhibited by this *Collegio*, no less than by the magistrate, in submitting to their examinations, whereupon depending on the result they should be permitted or forbidden to do so." Hoffmann-Axthelm points out that the edict made a sharp distinction between frauds and quacks and valid operators in stating that the former "should be tolerated nowhere and suppressed with unrelenting harsh punishment."

Unfortunately, these regulations established in France, Germany, and elsewhere were rarely enforced, and quacks and charlatans abounded. In France one of the most notorious of these was a huge man known far and wide as Le Grand Thomas (Great Thomas), who plied his trade in Paris on the Pont Neuf (fig. 128). His flamboyant showmanship attracted much attention, and many contemporary drawings of him exist. A writer of his period described his appearance vividly:

> The superb horse which had the honor of carrying the incomparable Thomas was adorned with a prodigious quantity of teeth strung one after another. A valet had the care of leading it by the bridle for fear that the joy and exclamations of the people would make it forsake the seriousness which befits such a ceremony. The adjustments of the Gros Thomas were new and extraordinary. His bonnet of solid silver had at its summit a globe surmounted by a singing cock. The lower part of his headpiece was terminated with a coat-of-arms in the middle of which could be seen the arms of France and of Navarre and, on the left side, a sun and these words: *nec pluribus impar*. His scarlet coat, made Turkish-wise, was adorned with teeth, jaws, and stones of the Temple; furthermore, he had a silver breastplate representing the sun, but so luminous that it could only be viewed from the side. His saber was six feet long. His retinue was composed of a drum, a trumpet and a standard-bearer who walked before him; at his sides were an infusion-maker and a baker.

128

This engraving of 1730 depicts one of the bizarre attractions of the Paris scene, "Le Grand Thomas en son Académie d'Operations." The charlatan Thomas presides at his outdoor "office" on the Pont Neuf, near the equestrian statue of Henry IV, at the middle of the bridge. Several of his assistants are probing the mouths of potential customers to see what teeth are to be extracted and to establish a fee. Library of Congress, Washington, D.C.

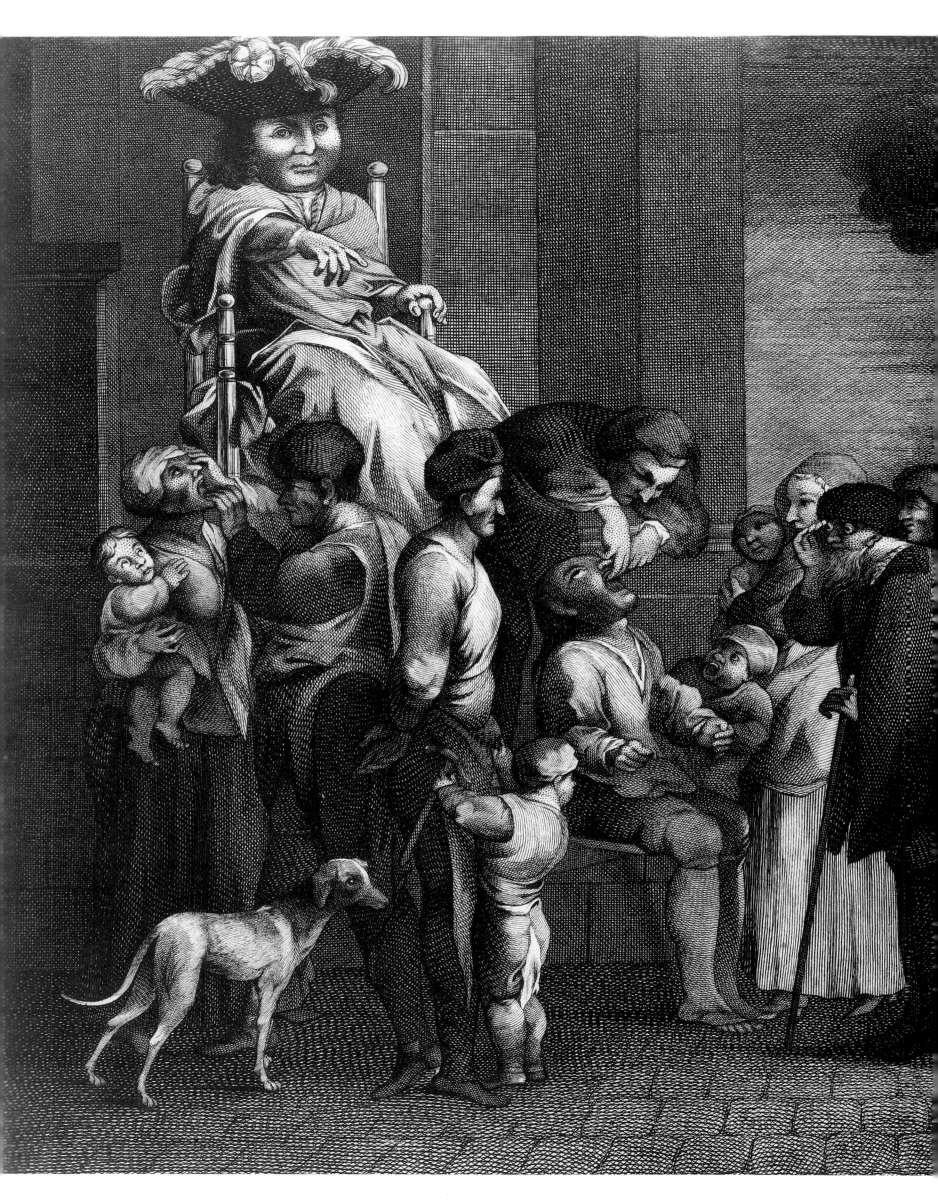

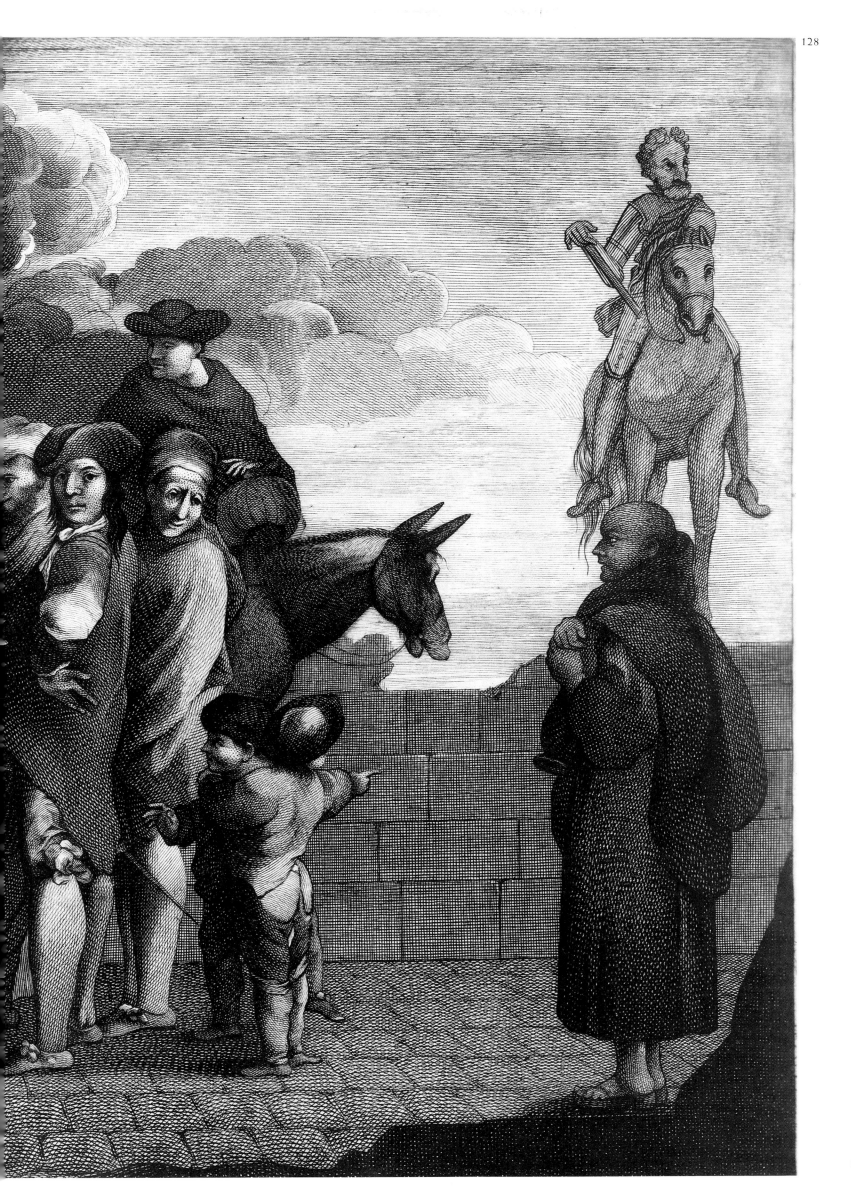

It is difficult to imagine that there were many quacks in Europe with such panache as Thomas, but certain it is that many thousands of equally unqualified specialists had no difficulty in attracting customers. It was still an age when only the rich could command the services of an adequately trained dentist.

Pierre Fauchard

Modern dentistry owes its greatest debt to a remarkable Frenchman who synthesized what was known in the West about dentistry and who presented it in an organized form so that all practitioners could benefit. Pierre Fauchard (fig. 129) was born in Brittany in 1678. After training as a military surgeon, he settled about 1719 in Paris, where he remained until his death in 1761.

In 1723 he completed his epic work, *Le chirurgien dentiste; ou, traité des dents* (*The Surgeon-Dentist; or, Treatise on the Teeth*), which, however, was not published until five years later, in 1728. A second edition was brought out in 1746, and it contained more material and more and better illustrations than the first. *Le chirurgien dentiste*, 863 pages in two small volumes, was the most important book on dentistry to appear and it was to remain the authoritative work in the field during the next century. Issued in German translation in 1733, it became available in English only in 1946, when the great dental historian Lilian Lindsay completed a translation.

In Fauchard's day it was customary for practitioners of any of the healing arts to guard their knowledge and skills jealously. But Fauchard despised such secrecy and, to his own financial detriment, made his methods public saying, "I have perfected and also invented several artificial pieces both for substituting a part of the teeth and for remedying their entire loss . . . and to the prejudice of my own interests, I now give the most exact description possible of them."

A number of his colleagues became jealous of Fauchard and spread the rumor that he was giving up his practice. Fauchard responded in his book: "The rumor having been falsely set about that he has abandoned the profession, which rumor cannot have been invented otherwise than by those individuals who, sacrificing honor to interest, would attract to themselves the persons who honor the author with their confidence; he therefore finds it necessary to give warning that he still continues the practice of his art in Paris, in the Rue de la Comédie Française, together with his brother-in-law and sole student, M. Duchemin."

Aware of weaknesses in the training of dentists in France, Fauchard decried the fact that the examining commission set up by the edict of 1699 lacked "a skillful and experienced dentist," noting that most "dental experts are only equipped with less than average knowledge." Unfortunately, his suggestion that a dentist also be on the examining board was not adopted.

In his great book Fauchard covered the entire field of dentistry, and many of the ideas and procedures he advocated or described are still current today, two and a half centuries later! He covered dental anatomy and morphology as well as anomalies of the teeth. He discussed tooth decay, its causes and prevention, and rejected the toothworm theory, claiming that he had never seen such worms either with the naked eye or with the microscope; rather he believed that caries were the result of a "humoral imbalance."

Oral pathology he investigated in great detail, citing numerous case histories and the treatment he had rendered. Teething problems interested him greatly, and he stressed how essential it is to retain the primary teeth until it is time for them to be shed. He dealt with replantation of avulsed teeth and transplantation of teeth from one individual to another, anticipating John Hunter's work by about forty years.

J. Le Bel painted this portrait of Pierre Fauchard between about 1723 and 1728, when the eminent surgeon-dentist was between forty-five and fifty years of age. The only likeness of Fauchard definitely known to have been drawn from life, it remained in the possession of his descendants until 1982. Fauchard's dress establishes him as a Frenchman of the upper middle class; his alert, intelligent gaze indicates that he arrived there by his own efforts and talent. This portrait served as the model for the engraved frontispiece by Scotin for Fauchard's famous treatise *Le chirurgien dentiste*. Private collection, France.

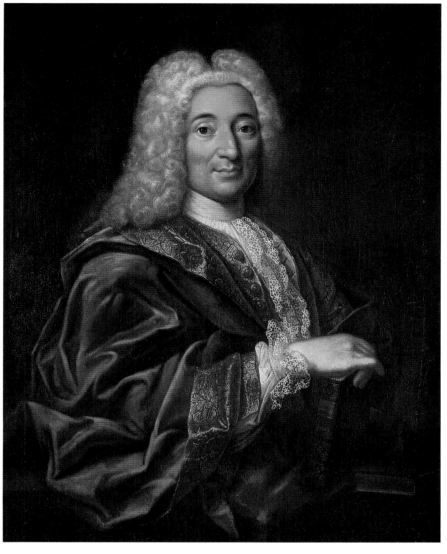

129

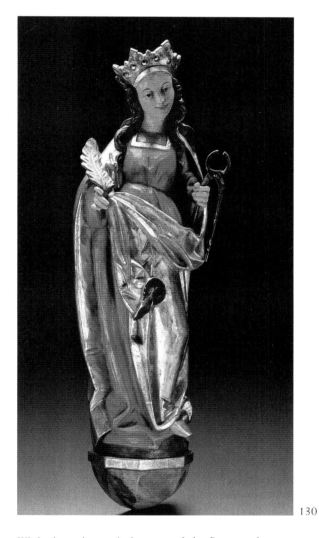

130

With the cultivated elegance of the Bavarian baroque style, this eighteenth-century Saint Apollonia, carved of wood, balances gracefully on a globe. The forceps she carries are of formidable size, but her smile and the palm of victory in her left hand offer the promise of recovery from the torments of toothache. Kulturhistorische Sammlung des Bundesverbandes der Deutschen Zahnärzte, Cologne.

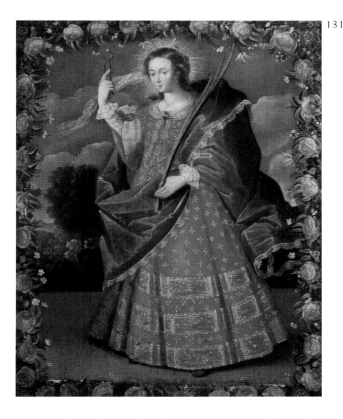

131

An unknown South American artist of the eighteenth century has depicted Apollonia, patron saint of dentists, dressed in the charming costume of the day. She stands in a landscape framed by a spray of roses that from a distance bear an amusing resemblance to a set of molar teeth. Museo Nacional de Bellas Artes, Santiago, Chile.

Figures 132–39 are plates from Pierre Fauchard's *Le chirurgien dentiste; ou, traité des dents* (1728).

132

Tooth replacements. Figures 1–4 and 8 show bridges made of human teeth drilled to accommodate threads by which they will be bound to adjacent natural teeth still in place. The backs of the teeth are joined and reinforced with a silver bar, as can be seen in figures 5–7. Figures 9–11 show a natural tooth crown on a silver post, which will be inserted into a root canal like a modern dowel crown.

133

The partial dentures shown in figures 1 and 2 are held in place by threads bound to natural teeth still in place. Figures 3 and 4 show a fixed bridge held in place by dowels inserted in the root canals of remaining teeth.

134

Fauchard's method of retaining a full upper denture in the mouth when the natural lower teeth are present is illustrated here.

135

Steel strips which act as springs will retain these full dentures in the mouth. The teeth are made of ivory. Those shown in figure 3 are set on an enameled metal base.

136

This rather complicated obturator has two wings that can be inserted through a palatal defect and raised or lowered as needed by means of the key shown in figure 16.

137

Fauchard designed this bow drill to cut into the enamel of natural teeth.

138

The pelican, an extraction instrument that dates back probably to the time of John of Gaddesden, consists of a fixed part and a movable arm with a hooked end. The hooked end engages the tooth to be extracted while the fixed end presses against adjacent teeth, acting as a brace and fulcrum. Two of Fauchard's pelicans are shown here (the one on the right is double-ended). The ends that press against the fulcrum teeth are covered with leather to protect the dentition.

139

Fauchard regarded the forceps, two of which are illustrated here, as less effective but also less risky for the patient than the pelican.

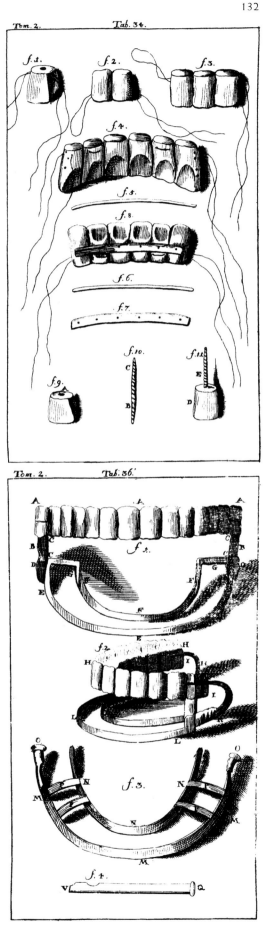

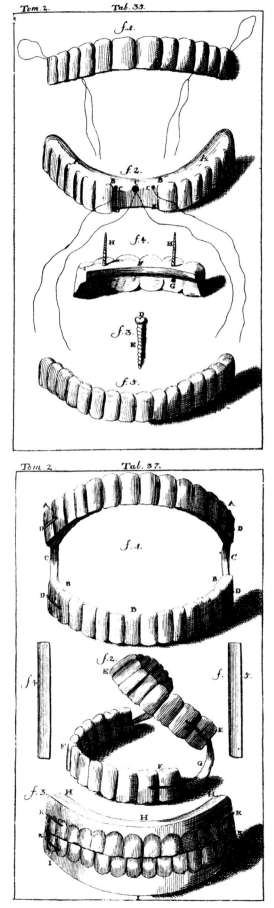

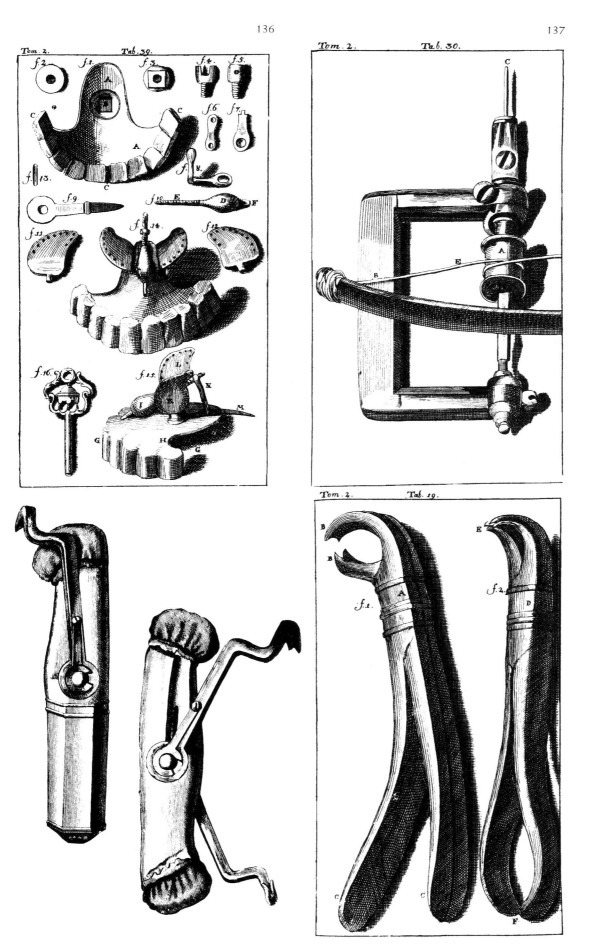

Tom. 2.   Tab. 39.

Tom. 2.   Tab. 30.

Tom. 2.   Tab. 19.

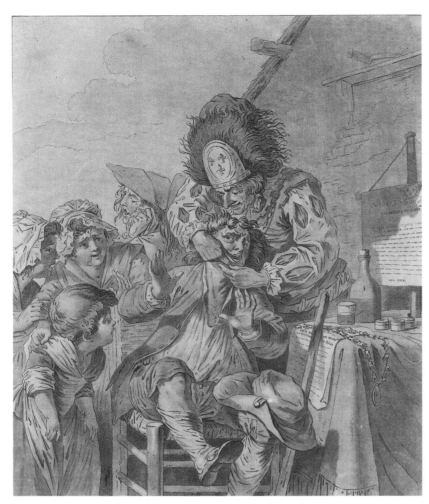

140

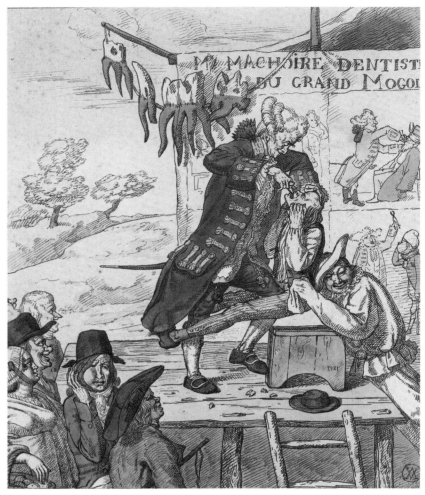

141

Like many a quack, this itinerant French tooth-drawer plies his trade in the street, and his flamboyant garb is calculated to attract attention. However, on the table, underneath a chain of extracted molar teeth, he displays the governmental certificate that allows him to practice. Colored aquatint by Wille the Younger, dated 1788. National Library of Medicine, Bethesda.

In this colored engraving by Adrien-Victor Auger (b. 1787), a gorgeously dressed charlatan who advertised himself as dentist to the Great Mogul is pulling the tooth of a struggling patient restrained by an assistant. Although it dates from 1817, the scene has not essentially changed since Fauchard's day, or even Paré's. National Library of Medicine, Bethesda.

Before the discovery of anesthesia, champagne and less expensive alcoholic beverages were used to deaden the pain of dental surgery, as this British cartoon of 1780 indicates. Northwestern University Dental School, Chicago.

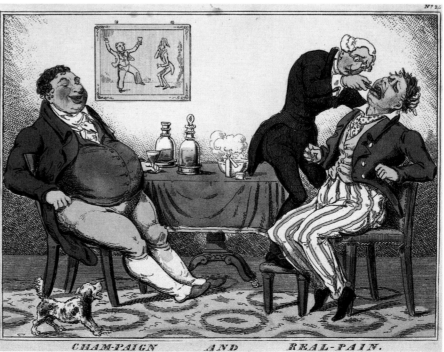

142

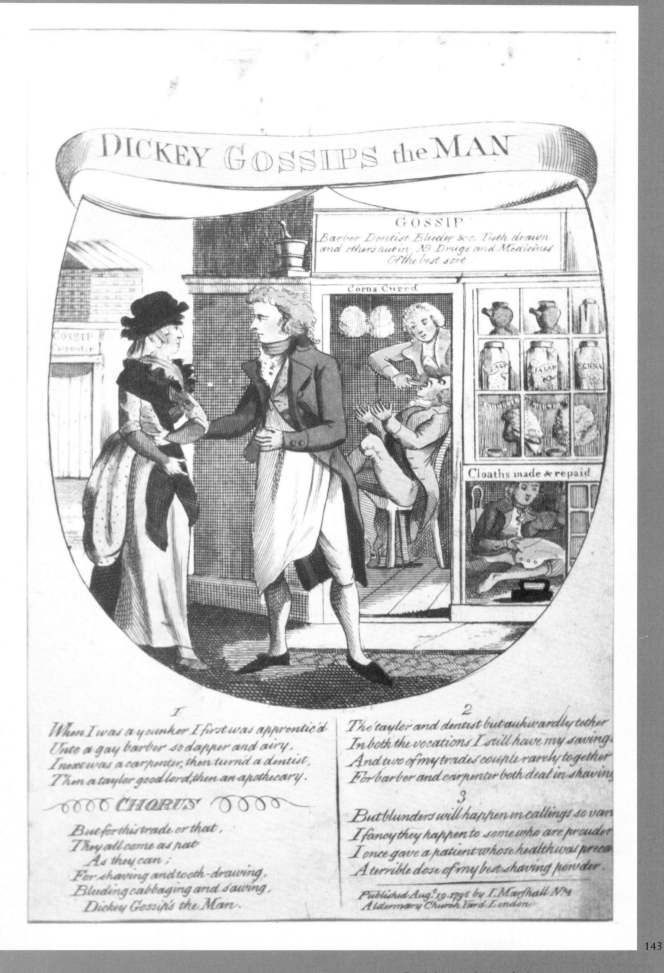

An English broadside of about 1796 advertises the services of "Dickey" Gossip, whose chief occupations are recorded above his door. Ancillary services are mentioned on signs here and there about his establishment. Collection Dr. Bernard S. Moskow.

A large portion of *Le chirurgien dentiste* is devoted to practical operative dentistry. Here Fauchard detailed his method of removing caries from a tooth and filling the cavity with lead or tin. He also devoted keen attention to prosthetic dentistry, describing how individual bridges (fig. 132) as well as partial and complete dentures (figs. 133–35) were to be constructed. He advocated using either human teeth or teeth carved from hippopotamus or elephant ivory in dentures, and he devised methods of retaining upper and lower dentures in place by joining them either with thin strips of steel or by spiral springs. He also constructed three springless dentures held in place by atmospheric pressure. He failed to appreciate this principle of retention, which keeps modern dentures in place during use, and did not pursue what would have been a monumental step forward. But his pioneering work in coloring and enameling denture bases to simulate the natural gums inspired those who followed him to make artificial replacements more lifelike and pleasing to wear.

Fauchard's understanding of periodontal disease was well in advance of his time. He was a firm believer in scaling the teeth and debridement of root surfaces to prevent gingival disease. A strong advocate of preventive dentistry, he recommended the use of mouthwashes as part of home care and gave many formulas for concocting them. (It astounds us to read that this advanced thinker firmly believed that one should rinse one's mouth every morning with several spoons of one's own freshly voided urine in order to insure good health.)

Fauchard gave much practical advice and illustrated his book with excellent drawings both of the instruments he devised and of his prosthetic appliances. And he brought a new dignity and decorum to the dentist's office by insisting that instead of sitting on the floor with the dentist standing over him (fig. 144) the patient be seated "in an armchair which is steady and firm, suitable and comfortable, the back of which should be of horsehair or with a soft pillow raised more or less according to the stature of the patient and particularly to that of the dentist" (fig. 145).

Fauchard won great fame and respect in his lifetime. He effectively separated dentistry from the larger field of surgery, even more emphatically from the trade of the tooth-drawers, and set it on its own feet as an independent profession, with its own circumscribed field of duties and services and its own name. (It was Fauchard who coined the term "surgeon-dentist," which is what the French call their dentists to this day.)

No one has made a more perceptive evaluation of Pierre Fauchard's achievement than the great American dentist Chapin A. Harris: "Considering the circumstances under which he lived, Fauchard deserves to be remembered as a noble pioneer and sure founder of dental science. That his practice was crude was due to his times; that it was scientific and comparatively superior and successful, was due to himself."

144, 145

In the eighteenth century it was considered best to position the patient considerably lower than the dentist during a tooth extraction. Ludwig Cron preferred to operate with the patient on the floor firmly holding the dentist's leg, as he demonstrates in figure 144, a print from his book *Aderlassen und Zahn-ausziehen* (*Bloodletting and Tooth-drawing*, 1717). In figure 145 a French dentist of the ancien régime extracts the tooth of a nobleman seated in a chair. With aristocratic composure the patient clutches neither the operator nor even the chair arm, but with his right hand gracefully registers mild shock.

146 (pages 168–69)

Thomas Rowlandson ridiculed the English vogue for tooth transplantation in this etching of 1787. A rich dowager looks on with distaste as a tooth destined for her mouth is removed from the jaw of a pauper. A poor girl who has just sold a tooth holds her painful cheek while looking at the pittance she has received for it. National Library of Medicine, Bethesda.

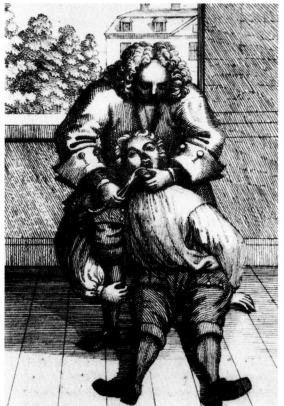

144

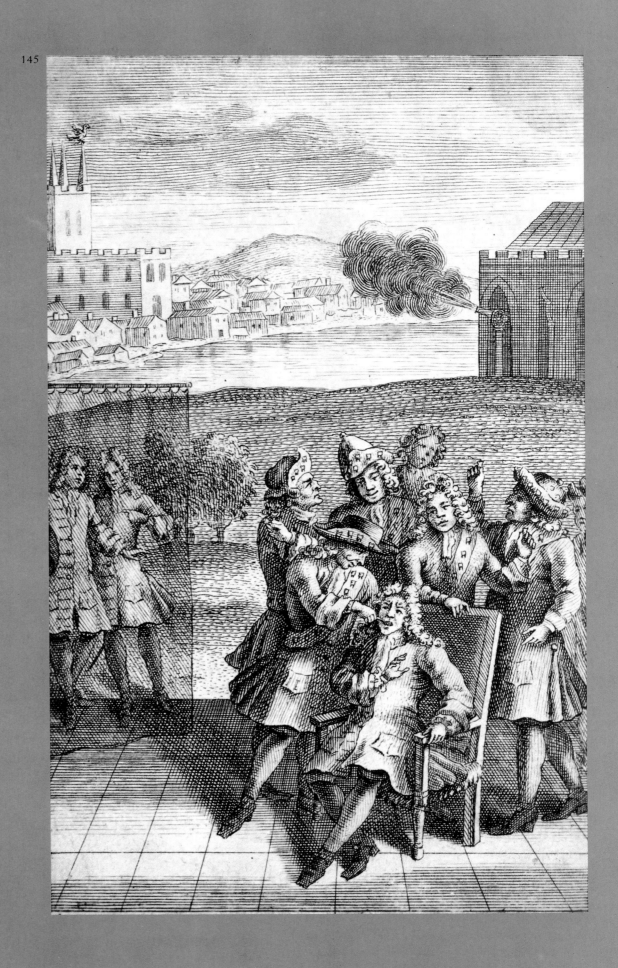

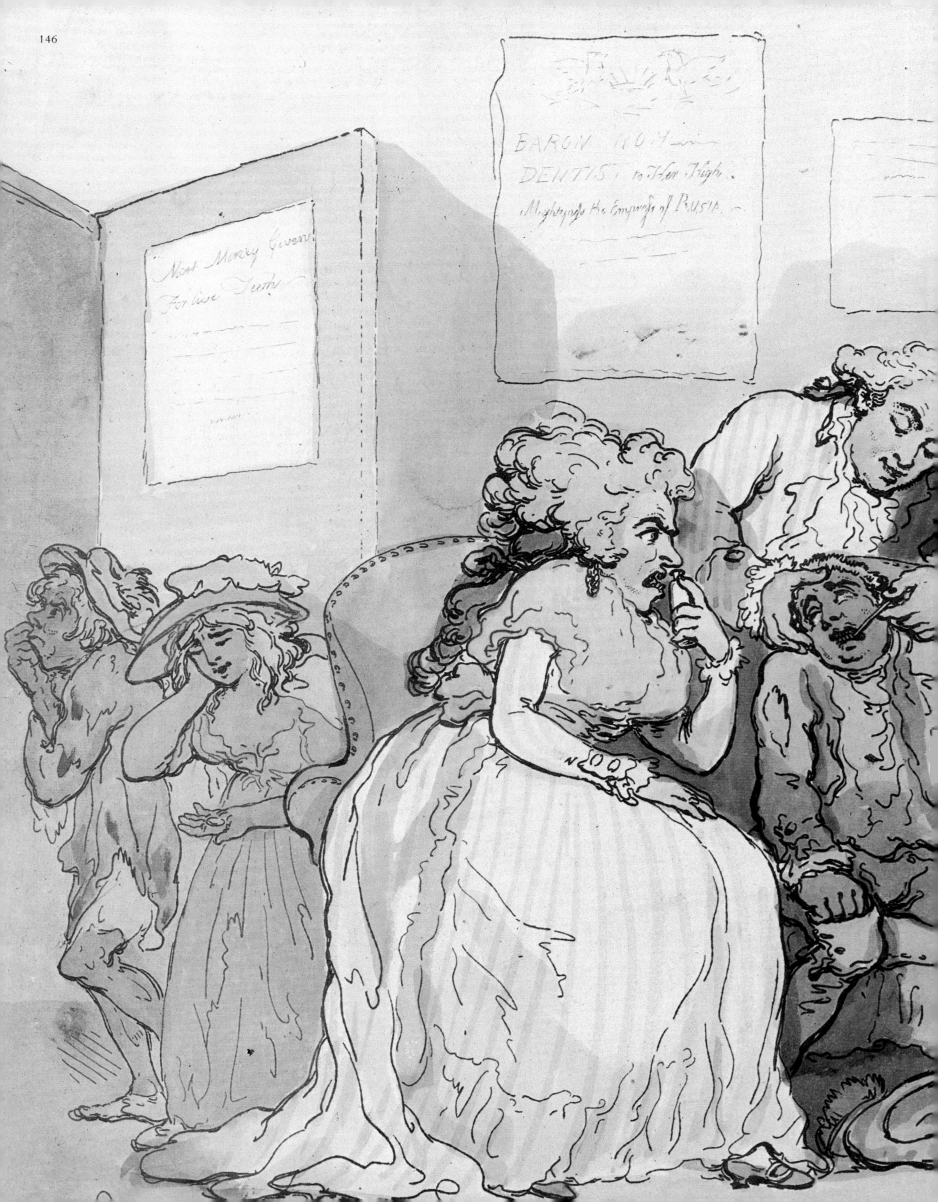

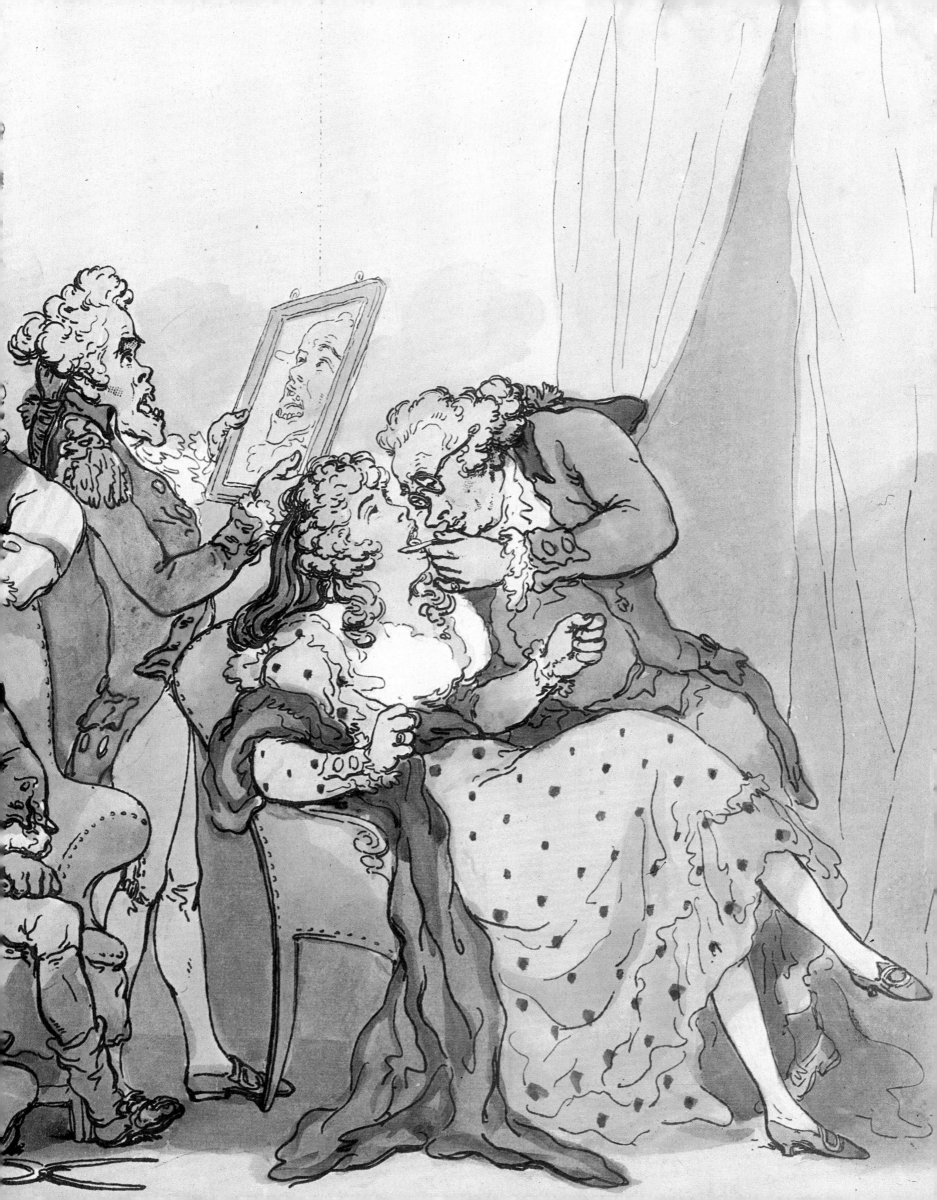

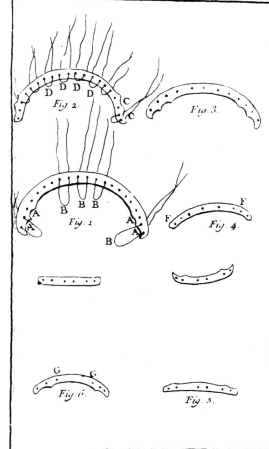

Etienne Bourdet was a progressive French dentist with an inventive mind. He used the ivory splints illustrated above to pull misplaced teeth into correct alignment. Shown below are two metal dentures of his devising. The first has sockets for natural human teeth (the latter to be held in place by metal pins). In the second version, natural teeth are impaled on pins fixed directly in the metal base. From volume two of *Recherches et observations* (1757).

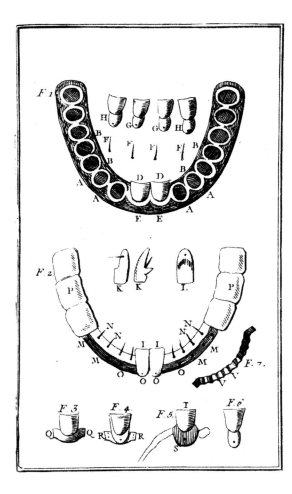

Fauchard's Followers in France and Germany

Fauchard's initiative in offering the public the benefit of his experience led other dental surgeons to follow his example, and soon the dentists of France and other lands were freely publishing their knowledge and techniques. Robert Bunon (1702–1748), who also practiced in Paris, wrote a number of tracts during the 1740s in which he challenged the widely held belief that maxillary cuspids should not be extracted because this would damage the eyes. He also refuted the notion that pregnant women should not be given dental treatment, insisting instead that it was at precisely this time that they most needed care.

Claude Mouton (died 1786), later to become dentist to the king of France, published in 1746 his *Essay d'odontotechnie*, the first book dealing exclusively with "mechanical dentistry," as dental technology was then called. He devised a gold crown with a gold post designed to be retained in the root canal, and described for the first time since the early Romans gold shell crowns, which he used to prevent broken-down molars from deteriorating further. To render crowns on anterior teeth more esthetically pleasing, he suggested enameling their labial surfaces in natural tooth colors. Another of his inventions was two small gold springs that fastened at either end of a removable bridge to hold it in place—the first use of a clasp to retain an artificial tooth.

One of the most important of Fauchard's followers (who gives Fauchard credit for having led the way, and who quotes him extensively in his own work) was Etienne Bourdet (1722–1789), who succeeded Mouton as royal dentist. His *Recherches et observations sur toutes les parties de l'art du dentiste* appeared in 1757 and went through numerous printings. Among the most important of his contributions were a detailed description of severe periodontoclasia and his treatment of the condition, which was, in essence, the modern gingivectomy. He also advocated extraction of the first bicuspids to alleviate overcrowding of the mouth—the modern practice—and described how misaligned teeth could be shifted into place by attaching them with threads to a splint of ivory (fig. 147).

One of his novel constructions was a denture base of gold punctuated with small holes much like the sockets of teeth (fig. 147). Projecting upward in these sockets were pins onto which natural human teeth, cut off slightly below the necks, were impaled. Unlike Fauchard, who used steel springs for denture retention, Bourdet used gold springs because they do not rust or corrode.

Until the mid-1700s, the pelican was the principal instrument used in extracting teeth. Bourdet was the first to describe in detail a new instrument called a key (whose invention was widely, and falsely, attributed to a dentist named Garangeot), which subsequently became very popular. Bourdet devised keys with interchangeable ends for use in extracting different teeth.

The publication of the German edition of Fauchard's work brought about a resurgence of dental literature in Germany. Before 1742, 150 German dental treatises had been issued, yet none was written by a dentist, being instead the work of physicians, surgeons, or barbers. In 1755 *Abhandlung von den Zahnen des menschlichen Körpers und deren Krankheiten (Treatise on the Teeth of the Human Body and Their Diseases)* was brought out by Philip Pfaff (1716–1780), dentist to Frederick the Great of Prussia. It was based in large part on Fauchard's work but also contained some things that were new, including a detailed description of taking impressions with softened wax and constructing from them models made of plaster of paris and capping vital pulp exposures with small sheets of gold, without first cauterizing, and killing, the pulp.

Several other Germans made significant contributions to dental literature, notably Johann Bücking (1749–1838), who in 1782 wrote *Complete Handbook on Tooth Extraction for Practicing Surgeons*, and Adam Brunner, from whose *Introduction to the Knowledge Necessary for a Dentist* (1765) we learn that the construction of dental prostheses was commonly left to turners and other craftsmen, while operative dentistry was the province of the dentist. (American dentists made their own prostheses until the late nineteenth century, and many began their careers as

An English quack's poster, dated 1757, advertises a surprising cure for the toothache, which, after one reads the copy, turns out to be a perfumed letter.

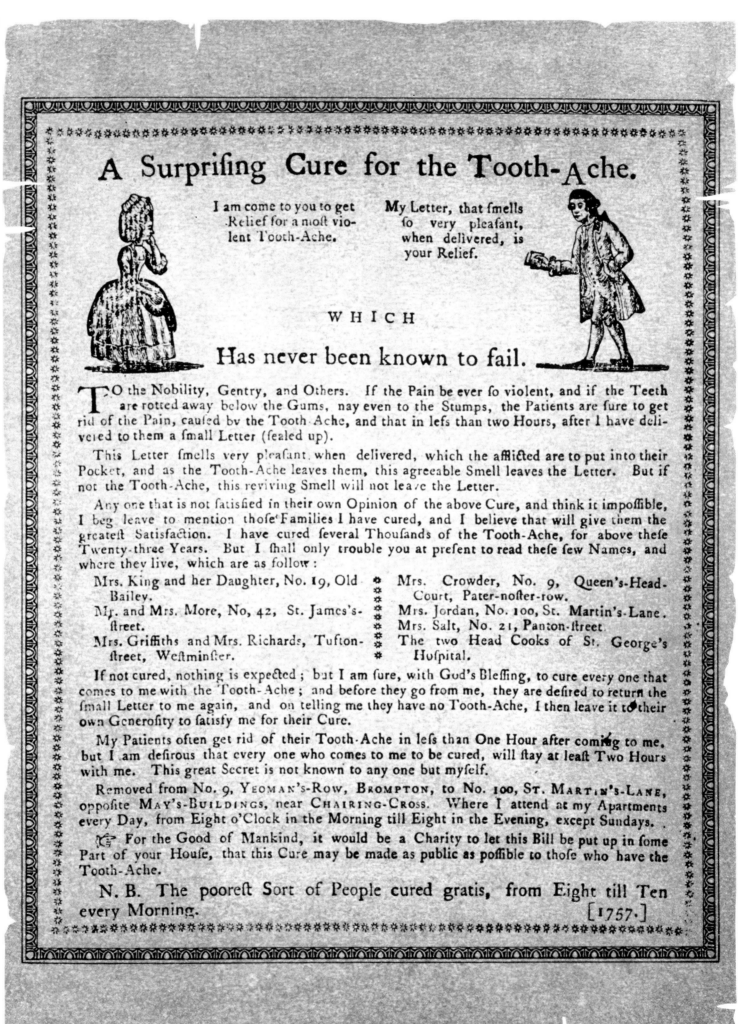

A Surprising Cure for the Tooth-Ache.

I am come to you to get Relief for a most violent Tooth-Ache.

My Letter, that smells so very pleasant, when delivered, is your Relief.

WHICH

Has never been known to fail.

TO the Nobility, Gentry, and Others. If the Pain be ever so violent, and if the Teeth are rotted away below the Gums, nay even to the Stumps, the Patients are sure to get rid of the Pain, caused by the Tooth-Ache, and that in less than two Hours, after I have delivered to them a small Letter (sealed up).

This Letter smells very pleasant when delivered, which the afflicted are to put into their Pocket, and as the Tooth-Ache leaves them, this agreeable Smell leaves the Letter. But if not the Tooth-Ache, this reviving Smell will not leave the Letter.

Any one that is not satisfied in their own Opinion of the above Cure, and think it impossible, I beg leave to mention those Families I have cured, and I believe that will give them the greatest Satisfaction. I have cured several Thousands of the Tooth-Ache, for above these Twenty-three Years. But I shall only trouble you at present to read these few Names, and where they live, which are as follow:

Mrs. King and her Daughter, No. 19, Old Bailey.

Mr. and Mrs. More, No. 42, St. James's-street.

Mrs. Griffiths and Mrs. Richards, Tufton-street, Westminster.

Mrs. Crowder, No. 9, Queen's-Head-Court, Pater-noster-row.

Mrs. Jordan, No. 100, St. Martin's-Lane.

Mrs. Salt, No. 21, Panton-street.

The two Head Cooks of St. George's Hospital.

If not cured, nothing is expected; but I am sure, with God's Blessing, to cure every one that comes to me with the Tooth-Ache; and before they go from me, they are desired to return the small Letter to me again, and on telling me they have no Tooth-Ache, I then leave it to their own Generosity to satisfy me for their Cure.

My Patients often get rid of their Tooth-Ache in less than One Hour after coming to me, but I am desirous that every one who comes to me to be cured, will stay at least Two Hours with me. This great Secret is not known to any one but myself.

Removed from No. 9, YEOMAN'S-ROW, BROMPTON, to No. 100, ST. MARTIN'S-LANE, opposite MAY'S-BUILDINGS, near CHAIRING-CROSS. Where I attend at my Apartments every Day, from Eight o'Clock in the Morning till Eight in the Evening, except Sundays.

☞ For the Good of Mankind, it would be a Charity to let this Bill be put up in some Part of your House, that this Cure may be made as public as possible to those who have the Tooth-Ache.

N. B. The poorest Sort of People cured gratis, from Eight till Ten every Morning.

[1757.]

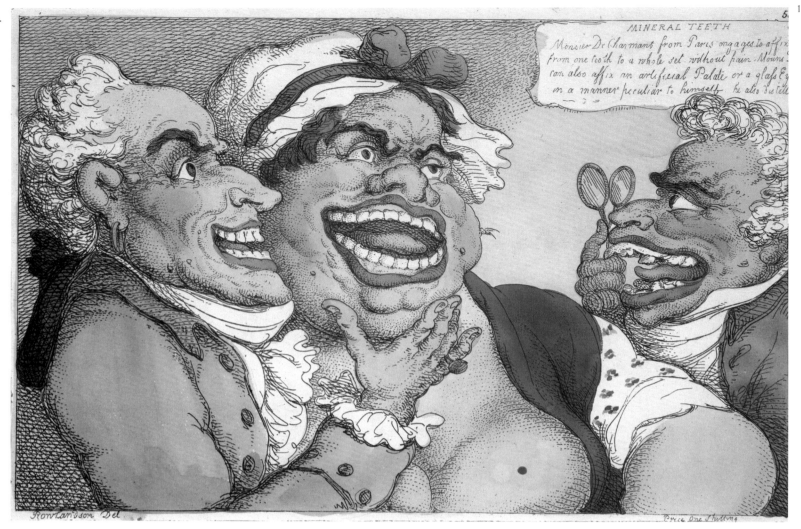

MINERAL TEETH

Monsieur De Charmant from Paris engages to affix
from one tooth to a whole set without pain. Monsu
can also affix an artificial Palate or a glass Ey
in a manner peculiar to himself he also distills

Rowlandson Del

Price One Shilling

When Nicolas Dubois de Chémant (see page 180) brought his porcelain dentures to England in the 1790s they were eagerly sought after by the gentry. This contemporary cartoon is by the great satirist Thomas Rowlandson. The Francis A. Countway Library of Medicine, Harvard Medical Library/Boston Medical Library, Rare Book Collection, Boston.

wood or ivory turners. Probably for this reason dentistry was for many years considered only a craft in the United States.) Brunner advised against the use of tobacco and clay pipes (which abraded the teeth) and included a comprehensive bibliography in his book—a real rarity in those days.

England

English dentistry did not advance as far as Continental dentistry during the eighteenth century. The guild that had united the barbers and the surgeons since 1540 was sundered in 1745, when the surgeons broke away and formed a Surgeons' Company. (This organization was dissolved in 1796, to be reorganized in 1800 as the Royal College of Surgeons of England.) Some of the barbers, intent on improving their status, associated with the surgeons, and these continued to be called "tooth-drawers." However, the designation "dentist," apparently as a result of French influence, was applied to some others, while a third group, which included those who did all kinds of dentistry, chose the term "operators for the teeth."

Between 1687, when Charles Allen's *Operator for the Teeth* was released, and 1742, no book on dentistry in English was published. Then Joseph Hurlock, a London surgeon, brought out a book, *A Practical Treatise upon Dentition*, in which he advocated lancing the gums of children to facilitate teething. This pernicious practice might never have taken such hold had it not been for Hurlock's convincing arguments, but it did indeed become very popular. As late as 1853, an American dentist, J. L. Levison, reported in the *American Journal of Dental Science* that he had been treating a child nine or ten months old when he noticed

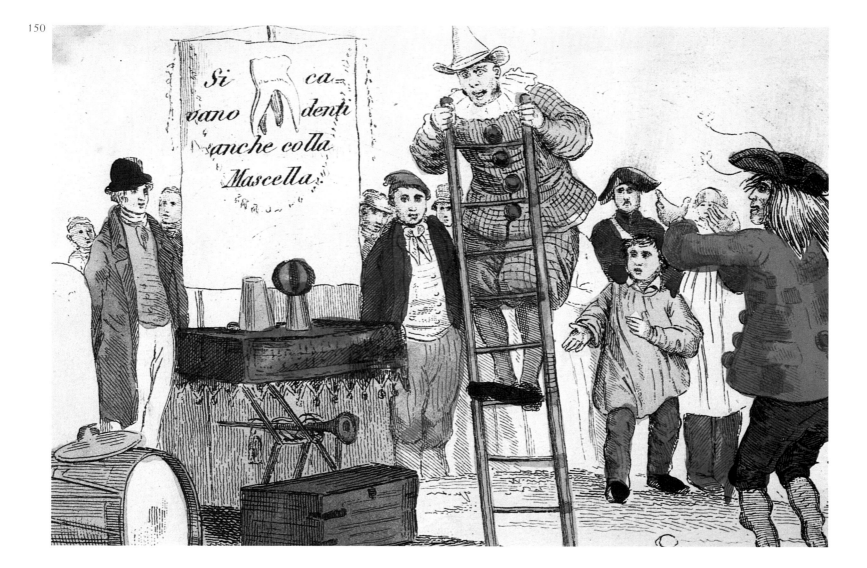

Si cavano denti anche colla Mascella.

symptoms of strabismus [crossed eyes] in the little fellow, and pointed out the appearance of his eyes to his mother, urging her to leave the room that I might lance his gums and save him from worse consequences. But she peremptorily refused "as the child was feverish." Within a few days, acute symptoms of cerebral disease were indicated, and when her usual [doctor] was summoned, he admitted that there existed *hydrocephalus internus*, and although he adopted...active [measures], yet nevertheless this lovely boy died within a week of my first seeing him.

In 1768 Thomas Berdmore's *Treatise on the Disorders and Deformities of the Teeth and the Gums* was published. Berdmore (1740–1785), dentist to King George III, boasted that he based his writings exclusively on his own personal observations, claiming he "could only have quoted a few French authors, who have written to make their names known." His poor opinion of his readers' education emerges quite soon, when he remarks kindly that he has designed his book "for artists who are not much given to reading."

Despite his high self-opinion, Berdmore added little new to dental knowledge, for in fact his own experience was not wide. He treated toothache principally with medicaments, sometimes by cautery, and, as a heroic measure, by extracting the tooth, filling the cavity with lead or gold, and then replanting it in its socket. He discusses the correction of poorly aligned teeth by means of threads, but is conspicuously vague about prosthetic treatment, leading us to conclude that he probably did little of that type of work.

This Italian painting of about 1800 pokes fun at the practice of street dentistry, still quite common at that time. A juggler-acrobat attracts a crowd from a ladder and his sign reads "We pull teeth and also the jaw." University of Maryland Health Sciences Library, Baltimore.

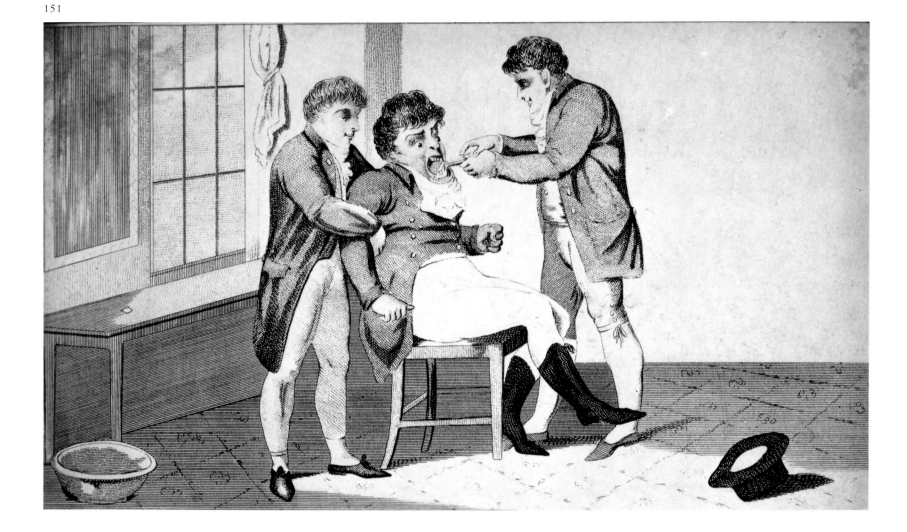

151, 152

In figure 151, a print of about 1750, an English dentist extracts a tooth using a new instrument called a key. In figure 152, a print in the collection of the Bundesverband der Deutschen Zahnärzte, Cologne, an eighteenth-century charlatan in soldier's uniform is about to extract a tooth with his sword. This method, which seems by contrast exceedingly barbaric, was very popular. As Pierre Dionis, surgeon to the family of Louis XIV, remarked, the street dentists used a sword in order to make the public believe they needed nothing more elaborate to make a tooth fly effortlessly out.

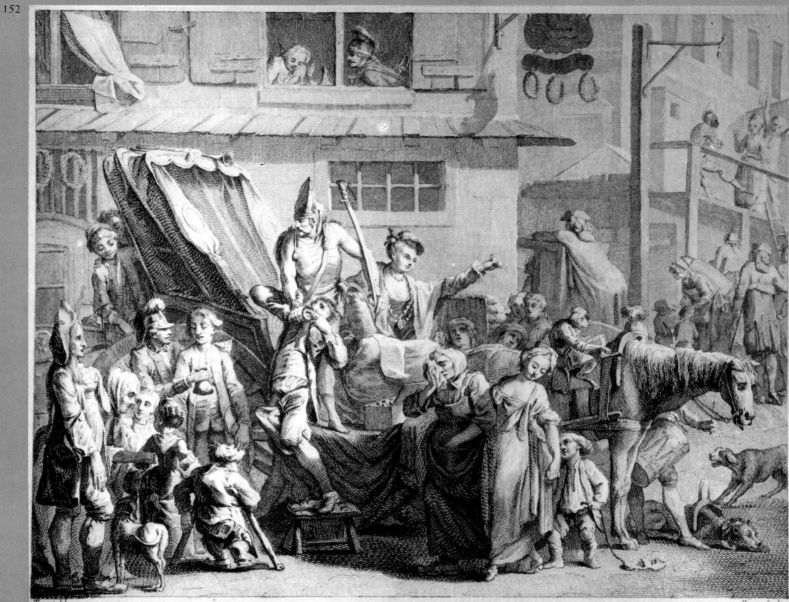

Touzet del.

Miger Sculp.

L'argent fait à chacun jouer ici son rôle,
Pendant que sur son char cet hardi Charlatan
Enleve avec son sabre, une dent à ce drôle,
Sa belle, à ses cotés, vend son orvietan
Un nouveau débarque qu'un grenadier engage
Par l'appas des ... s perdant sa liberté,

LE CHARLATAN.

à Paris,
Se vend chez Miger Graveur, Rue Montmartre
à coté de celle des Vieux Augustins.

Du metier des héros va faire apprentissage.
Avec sa Colombine Arlequin en gaieté,
Faisant sur leurs treteaux mille bouffonneries
Excitent des passants la curiosité
Pour se faire payer leurs plates Comedies

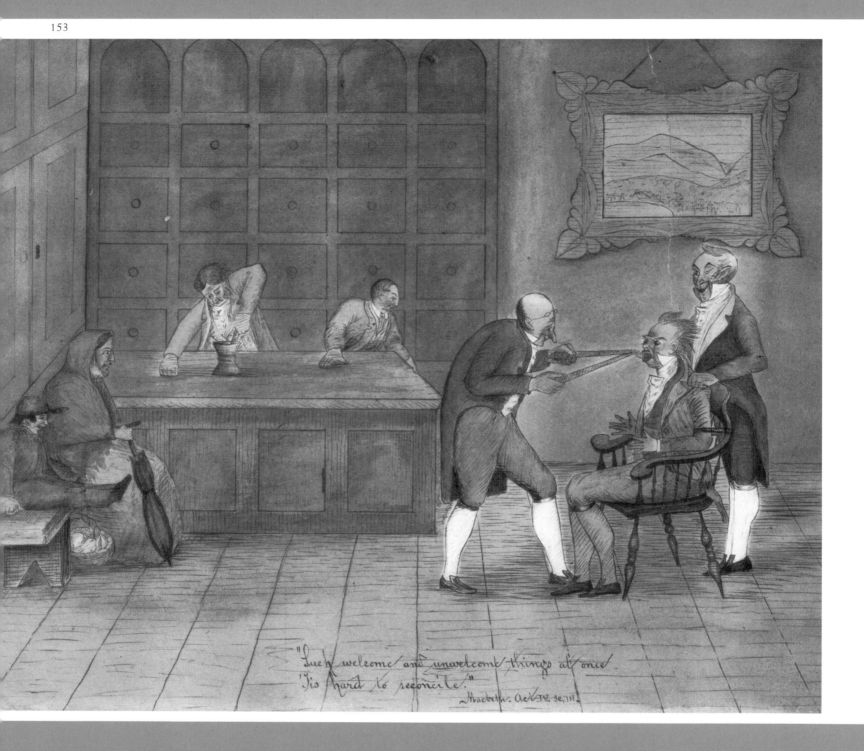

"Such welcome and unwelcome things at once
'Tis hard to reconcile."

Macbeth. Act. IV. se. III.

This pen and ink and watercolor cartoon by J. Smith depicts a dental waiting and examination room of about 1780. The caption, a quotation from *Macbeth*, must have struck a sympathetic chord in contemporary ears.

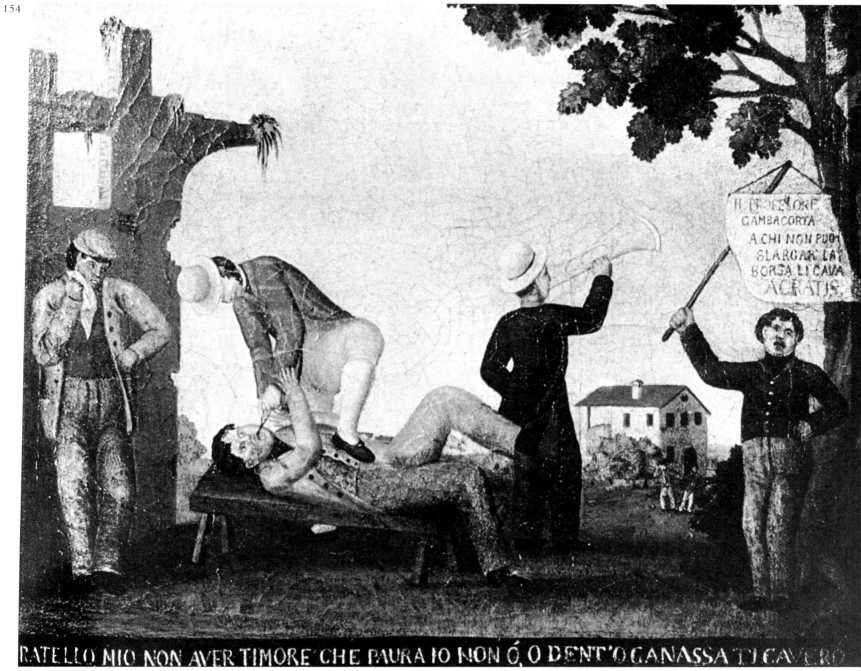

RATELLO MIO NON AVER TIMORE CHE PAURA IO NON Ó, O DENT'O GANASSA TI GAVERO

A self-styled "professor" threatens to extract all the teeth of his patients if his fee is not paid, in this Italian painting of about 1800. Ospedale S. Spirito, Rome.

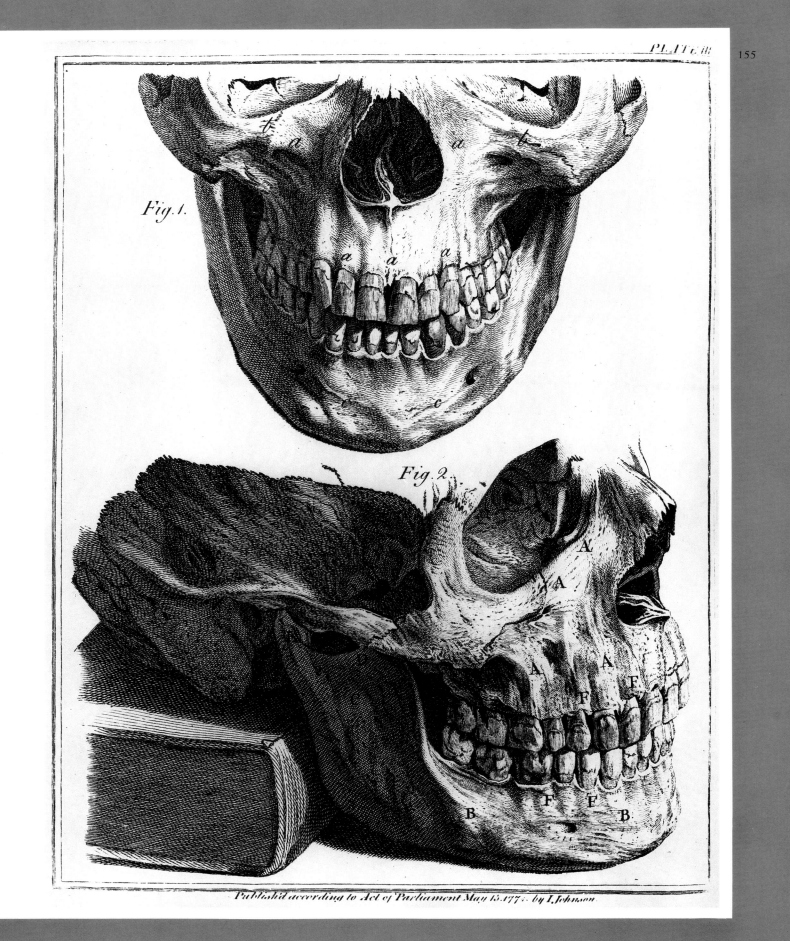

Plate 3 from John Hunter's *Natural History of the Human Teeth* shows the lower half of the human skull in front and side views. National Library of Medicine, Bethesda.

John Hunter

In the annals of English medicine there is no more illustrious name than John Hunter (1728–1793), greatest surgeon of the eighteenth century, who early in his career studied the practice of dentistry and made the teeth the subject of his first major publication (fig. 156).

Hunter, the youngest of ten children, was born near Glasgow, Scotland. His father died when he was only thirteen, and because his mother was left badly off financially, he received only the most rudimentary education. His brother William, however, ten years his senior, was able to go to London and there achieved renown as a distinguished anatomist and obstetrician and established a successful school of anatomy at which surgeons studied. At the age of twenty John went to London to work and study with his brother. In time he took work at a London hospital, dressing wounds, observing surgical practice, and eventually becoming a pupil of the renowned surgeon Percivall Pott. In 1768 he was granted the diploma of membership in the Surgeons' Company. Earlier in his professional career Hunter had become a close friend of a number of successful dentists, especially James Spence and his two sons and Martin van Butchell, the most fashionable, albeit the most flamboyantly eccentric, dentist of London at that time. He also was a friend to William Rae, a progressive dentist who, at Hunter's invitation, in 1785 delivered a series of lectures on the teeth in Hunter's house.

Hunter observed these men with their patients. Then, working with cadavers supplied to him by "resurrectionists" (people who obtained corpses surreptitiously, through grave-robbing), he made a detailed study of the mouth and jaws that culminated in the publication in 1771 of his first major work, *The Natural History of the Human Teeth: Explaining Their Structure, Use, Formation, Growth and Diseases*. This book received almost immediate acclaim, and German, Dutch, Italian, and Latin translations were issued within a few years. (An American edition, with notes by Eleazar Parmly, appeared serially in the *American Journal of Dental Science* in 1839.)

Hunter's book is remarkable for its exceptionally accurate plates (fig. 155), and most of his statements on dental anatomy hold true today. His understanding of the growth and development of the jaws and their relation to the muscles of mastication was perfect. He made several valuable contributions to scientific nomenclature, coining the terms incisors, cuspids, and bicuspids. He correctly disapproved of extracting primary teeth to permit permanent teeth to erupt, yet made the incorrect recommendation that the first permanent molar was the tooth to sacrifice should there be insufficient room in the jaw for all the teeth. He also maintained that teeth do not grow throughout a lifetime, explaining that an extruded tooth only appears to grow longer because its antagonist is missing.

In 1778 Hunter brought out his second major book, *A Practical Treatise on the Diseases of the Teeth*. This is a far less significant work than *The Natural History of the Human Teeth*, primarily because it was not based on personal experience. Many of the procedures Hunter mentions are superficially treated, no doubt because he either never performed them or never saw them performed. He recommends treating an abscessed molar by extracting it, boiling it, and immediately replacing it in its socket, for he reasoned that the tooth, being "dead," was therefore free from disease!

Nevertheless, there is much in this work that is sound. Hunter offers an excellent clinical picture of the various stages of inflammation of affected teeth and of "decay of the teeth arising from rottenness," though he incorrectly assumed that caries can proceed from within a tooth outward. His description of periodontal disease is accurate, although he linked the condition to scurvy, failing to discern it as a local condition. But Hunter's recommended treatment, not unlike a gingivectomy, is commendable.

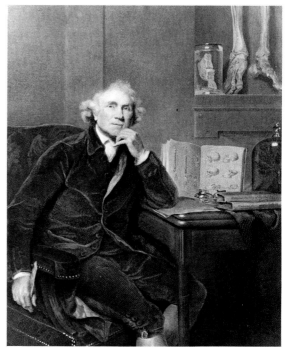

John Hunter, often called the father of modern surgery, wrote his first major book in 1771. *Natural History of the Human Teeth* was considered a milestone in the history of dental anatomy. After a painting by Sir Joshua Reynolds. National Library of Medicine, Bethesda.

Prosthetic Dentistry

Tooth Transplantation

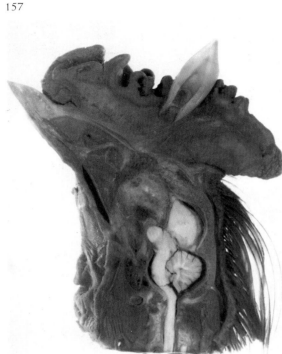

From the earliest times, artificial replacements for missing teeth were either made from animal products, such as ivory, teeth, or bone, or taken from the mouth of a dead person. The former were generally unsatisfactory because they absorbed odors and became discolored. As for human teeth, they were both scarce and expensive, and most people felt a natural repugnance to putting a corpse's tooth into their mouths. In the eighteenth century John Hunter argued the advantages of transplanting the teeth of a living human directly in the jaw of another human (which Berdmore, to his credit, resolutely opposed), and his outstanding reputation made this dubious procedure more widely accepted than it should have been. Such a strong believer was he in the novel idea that he implanted a human tooth whose root end had not yet completely developed into a living cock's comb; he saw the fowl's blood vessels grow into the pulp canal of the tooth and the tooth itself become firmly rooted in the comb (fig. 157). This led him to recommend that a "scion" human tooth (his term for the one to be implanted) be secured from a young person, and he made what to us today seems an unconscionable recommendation: that the dentist have several donors in attendance when transplanting teeth; if the first tooth did not fit the socket, one from the next person was to be tried, and so on until a proper fit was achieved! It is surprising that the father of modern surgery, whose considerable knowledge was based on scientific research and practical experience, should have supported such an objectionable procedure.

Transplantation died out in time (although it did persist well into the nineteenth century), after repeated failures had been publicized; after the risk of transmitting disease, especially syphilis, had been recognized; after the satirists of the day, especially Rowlandson, had heaped ridicule upon the practice (fig. 146); and, most important, after "mineral," or porcelain, teeth had been introduced.

"Mineral" Teeth

A Parisian apothecary, Alexis Duchâteau (1714–1792), found that his own ivory dentures became stained and malodorous after he tasted the concoctions he prepared. Seeking a solution, he attempted to make a denture from porcelain at the Guerhard porcelain factory. Since he was not a dentist and was unfamiliar with taking impressions, his efforts failed. Only after he teamed up with a Parisian dentist, Nicolas Dubois de Chémant, were his efforts eventually successful.

Satisfied with his new dentures, Duchâteau abandoned his interest in porcelain teeth and went back to his apothecary shop. Dubois de Chémant, however, worked diligently at perfecting the invention—a very difficult achievement because the one-piece dentures had to resist distortion during firing. In the course of his experiments, Dubois de Chémant twice modified the composition of the original mineral paste in order to improve its color and dimensional stability, and to improve the attachment of the porcelain teeth to the porcelain base. In time the results were to his satisfaction and in 1788 he published his findings in pamphlet form (his definitive *A Dissertation on Artificial Teeth* was eventually published in 1797). In 1789 Dubois de Chémant presented his invention to the Académie des Sciences and the faculty of medicine of Paris University, and both bodies applauded his efforts. He then received a royal patent from Louis XVI.

At this point, Duchâteau came back into the picture and, claiming that Dubois de Chémant had pirated his invention, asked that the patent be revoked, a request that was denied. Nevertheless, many of Dubois de Chémant's colleagues, probably acting out of jealousy, sided with Duchâteau and accused Dubois de Chémant in court of stealing his ideas. The law, however, upheld Dubois de Chémant and recognized his patent as valid.

Illustrated here is a cross section of the head of the rooster into whose comb John Hunter implanted an incompletely formed human tooth. The tooth became firmly rooted and the blood vessels of the comb grew into the tooth. This experiment convinced Hunter of the practicability of transplanting human teeth. Hunterian Museum, Royal College of Surgeons of England, London.

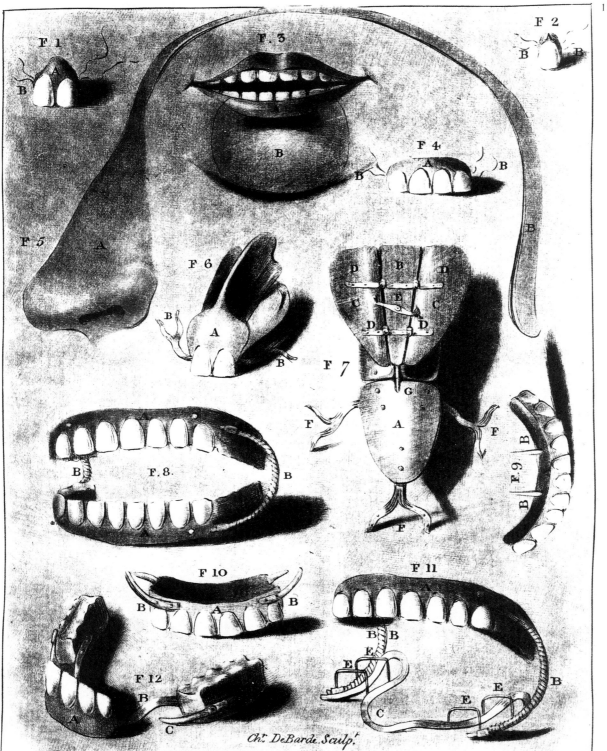

Ch.ᵉ DeBarde. Sculp.ᵗ

Dubois de Chémant left for England in 1792 to escape the French Revolution, and there he applied for and received a fourteen-year English patent for the exclusive manufacture of what he termed "mineral paste dentures." He also called them "incorruptible teeth," a term that gained wide currency. In fact, the term "incorruptibles" was for many years synonymous with porcelain teeth.

Dubois de Chémant played a major role in the advancement of prosthetic dentistry. His dentures remained popular until the introduction of individually baked porcelain teeth by Giuseppangelo Fonzi in the next century.

This page from Nicolas Dubois de Chémant's *Dissertation on Artificial Teeth* (1797) shows some of the earliest porcelain teeth and a porcelain nose. National Library of Medicine, Bethesda.

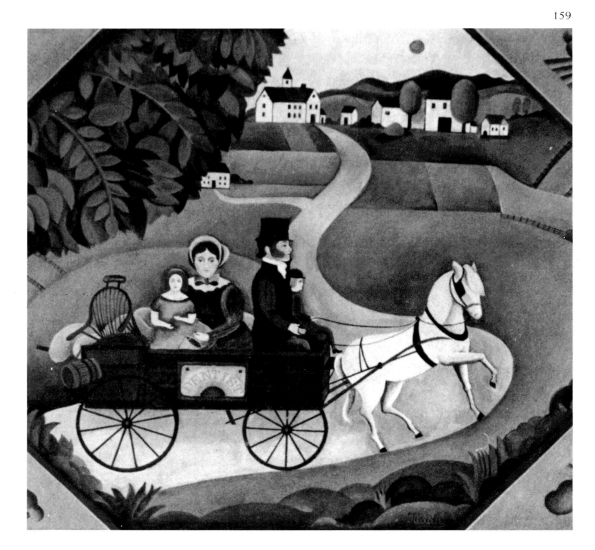

An American primitive artist named Hedda painted this itinerant dentist and his family about 1800.

XI
AMERICA:
FROM THE EARLIEST TIMES TO
THE MID-NINETEENTH CENTURY

"Torments of the Toothache Unrelieved"

In the very earliest days, life in America was difficult indeed. Housing was primitive and afforded scant protection from severe winters and stifling summers. Public-health measures were nonexistent, and disease was largely uncontrolled. Agues and fevers were common, and the swamps, bogs, and marshes that dotted the land encouraged the spread of mosquito-borne diseases, such as yellow fever. Poor sanitation favored the spread of typhus and typhoid fever, and death at a young age was the common lot. Professional medical and dental care was a luxury most colonists never enjoyed.

Because there were so few medical specialists in the colonies during the seventeenth and early eighteenth centuries, clergymen often were called upon to minister to the sick since they were among the few who could read and write and had had some advanced education. (Medical knowledge in the 1600s was so scant that literacy alone enabled a man to learn enough to practice simple medicine quite respectably.)

It was Cotton Mather (1663–1728), prominent Congregational clergyman of Boston and a man of great intellect and learning, who produced in 1724 the first medical tract recorded in this country, *The Angel of Bethesda*. Among other things, Mather wrote about diseases of the mouth, reminding his readers that Adam's and Eve's sin was occasioned by that organ, describing its afflictions as the result of an improper balance of humors. He listed numerous folk remedies for the relief of toothache and castigated the medical profession for its inability to cure this all too common complaint: "It looks like some disgrace to the physician, that so many people, even of their own dearest or nearest relatives, do so commonly, whole days, perhaps weeks, [remain] under the torments of the toothache unrelieved. It seems to say, Sire, you are physicians of how little value. You can't so much as cure the toothache."

John Wesley (1703–1791), the great English cleric and founder of Methodism, authored a tract called *Primitive Physic; or an Easy Method of Curing Most Diseases*, which was published in numerous editions between 1764 and 1795. In an edition of 1788, which was published in America, Wesley advised the colonists how best to care for themselves in the absence of adequate medical help.

Wesley was a firm believer in the value of simple, natural remedies and opposed the use of potentially dangerous drugs. His book contained information on the teeth: a description of their anatomy and their diseases (Wesley did not subscribe to the toothworm theory); basic oral hygiene; and simple rules for preventing toothache. Among his recommendations were keeping the mouth full of warm water to insulate an aching tooth from the cold air and gargling three times a day with salt and water "to kill the animalculae that cause the gums to waste away from the teeth." To relieve "palsy of the mouth" (paralysis of the facial nerve), he prescribed "purging well. [Then] chew mustard-seed often. Or gargle with juice of wood sage."

Among the first medical specialists in America were three barber-surgeons sent by the Massachusetts Bay Company to Plymouth to serve the needs of the settlers. In addition to simple medical treatment, they also provided minimal dental care—extractions. In fact, one of the three, William Dinly, perished in a snowstorm while on his way to a settler's cabin to extract an aching tooth.

Most physicians in colonial times included dental treatment in their practice. During the late eighteenth century, most of them became proficient in the use of the key for tooth extraction but rendered no other dental service except to prescribe medicines of dubious value. Extracting teeth became such a common practice among physicians that the New Jersey Medical Society in its fee schedule established in 1766 listed "Extracting a tooth—one shilling, sixpence."

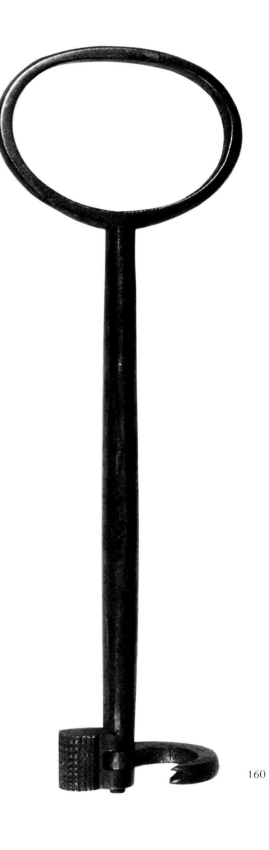

160

This early American extraction instrument known as a key was probably made by a New England blacksmith. It is the forerunner of more elaborate nineteenth-century models with ivory or bone handles. Harvard University Medical Museum, Boston.

CHARLES WALKER, M.D.
DENTIST.
ROOMS AT HIS RESIDENCE IN KING STREET,
NORTHAMPTON, MASS.

PERFECTION will be the first desideratum in all his dental operations; to make his prices reason able and to be ready with promptness to attend to the calls of those who require his advice or professional services WILL BE HIS NEXT CARE.

O H Throop, Del. & Sc.

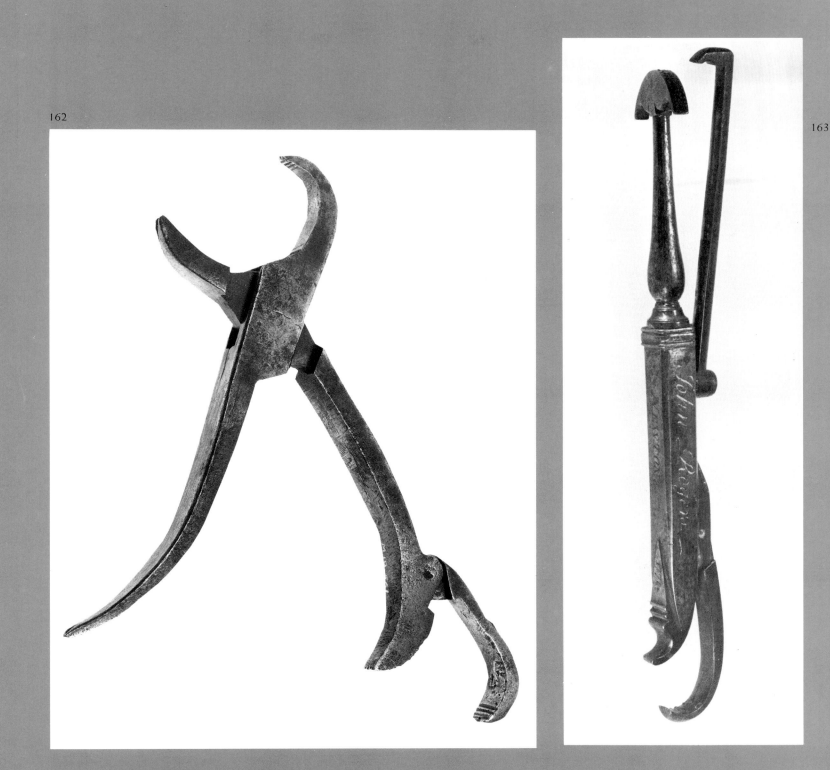

Many colonial dentists traveled considerable distances to visit patients. This instrument, dating from about 1700, combined the functions of pelican and forceps, thereby reducing the weight of the doctor's equipment case. National Museum of American History, Smithsonian Institution, Washington, D.C.

John Rogers of Newton, Massachusetts, skillfully hand-crafted and proudly signed this double-ended pelican in 1774. Harvard University Medical Museum, Boston.

161

About 1840 Charles Walker, a physician in Northampton, Massachusetts, announced his intention of practicing dentistry on this trade card now in the New-York Historical Society, New York City. Bella Landauer Collection.

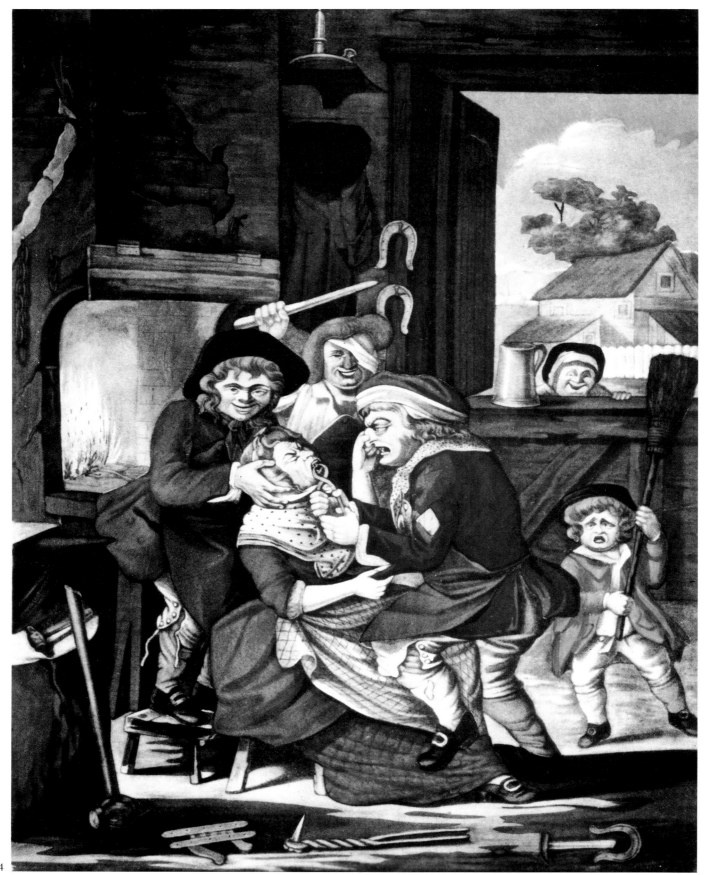

164

Because formal university training was very difficult to get, early physicians in America attended lectures to improve their skills. In 1787 a Dr. Fowlke advertised in a Baltimore newspaper that he "would conduct lectures on anatomy, surgery, dissection and midwifery...and five lectures will be given on the formation, diseases and operations of the teeth in order to enable country practitioners to become useful and expert dentists."

Most Americans relied on simples and home remedies to alleviate or cure dental ills. The recipes were passed down from generation to generation or could be found in the almanacs that circulated widely in the colonies. The title page of one of the popular home-remedy books, a typical compendium of its kind, published by Benjamin Franklin in Philadelphia in 1736, read: "Every Man his own Doctor, or, the Poor Planter's Physician. Prescribing Plain and Easy Means for Persons to cure themselves of all, or most of the Distempers, incident to this Climate, and with very little Charge, the Medicines being chiefly of the Growth and Production of this Country." Popular remedies listed in these publications were, among many others, "the juice of rue," which was to be dropped into the ear of the side of the head affected with the toothache, and tobacco ash rubbed on the teeth to prevent toothache. Toothache must have plagued our ancestors, for, as Peter Kalm, a Swedish botanist who spent the years 1747 to 1751 in the colonies on a scientific mission for his government, observed in the *Travels into North America* he later published: "The remedies against the toothache are almost as numerous as the days in a year. There is hardly an old woman but can tell you three or four score of them, of which she is perfectly certain that they are as infallible and speedy in giving relief as a month's fasting, by bread and water, is to a burdensome paunch."

When all of these home remedies failed, extraction was the only recourse. This operation was performed by either an itinerant tooth-drawer, the neighborhood doctor or barber, or, in many cases, the local blacksmith. As the country grew, however, a new class of dental practitioners became prominent in the colonies. They came chiefly from the ranks of native craftsmen and artisans who, skilled in fine work, had decided to try their hand at dentistry. A few were emigrants from England or France, where they had received varying amounts of training before embarking for the New World.

Professional Dentists Arrive in the Colonies

The first professional dentist to travel to the colonies and set up a practice was Robert Woofendale, who claimed to have been a preceptorial student of Thomas Berdmore's, the dentist to King George III whom we have already met. In 1766 Woofendale arrived in New York, and an advertisement in the *New York Mercury* for November 17, 1766, states that he "performs all operations upon the teeth, sockets, gums and palate; likewise fixes artificial teeth, so as to escape discernment." We should note in passing that the daily newspapers had become the principal vehicle for advertising the services of all health practitioners by the mid-1700s. The first advertisement placed by a dentist that we know of appeared in the *New York Weekly Journal* on January 6, 1735; James Mills, a wigmaker by trade, announced, "teeth drawn...old broken stumps taken out very safely and with much ease." Somewhat later (from 1738 to 1742) William Whitebread advertised in Philadelphia that he was an "operator for the teeth."

After only two years in New York, when it is claimed he made the first set of artificial teeth constructed in this country, Woofendale returned to England, where he was to remain for the next twenty-seven years. During this time he published *Practical Observations on the Human Teeth* (1783), the most important dental text of the time after Berdmore's. The publication gives us an excellent picture of the type of dentistry that was brought from England to America in the eighteenth century. In 1795 Woofendale returned to New York but retired after only two years, turning the practice over to his son.

164

In rural areas of England and the American colonies the local blacksmith frequently served as the local dentist. Surrounded by the tools of his trade, a country tooth-drawer treats a patient in a painting of 1784, by Robert Dighton. Kulturhistorische Sammlung des Bundesverbandes der Deutschen Zahnärzte, Cologne.

John Baker, who arrived in the colonies very shortly after Woofendale, placed his advertisements in Boston newspapers beginning in the late 1760s. He apparently hailed from county Cork, Ireland, and it is probable that he had studied some dentistry there, for he claimed he "displaced teeth and stumps after the easiest manner, be they ever so deep in the socket of the gums," and also filled teeth with gold or lead, cured "scurvy" (probably periodontal disease), and made "artificial teeth . . . fix[ing] them with pure gold so that they will remain fast for many years." He always listed himself in his advertisements as John Baker, M.D., but whether he had ever formally secured a medical degree is questionable; probably he appended the letters to his name in order to enhance his professional standing.

Baker traveled frequently; from 1767 to 1786 his notices appeared in newspapers in Boston, New York, Williamsburg, and Annapolis. He attracted a distinguished clientele—George Washington's account books carry notices of payments to Baker for professional services rendered—and he had amassed a fortune by the time he died, in 1796.

While living in Boston, Baker accepted as a student the silversmith Paul Revere, who probably decided to try his hand at dentistry when unfavorable economic conditions after the French and Indian War made the trade in luxuries sluggish. On September 5, 1768, there appeared in the *Boston Gazette* a notice that Revere offered his services to all those who had been "so unfortunate as to lose their fore-teeth." The advertisement noted that Revere had learned his trade from Mr. John Baker, "Surgeon-Dentist" (fig. 165).

Revere practiced dentistry for about seven years, and his journals, ledgers, and cash books of that period itemize the manifold dental operations he performed—fillings, cleanings, and tooth replacements—as well as the fees he secured for each. One of Revere's most singular contributions to dentistry was his postmortem identification of a two-unit bridge that he had constructed for Dr. Joseph Warren of Boston. Warren was killed at the Battle of Bunker Hill in 1775 and was buried by the British in a mass grave. A year later, when the British withdrew from Boston, the people of Massachusetts wished to give the doctor a proper burial. The grave was accordingly opened and the bodies exhumed, but they were so decomposed as to make recognition impossible. Revere, however, studied the skulls and identified Warren's body on the basis of the bridge he had made. This was the first medicolegal identification of a corpse based on dental evidence.

165

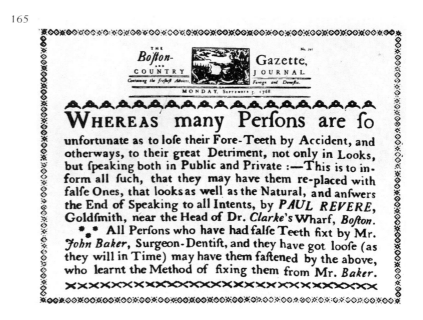

On September 5, 1768, Paul Revere advertised his services as dentist in the *Boston Gazette*.

Among Benjamin Franklin's personal papers was discovered a letter of 1789 from a young English immigrant appealing to the great man for a loan of twenty dollars to "keep an impecunious young dentist out of jail" and to help him get established in the practice of dentistry. We do not know what Franklin's response to this appeal was, but its author, who signed himself R. C. Skinner and made known that he had been a preceptorial student of the eminent London dentist called Chevalier Bartholomew Ruspini, succeeded about 1790 in establishing a practice in New York City, where he remained for about forty-five years. Skinner also maintained an itinerant practice, stopping in a number of cities for several weeks at a time in order to provide much-needed dental care to the inhabitants. Among the places where he worked of which there is recorded evidence are Albany and Batavia, New York, and Hartford, Connecticut.

Skinner has gone down in history for three reasons. In September 1792 he applied to the recently founded New York Dispensary for an appointment as staff dentist. His offer was gladly accepted, and the answer he received signals the establishment of the first in-hospital dental clinic in the United States.

166

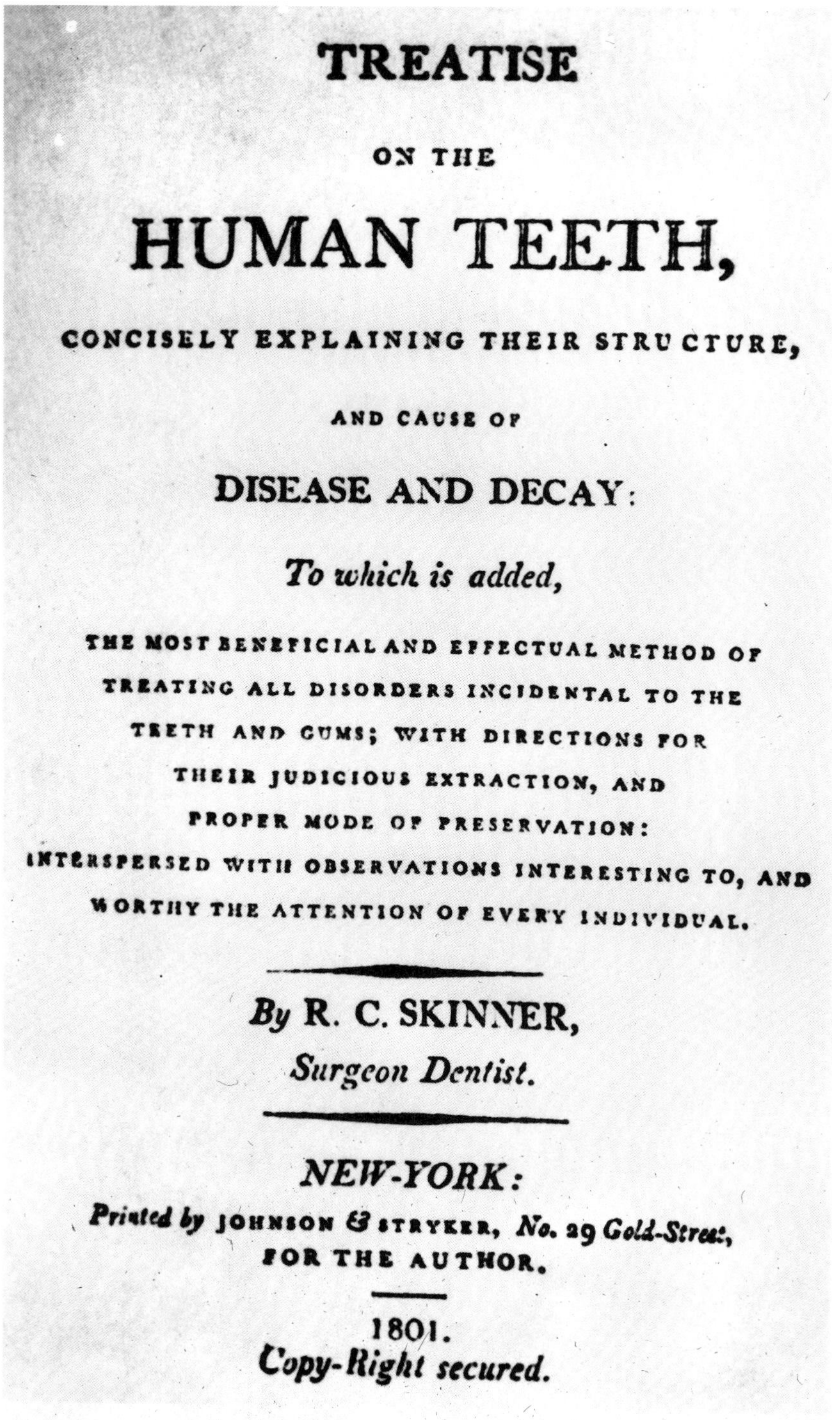

TREATISE

ON THE

HUMAN TEETH,

CONCISELY EXPLAINING THEIR STRUCTURE,

AND CAUSE OF

DISEASE AND DECAY:

To which is added,

THE MOST BENEFICIAL AND EFFECTUAL METHOD OF
TREATING ALL DISORDERS INCIDENTAL TO THE
TEETH AND GUMS; WITH DIRECTIONS FOR
THEIR JUDICIOUS EXTRACTION, AND
PROPER MODE OF PRESERVATION:
INTERSPERSED WITH OBSERVATIONS INTERESTING TO, AND
WORTHY THE ATTENTION OF EVERY INDIVIDUAL.

By R. C. SKINNER,

Surgeon Dentist.

NEW-YORK:

Printed by JOHNSON & STRYKER, No. 29 Gold-Street,
FOR THE AUTHOR.

1801.
Copy-Right secured.

R. C. Skinner's *Treatise on the Human Teeth,* of 1801, was the first book on dentistry published in America. Shown here is the title page.

Sir:

The Board of Managers of the Dispensary received yours addressed to them;—they directed me to acquaint you of the acceptance of your offers, in such cases as may be of avail to the Dispensary. It gives pleasure, Sir, to find that an institution founded upon such motives, will meet with your benevolent attention.

I am, Sir, with respect
Your obed't. Servant,
Wm. Cock, Secr'y.

Mr. Skinner
Surgeon-Dentist

Skinner also offered his professional services free of charge to the Hospital and Alms House of New York City, the first dental clinic for the indigent in America. His third important contribution was to write the first book on dentistry published in America. Entitled *A Treatise on the Human Teeth*, and published in 1801, it was a twenty-six-page pamphlet written for the general public (fig. 166). It listed sound rules of oral hygiene, explained the nature of dental diseases and the methods of dealing with them, and stressed to the patient the need for preventive maintenance of the teeth. Authorship of this booklet has earned for Skinner the title father of American dental literature.

A number of French dentists also chose to make America their home in the latter part of the eighteenth century, when France was the center of advanced dental practice. The first to arrive was Michael Poree, who, in the *Pennsylvania Gazette* for August 25, 1768, announced that he was an "operator for the teeth" in Philadelphia. After 1771 he began to move around the country, settling for a time in New York City, Baltimore, and Boston. Poree was followed by his compatriots Joseph Lebeaume, who arrived in Charleston in 1774; Frederick Raymond, who settled in Baltimore in 1792; and a man we know only by his surname, LeBreton, reputedly the first dentist in the colonies to fit his patients with complete dentures of porcelain, who arrived in Philadelphia in 1794. The two outstanding colonial dentists of French birth, however, were Jacques Gardette (1756–1831) and Jean Pierre LeMayeur (died 1806).

Gardette studied at the Royal Medical School in Paris from 1773 to 1775. He accepted a commission as a surgeon in the French navy and came to America in 1778, when France sent her ships to defend the cause of the American revolutionaries. Resigning his naval commission, Gardette first practiced in Newport, Rhode Island, but then in 1785 he moved to Philadelphia, took the oath of allegiance to the United States, and established practice in that city. After forty-five years in his adopted country, he returned to France, where he lived out his days.

Gardette was the author of the first scientific article on dentistry to appear in an American periodical. His "Remarks on the Diseases of the Teeth" was printed in *The American Museum; or, Universal Magazine* in May, 1790. Making a strong plea for properly trained practitioners, Gardette asked, "There are cases in which the dentist is absolutely necessary—when the teeth begin to make their appearance, or to shed—when they are carious or decayed—when they become troublesome by irregularity or looseness—when they are hollow, etc. Given these different cases, who but a skillful dentist—a master of the art—will be able to give the necessary and suitable assistance?"

LeMayeur practiced in London before embarking for New York. There he arrived in 1781, while the town was still occupied by the British, carrying a letter of introduction to Sir Henry Clinton, commander in chief of British forces. He was well received and was soon launched in a profitable practice. An anti-French statement made in his presence sent him off in a huff, however, and his departure from New York came to the attention of General Washington, who invited LeMayeur to come to his headquarters in Newburgh, New York, where he put himself in LeMayeur's professional care. LeMayeur continued to treat Washington until 1787. During those years, the Frenchman practiced in Philadelphia, Richmond, and New York. In 1789 he became a naturalized citizen and settled in Virginia, where he lived until his death in 1806.

Isaac Greenwood, a skilled ivory-turner in Boston who also made dentures of ivory, gradually began to practice dentistry as a sideline, and four of his sons became prominent dentists in their own right: Isaac Greenwood, Jr., Clark, William Pitt (who lived to see the formation of the American Society of Dental Surgeons), and John, most prominent of all. In an advertisement of 1789, Isaac Greenwood advised the public that "Delays are dangerous: attend to your teeth and preserve your health and beauty, and them from decay." He also listed the commodities he dealt in—toothbrushes and tooth powders, umbrellas, oil-silk bathing caps, musical instruments, walking sticks, whips, picture frames, chessmen, dice, and billiard balls! His last notice of practice appeared in 1796.

John Greenwood (1760–1819) first announced himself as a dentist ten years earlier, in 1786. He had settled in New York City, where he eventually became well enough known to attract George Washington's attention. Though he had little formal education, Greenwood (fig. 167) was a capable practitioner and ahead of his time. He was a strong believer in regularly cleaning the teeth and, although he wrongly concluded that the tartar deposited on the teeth came from the breath, he was nevertheless correct in advocating its regular removal. His reasoning was perceptive: he felt that the tartar accumulation would sever both blood vessels and supporting periodontal fibers, and the teeth, deprived of their blood supply and support, would become loose and fall out. He understood the importance of caring for children's teeth from an early age, offering parents the very forward-looking option of reduced fees in exchange for commitment to a full year of care.

On two counts Greenwood took issue with John Hunter: he opposed transplanting teeth, calling it a "miserable operation," and he did not agree that carious destruction sometimes originates within the tooth. Greenwood's practice was large and his reputation considerable. He was apparently the last and most trusted of George Washington's dentists.

167

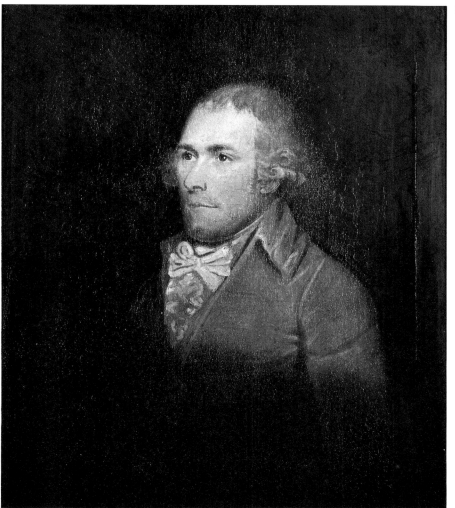

Will Lovett (1733–1801) painted this portrait of John Greenwood, who was George Washington's favorite dentist, now in the New-York Historical Society, New York City.

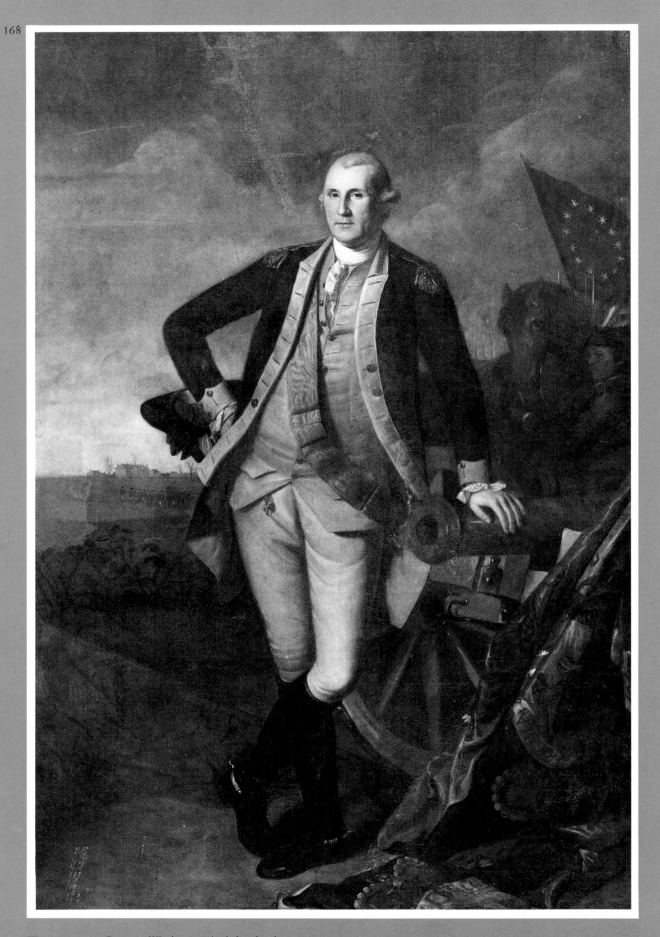

The scar on George Washington's left cheek, which can clearly be seen in this portrait of the general at Princeton, painted by Charles Willson Peale in 1779, was probably caused by a tooth abcess that had created a fistula. Pennsylvania Academy of the Fine Arts, Philadelphia.

George Washington: A Case History

Readers will by now have noticed that George Washington was at one time or another treated by most of the prominent dentists practicing in colonial and Federal America, among them Benjamin Fendall (who, records show, also made a partial denture for Martha Washington), John Baker, a Mr. Spencer, Jean Pierre LeMayeur, Jacques Gardette, Andrew Spence, Edward Whitlock, and John Greenwood. On one occasion Washington was even obliged to have his physician, James Craik, extract an aching tooth. All his adult life, the father of his country was plagued by toothache. At forty-seven, when he sat for his portrait to Charles Willson Peale, his face had a noticeable scar on the cheek as a result of a fistula, which had probably developed from an abscessed tooth (fig. 168). (Incidentally, Peale, who flirted with many vocations, at one time tried his hand at making porcelain dentures.) Washington's diaries contain numerous references to bouts of toothache, and the general's well-known hair-trigger temper may have been the result of a constant battle with pain. As he aged, Washington lost one tooth after another until, in 1790, at the time of his inauguration as president, he had only one tooth left, a lower left bicuspid.

His correspondence and that of his wife are a litany of continuing dental problems, and some contain singular requests. While commanding the Continental army at Newburgh in 1783, Washington wrote to John Baker, "I shall be obliged to you for some of the plaster of paris, or that white powder with which you take [in wax] the model of the mouth for your false teeth—and directions how to mix and make use of it—When you have done this, I can then give you back a model as will enable you to furnish me with what I want."

In 1799 Martha wrote rather urgently from Philadelphia to her dentist, saying she would be "much obliged to Mr. [Edward] Whitlock to make for her a set of teeth, something bigger and thicker in the front. . . . She will be very glad if he will do them soon, as those she has is almost broke."

John Greenwood made four sets of dentures for George Washington, fabricating them from a variety of materials such as gold, hippopotamus tusk, elephant ivory, and human teeth (fig. 184). (Contrary to the popular myth, Washington never had wooden teeth.) One of the sets was too short, and when Gilbert Stuart came to paint the president's portrait, he found Washington's face so sunken that he was obliged to pad his lips and cheeks with absorbent cotton, hoping to give it a more normal appearance. Unfortunately, Washington's countenance assumed a benign, grandmotherly appearance, in marked contrast to his portraits as a young and vigorous man with his own teeth.

In 1798 Washington must have complained to Greenwood that the dentures he had made for him were discolored. Returning the teeth, Greenwood advised him that the stains were "occasioned either by your soaking them in port-wine, or drinking it. Port, being sour, takes off all the polish . . . I advise you to either take them out after drinks and put them in clear water and put in another set, or to clean them with a brush and some chalk finely scraped."

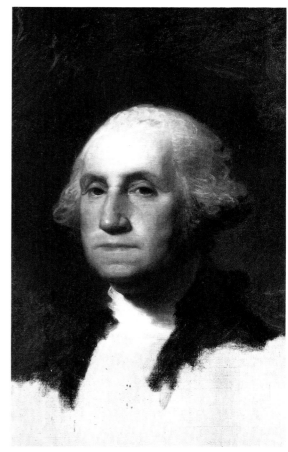

For this portrait of George Washington, painted in 1796 after he had lost all but one of his teeth, Gilbert Stuart padded out the president's lips with absorbent cotton to restore the natural lines of the mouth. Detail of a painting jointly owned by the Museum of Fine Arts, Boston, and the National Portrait Gallery, Smithsonian Institution, Washington, D.C.

A Notable Dentist of the Early Republic: Josiah Flagg

One of the few qualified dentists of the late 1700s who did not treat George Washington was Josiah Flagg, a highly progressive practitioner who may have been trained by Paul Revere, since his father was Revere's partner. His first advertisements—handbills announcing that he was available to treat dental ills in the small towns surrounding Boston—appeared in 1783; between 1785 and 1792 he was settled in Boston itself, where he returned in 1795 after practicing in Charleston, South Carolina, beginning in 1792. To judge from his advertisements, he was in advance of his times, practicing oral surgery on "hare lips," in

JOSIAH FLAGG,
Surgeon Dentift.

Informs the public, that he practifes in all the branches, with improvements. [*i. e.*] Traif-plants both live and dead Teeth with greater conveniency, and gives lefs pain than heretofore practifed in Europe or America ;---Sews up Hare Lips ;---Cures Ulcers ;---Extracts Teeth and ftumps, or roots with eafe ;---Reinftates Teeth and Gums, that are much depreciated by nature, careleffnefs, acids, or corroding medicine ;---Faftens thofe Teeth that are loofe ; (unlefs waft-ed at the roots) regulates Teeth from their firft cutting to prevent feavers and pain in Chil-dren ;---Affifts nature in the extenfion of the jaws, for the beautiful arrangement of the fecond Sett, and preferves them in their natural whitenefs entirely free from all fcorbutic complaints---and when thus put in order, and his directions followed, (which are fimple) he engages that the further care of a *Dentift* will be wholly unneceffary ;---Eafes pain in Teeth without draw-ing ;---Stops bleeding in the gums, jaws or arteries ;---Lines and plumbs Teeth with virgin GOLD, FOIL, or LEAD ;---Fixes *Gold Roofs and Palates,* and artificial Teeth of any quality, without injury to and independent of the natural ones, greatly affifting the pronunciation and the fwallow, when injured by natural, or other defects.---A room for the practice with every accomodation at his houfe, where may be had Dentifices Tinctures, Teeth and Gum Brufhes, Maftics, &c. warranted approved and adapted to the various ages and circumftan-ces :---Alfo Chew-fticks, particularly ufeful in cleanfing the fore Teeth and preferving a natural and beautiful whitenefs ; which Medicine and Chew-fticks are to be fold wholefale and re-tail, that they may be more extenfively ufefull.

** DR. *FLAGG,* has a method to furnifh thofe Ladies and Gentlemen, or Children with artificial Teeth, Gold Gums, Roofs, or Palates, that are at a diftance and cannot attend him perfonally.

☞ *C A S H* Given

for Handfome and Healthy Live TEETH,

At No. 47, Newbury-Street, BOSTON, (1796.)

Josiah Flagg was America's first native-born, full-time dentist. He offered a full range of dental ser-vices, from prosthetics to orthodontics. As this handbill of 1796 indicates, Flagg, like many of his colleagues, bought live teeth, either for transplan-tation or for use in dentures. Massachusetts His-torical Society, Boston.

addition to performing extractions. Orthodontics was among his skills, for he assisted "nature in the extension of the jaws for the beautiful arrangement of the second set of teeth." All part of Flagg's repertoire were endodontics ("Sensation of the nerves of the teeth in the head can be extracted by a simple, safe, easy process"), prosthetics ("Fixes gold roofs and palates"), and operative dentistry ("Lines and plumbs teeth with virgin gold, foil or lead").

Flagg volunteered for naval service in the War of 1812, but was captured by the British and sent to England, where he was released on parole for the duration of the war. While in England he practiced dentistry and continued his studies in the field. During that time we hear that he attended a lecture by the renowned surgeon Sir Astley Cooper. Cooper was having difficulty extracting a bicuspid root from a patient's mouth and asked Flagg if he would like to try his hand at it. Flagg, borrowing a jeweler's tool much like an elevator, inserted the instrument in the patient's mouth and in a moment the root flew across the room!

In 1816, on his return trip to America, Flagg was shipwrecked off New York. His health was undermined by the experience, so he returned to Charleston to take advantage of the warm climate. However, before the year was out he was dead at the age of fifty-three, a victim of yellow fever.

One of Josiah Flagg's contributions to the progress of dentistry was his construction, about 1790, of the first dental chair (fig. 171). He took an ordinary Windsor chair and, by adding an adjustable headrest and an extended armrest for holding instruments, converted it into a very practical piece of equipment.

171

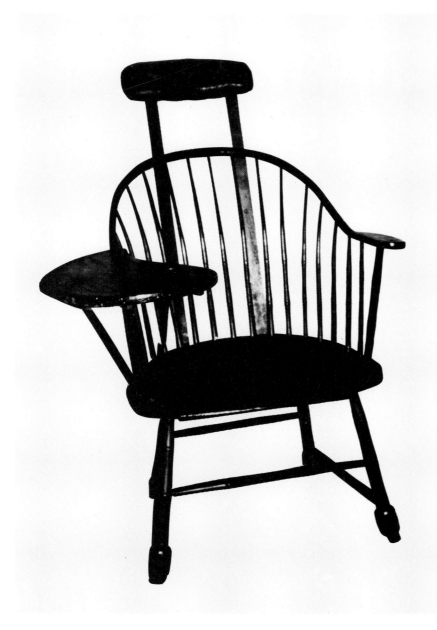

Josiah Flagg was the inventor of the first dental chair. With an adjustable headrest and an extension on the arm to hold instruments, it made a considerable advance in comfort and convenience over earlier arrangements (see, for example, figures 144, 145).

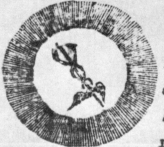 **D**IRECTIONS by **D**R. *J.*
FLAGG, to ufe his **D**ENTIFICES,
or **T**INCTURES, *(viz.)* Ufe *Cold
Water*, and a Brufh, every day after
rubbing the Gums hard with your
finger to make them bleed what you can rinfe them
clean with *Cold Water*, holding the water in your mouth
untill the keennefs of the air is off before you apply it to
your teeth : After which ufe with the Brufh the warranted and approved Antifcorbutic *Tincture*
But not rinfe it off for fome time :————It may be ufed
every day for the firft week or ten days, and once or twice
a week afterwards at difcretion :————When once in
good order, there is no further need of a **D**ENTIST or
Medicine. —*N.B.* Fear not the ftiffnefs
of the brufh;— And if your Tincture
is too potent for the Gums, add to it
Port Wine to your likeing; But
not mix the whole in the vial. —

Josiah Flagg

To Mr J. Green.

May, 1800

America Takes the Lead: 1800–1840

Although France had been the cradle of modern dentistry, during the nineteenth century leadership in the field passed to the United States for a variety of reasons. First, the turmoil wrought by the Revolution temporarily suspended advancement of the sciences in France, while the spirit of inquiry took hold in the fledgling United States upon the establishment of a popular democracy there. Second, the opportunity for personal advancement and monetary gain in the new nation lured to American shores some of the most able dental practitioners of the Old World. Consequently, dental literature increased greatly in volume and importance; between 1800 and 1840, forty-four treatises were published in the United States. Third, an expanding population that demanded goods to make life easier fostered the development of a generation of tinkerers and inventors, a number of whom turned their energies and talents to making dental procedures easier and more effective. Fourth, the growth of free public-school education resulted in time in a nation whose inhabitants read many newspapers and books and acquainted themselves with the advantages offered by dentistry rendered by reasonably well-trained specialists. By 1826 Leonard Koecker, a dentist who had practiced in Baltimore, Philadelphia, and London, felt himself able to assert in his important text, *Principles of Dental Surgery*, "In no part of the world has [the dental] art attained a more elevated station."

172

Josiah Flagg made available to his clients tinctures "sold wholesale and retail" that they might be "more extensively useful." Illustrated here is a prescription for such a preparation, which can be watered down should it prove "too potent for the gums."

This tooth-powder packet and accompanying booklet stressing the need for home dental care were distributed by a Parisian dentist in 1819. Medicinsk-Historisk Museum, University of Copenhagen.

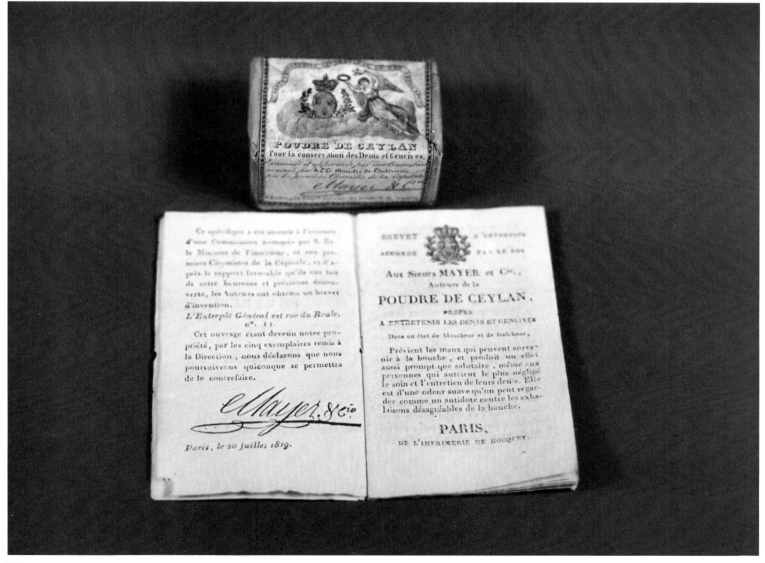

173

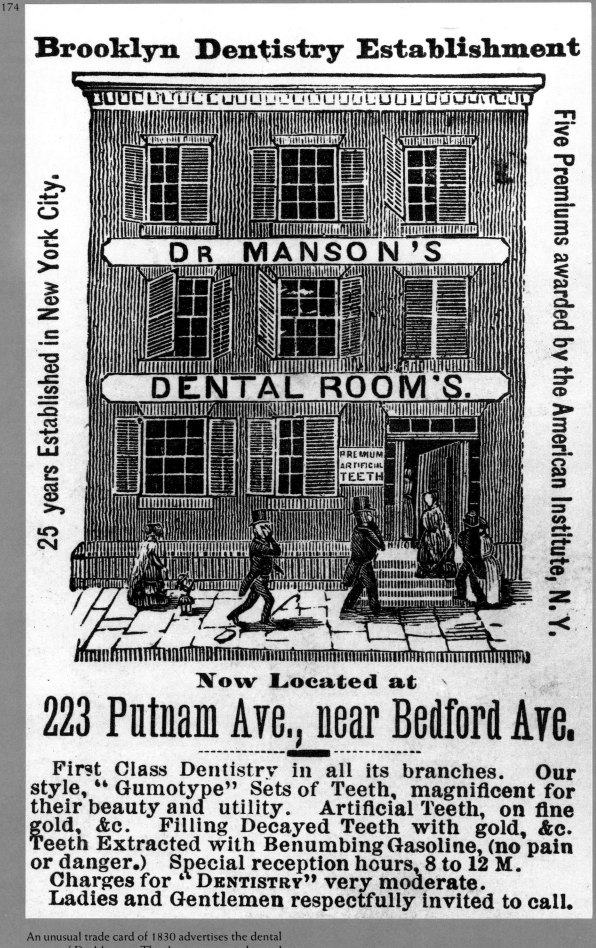

Brooklyn Dentistry Establishment

DR MANSON'S

DENTAL ROOM'S.

PREMIUM ARTIFICIAL TEETH

25 years Established in New York City.

Five Premiums awarded by the American Institute, N. Y.

Now Located at

223 Putnam Ave., near Bedford Ave.

First Class Dentistry in all its branches. Our style, "Gumotype" Sets of Teeth, magnificent for their beauty and utility. Artificial Teeth, on fine gold, &c. Filling Decayed Teeth with gold, &c. Teeth Extracted with Benumbing Gasoline, (no pain or danger.) Special reception hours, 8 to 12 M.

Charges for "DENTISTRY" very moderate.

Ladies and Gentlemen respectfully invited to call.

An unusual trade card of 1830 advertises the dental rooms of Dr. Manson. The doctor apparently used something akin to gasoline as a painkiller, for general anesthetics did not come into use until the second half of the nineteenth century. New-York Historical Society, New York City. Bella Landauer Collection.

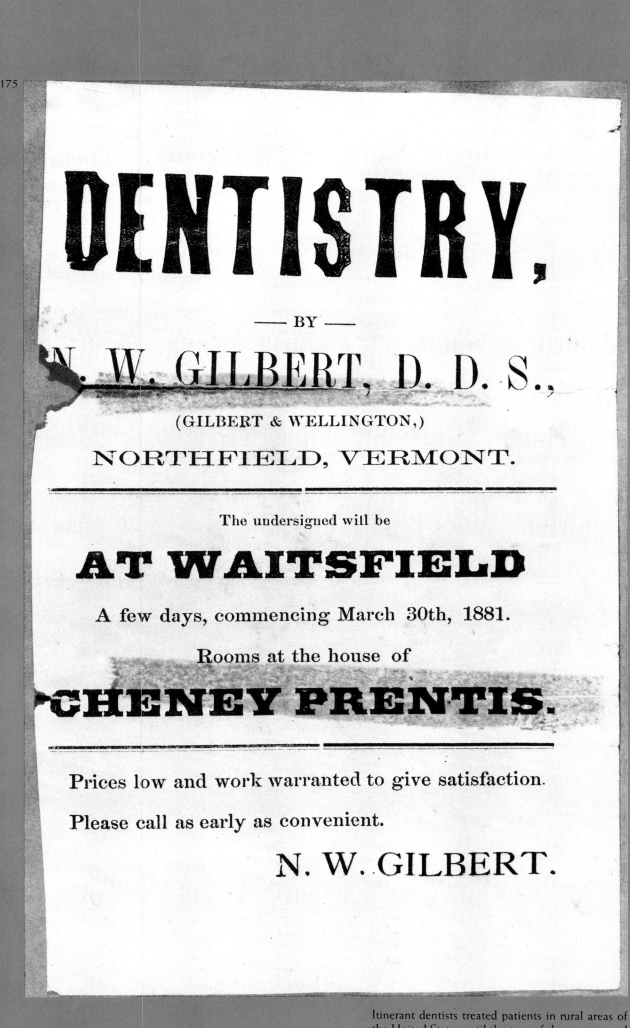

Itinerant dentists treated patients in rural areas of the United States until the turn of the century and even later. This poster announcing the arrival of Dr. N. W. Gilbert was hung up in Northfield, Vermont, in the spring of 1881. New-York Historical Society, New York City. Bella Landauer Collection.

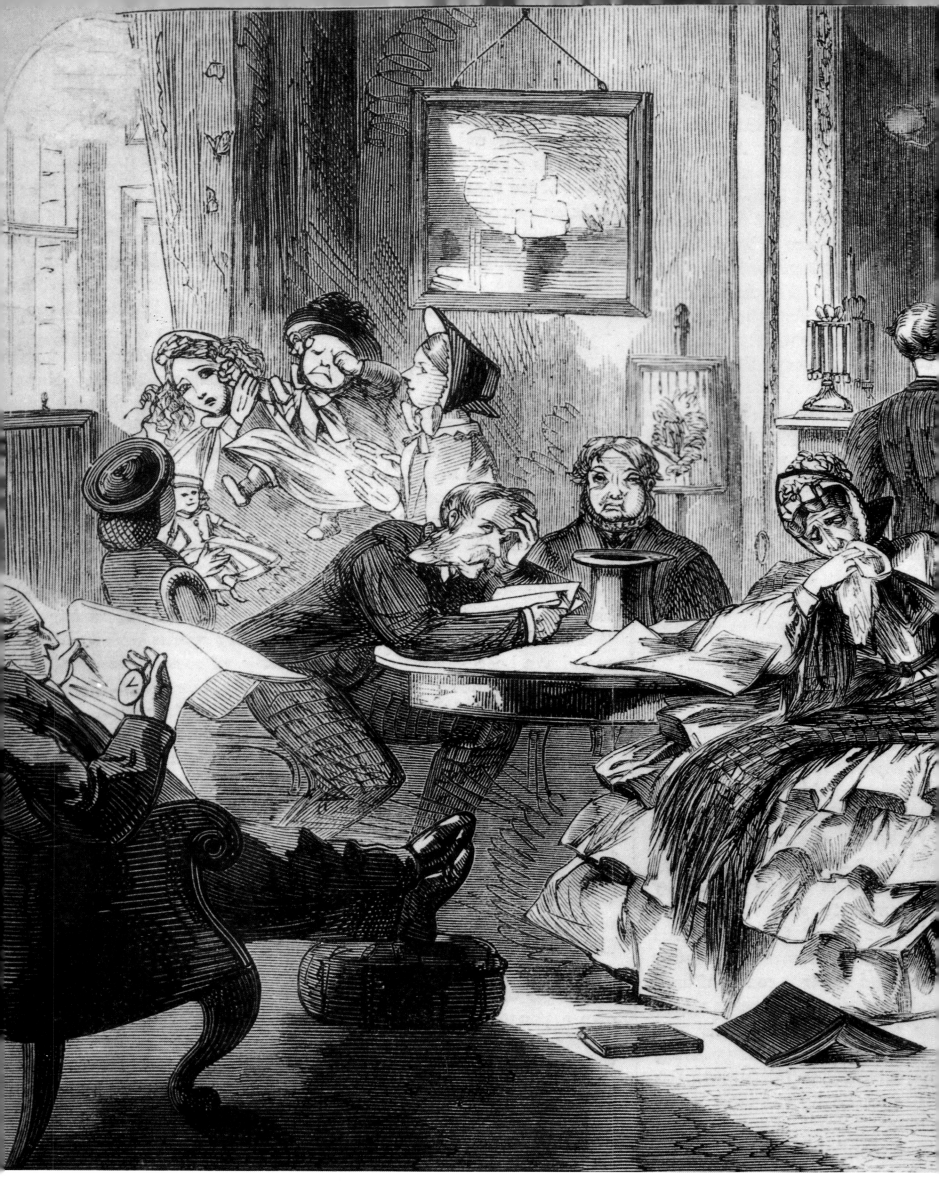

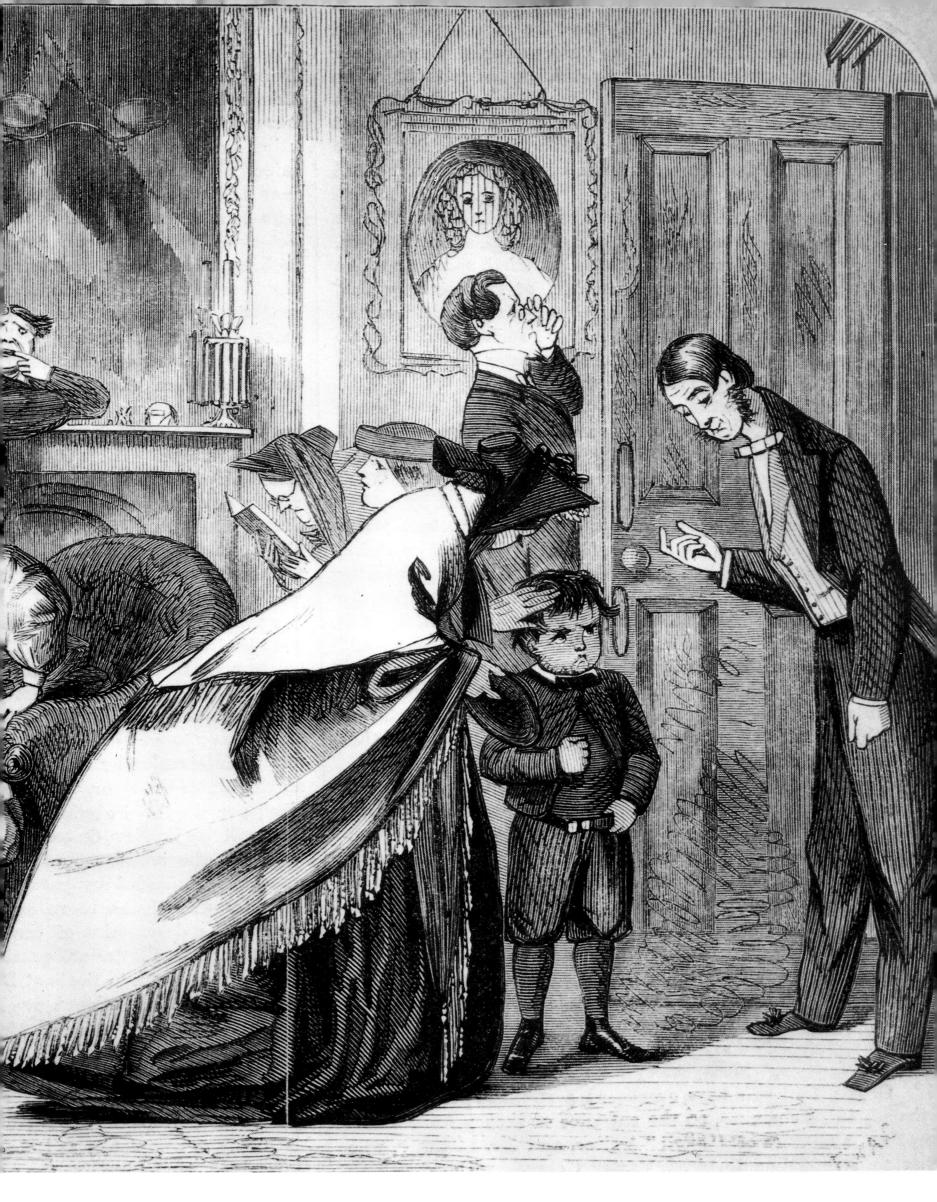

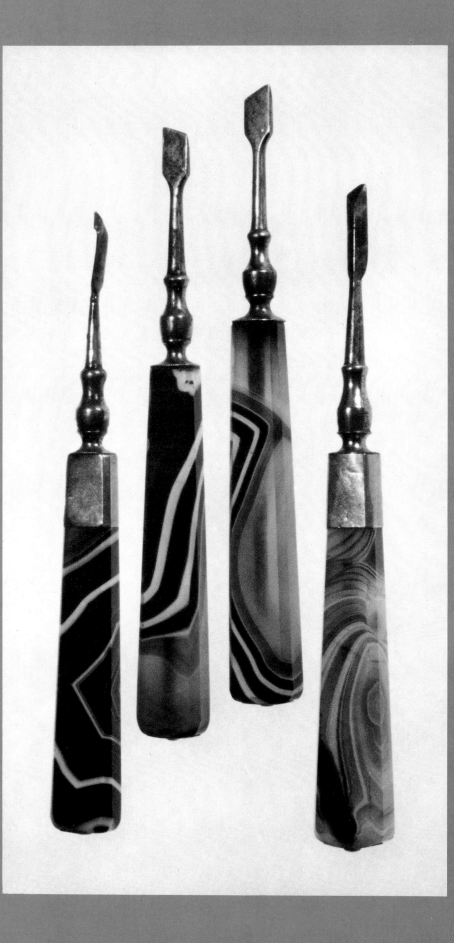

176 (pages 200–201)

About the time this cartoon was published, David Bates (1810–1876), a Philadelphian known as "Old Mortality," wrote the following lines:

Is Dr. Jones, the dentist in?
An aching tooth has made me fret;
But something seems to lull the pain—
Perhaps, sir, you can save it yet. . . .

The tooth is out; once more again
The throbbing, jumping nerves are stilled;
Reader, would you avoid this pain?
Then have your crumbling teeth well filled.

Though the print was not intended to illustrate Bates's stanzas, nevertheless the aesthetic intentions of the poet and the artist perfectly coincide.

Most dental instruments of the mid-nineteenth century had bone or ivory handles. These handsome chisels and excavators of about 1860 have handles of onyx. Harvard University Medical Museum, Boston.

At the beginning of the century, dental care was provided by four different groups of practitioners, and it varied greatly in quality. At the most elementary level, one doctored oneself—for in those early self-reliant days, home physicking was widely practiced. Popular home-remedy books and almanacs offered volumes of advice, but the results must often have failed to measure up to what was promised. Who today would have the courage to take up an extraction key and set to work on an aching tooth upon reading in his copy of a periodical like *The Family Physician and Guide to Health* (published in upstate New York in 1833), "Any person attending to the following directions will be as well qualified to extract teeth as the best surgeon in the Union." What are these directions? Merely that "the teeth may be turned [with a key] either out or in, but it will be found most convenient to turn the double teeth in and the single, or forward, teeth out."

Most people still turned to their local physician, whose skills included simple extractions, lancing, and bloodletting. Every physician had in his armamentarium at least one extraction key and one forceps, and these he probably learned to use by trial and error (figs. 160, 162).

There were specialists also—those who practiced dentistry as their principal occupation. Some had served an apprenticeship with an established dentist and then set up practice on their own. Others were physicians who had earned their degrees after studying with an established physician or by meeting the requirements of an accredited medical school. Until about 1850 almost all prominent dentists were medical doctors who had chosen dentistry rather than general medical practice as their vocation.

And of course there were still to be found the itinerants who extracted teeth, sold tooth powders and other nostrums, and occasionally filled carious teeth with questionable materials and questionable results. These itinerants had little if any professional training, having drifted into the trade for want of anything better and because the constant demand for dental treatment assured them of a steady income. The local blacksmith, barber, or apothecary might also occasionally practice a little dentistry. None of these individuals had any influence upon the development of the profession.

By 1830 most large cities in the United States, including New York, Boston, Hartford, Albany, Philadelphia, Baltimore, Richmond, and Charleston, had resident dentists. Smaller communities depended for responsible dental care on the qualified dentists who traveled from town to town. They would come into a village and secure lodgings in an inn, boardinghouse, or hotel; distribute handbills or put an advertisement in the local newspaper; and then, working with instruments they carried in a case, but with no dental chair or equipment that was not portable, extract or fill teeth, construct dentures, and render other necessary services. Many of these professionals were dentists of the highest caliber, and their work was as good as might be found anywhere at that time, though their resources were meager. They traveled partly to increase their incomes, but also certainly out of a genuine desire to help people.

In the main these early dentists were, in the words of J. Ben Robinson, "capable, well-trained, public-spirited dental surgeons who worked diligently to prepare themselves to meet fully the requirements of a competent dental practice, and who made a conscientious and determined effort to promote the science and art of dentistry and to elevate it in public esteem." Their struggle was uphill, for there were no regulations limiting dental practice to trained individuals. Anyone could buy a key or forceps and hang out a shingle, even though he lacked the most elementary knowledge of anatomy or therapeutics. Nevertheless, skilled, properly trained dentists, the leaders of the profession, exerted a great deal of effort to inform the public that there was a huge difference between the quacks who preyed on them and trained operators. B. T. Longbothom, author of the second book on dentistry published in America (*A Treatise on Dentistry*, of 1802), gave an excellent description in his preface of the latter, incidentally showing that the profession had gone far beyond mere tooth drawing and tooth scraping:

The word Dentist has been so infamously abused by ignorant pretenders, and is in general so indifferently understood, that I cannot forbear giving what I conceive to be its original meaning: viz., the profession of one who undertakes and is capable not only of cleaning, extracting, replacing by transplantation and making artificial teeth, but can also from his knowledge of dentistry, preserve those that remain in good condition, prevent in a very great degree, those that are loose, or in a decayed state, from being further injured, and can guard against the several diseases, to which the teeth, gums, and mouth are liable; a knowledge none but those regularly instructed, and who have had a long, and extensive practice, can possibly attain; but which is absolutely necessary, to complete the character of a Surgeon Dentist.

More than thirty years later, untrained practitioners were as prevalent as ever, and one of the leading dentists of the time, Shearjashub Spooner, in his *Guide to Sound Teeth; or, A Popular Treatise on the Teeth* (1836), warned the public:

One thing is certain, this profession must either rise or sink. If means are not taken to suppress and discountenance the malpractices of the multitude of incompetent persons, who are pressing into it, merely for the sake of its emoluments, it must sink;—for the few competent and well-educated men, who are now upholding it, will abandon a disreputable profession, in a country of enterprise like ours, and turn their attention to some other calling more congenial to the feelings of honorable and enlightened men.

Advances in Prosthetic Dentistry

Nicolas Dubois de Chémant's revolutionary all-porcelain dentures were a great improvement over earlier dentures made of organic materials, which had a tendency to deteriorate and disintegrate in the mouth and to absorb stains and odors. But Dubois de Chémant's dentures, baked of one piece of porcelain, were susceptible to shrinkage and distortion. During the first years of the nineteenth century, an invention by Giuseppangelo Fonzi (1768–1840) made modern prostheses possible.

In 1808 Fonzi presented his "terro-metallic incorruptibles"—as he named them—to a scientific commission of representatives of the Athenaeum of Arts and the Academy of Medicine of Paris, and these bodies gave the invention their unqualified endorsement. Fonzi created molds in which he constructed individual porcelain teeth (fig. 183). Before firing, a pin of platinum was embedded in the back of each tooth, and this pin was later soldered to a gold or silver denture base. Subsequently, other technicians improved Fonzi's artificial teeth, making their color more lifelike by baking them of different earths and perfecting their shape by carving the molds more skillfully. In England Claudius Ash, a goldsmith who began producing fine porcelain teeth in 1837, a few years later introduced the "tube tooth," which could be inserted over a post in a denture; it became widely accepted for use in bridges as well as in full dentures. Somewhat later, in 1851, John Allen of Cincinnati patented "continuous-gum teeth," a prosthesis consisting of two or three porcelain teeth fused to a small block of porcelain colored like the gingivae. These blocks could be attached to a denture base as needed. But the method by which porcelain teeth were made was laborious and their production was very limited. Natural human teeth continued to serve as replacements in dentures for some years.

Individual porcelain teeth were introduced in America in 1817 by a French immigrant dentist, Antoine Plantou, who offered, for a fee, to teach dentists in the New World his method of producing them. We have a letter of August 11, 1827, from him to Nathan Keep, Boston's most prominent dentist, in which Plantou

178

The S. S. White Company, founded in Philadelphia in the 1840s, eventually became the largest dental manufacturing company in the world. S. S. White supply houses, such as this one in New York City, were established in the nineteenth century in most major American cities and also abroad. The Francis A. Countway Library of Medicine, Harvard Medical Library/Boston Medical Library, Rare Book Collection, Boston.

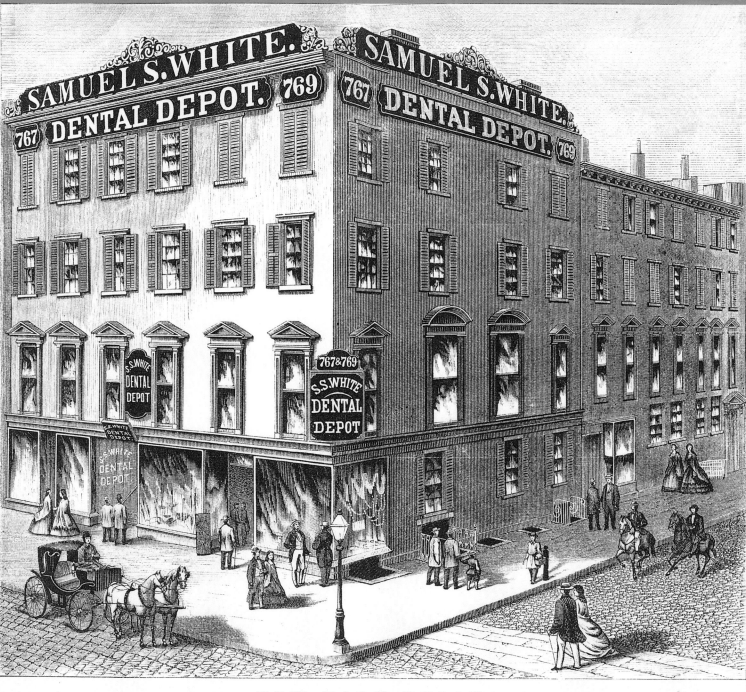

NEW YORK DEPOT.

advised that six hundred dollars would suffice to purchase "not only the receipt but also material already prepared to make teeth."

A number of Americans tried their hands at improving and producing mineral teeth, but Samuel W. Stockton, a Philadelphia jeweler, was the first to produce porcelain teeth in quantity, at a small factory. He had taken as an assistant his nephew, Samuel S. White, who learned from his uncle both the process of making teeth and the other arts of dentistry. In 1843 White left his uncle's employ and founded his own business, which eventually became the leading dental manufacturing company in the world. In 1846 White gave up his dental practice in order to devote his time to manufacturing.

Advances in Restorative Dentistry

"It is the opinion of scientific dentists of the present day, that the teeth of most persons may, by proper management, be preserved to the end of their lives." Shearjashub Spooner's observation in his *Guide to Sound Teeth* is in marked contrast to the attitude held by most people during the preceding centuries, including that of the medical profession, who viewed extraction as an inevitable part of dental treatment. By Spooner's day, however, the dental profession was seeking improved ways to fill carious teeth and restore them to useful function. Over the centuries a variety of improbable materials ranging from cobwebs to rosin had been tried. About 1850 gutta-percha, made from the exudate of trees of the sapodilla family, was introduced; mixed with lime, quartz, and feldspar, it was first marketed under the name of Hill's Stopping. Gutta-percha became immensely popular and was used not only as a temporary filling material but also as a nonpermanent restorative in teeth too weak to be filled with metal.

The technique of pouring low-fusing molten metal into the tooth cavity was soon discarded because the extreme heat of the metal often destroyed the pulp, and because gaps appeared around the edges of the cooling metal that would trap decay-producing material. Silver foil and tin foil were also tried, with but modest success. Cements of various kinds also had their vogue and then in time were also discarded or, like gutta-percha, were retained as temporary filling materials. Most reputable dentists used only gold foil; the eminent Leonard Koecker insisted that this was the *only* material to be used.

In 1833 two Frenchmen by the name of Crawcour came to America with what they claimed was a new material for filling teeth. A crude amalgam, their so-called Royal Mineral Succedaneum was prepared from shavings of silver cut from coins and mixed with enough mercury to make a sloppy paste. The Crawcours' blatant advertising and reprehensible habit of leaving carious matter in the teeth they filled brought down upon them the wrath of many of the most prominent members of the profession, and after a few months they were forced to return to France. Nevertheless, during their short stay they traveled widely, touting Royal Mineral Succedaneum and placing fillings in a great many mouths. Many American dentists saw in the material an answer to their problems with gold foil, which was very difficult and time-consuming to use, and many began to experiment with silver amalgam, though the leaders of the profession did not.

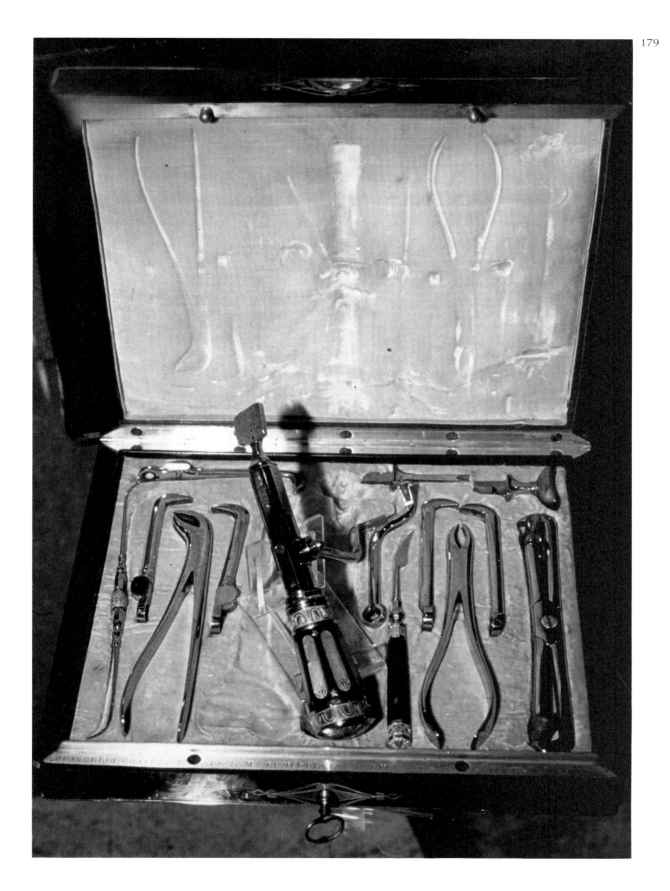

This instrument case was used to treat the dental ailments of Napoleon I. Musée de la Chirurgie Dentaire, Lyons.

Rembrandt Peale painted this portrait of Horace Hayden, one of the founders of professional dentistry in America, now in the collection of the Medical and Chirurgical Faculty of Maryland, University of Baltimore.

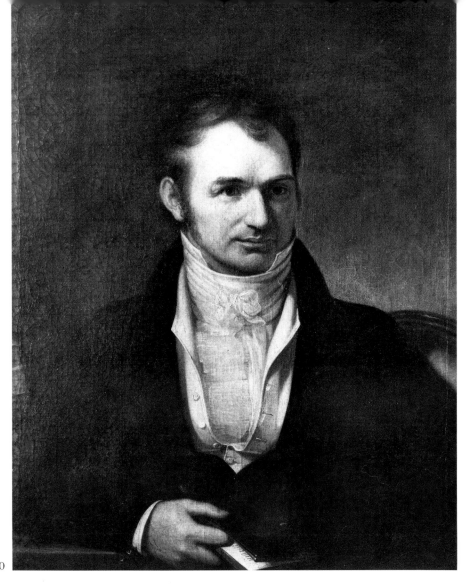

180

181

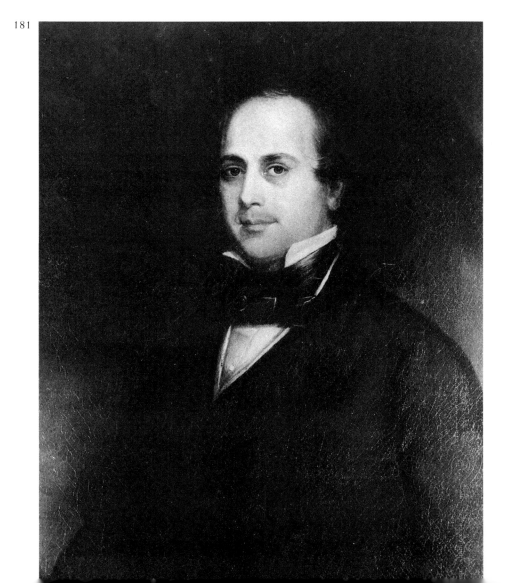

Chapin Harris was instrumental in establishing the first dental college in the world, the first nationwide association of dentists in the United States, and the first authoritative dental periodical. His portrait, painted by David Acheson Woodward, is in the collection of the Baltimore College of Dental Surgery, Dental School, University of Maryland.

The Foundations of Professional Dentistry

Professional dentistry rests upon a threefold base: education, organization, and literature. During the years 1839 and 1840 in the United States the tripod of dental professionalism was established for the very first time anywhere, and dentistry was elevated to the high level of excellence at which it has since remained. Although about a dozen dentists contributed to this remarkable advance, two in particular stand above all the others, Horace H. Hayden and Chapin A. Harris.

The Architects

Born in Connecticut into an educated family, Horace H. Hayden (1769–1844, fig. 180) early showed an aptitude for the natural and biological sciences. He began his working career as a geologist and authored a highly regarded text on that subject. In 1792 he was in New York City and, in need of dental treatment, put himself in the care of John Greenwood, who inspired the younger man to take up dentistry as a vocation. Whether he became Greenwood's student is not known; in a short time, however, Hayden evidenced a firm grasp not only of dentistry but of medicine.

He began to practice his new profession in upstate New York, but by 1800 he was in Baltimore, first as an assistant to Thomas Hamilton, one of the city's leading dentists, then before long practicing on his own in the city and its surrounding communities. Hayden soon developed a reputation and contributed articles to professional journals on such medical topics as ulcerated tonsils and such dental subjects as anatomical and pathological aspects of the teething of infants. In 1810 Hayden was granted a license to practice dentistry—the first ever issued in America—by the Medical and Chirurgical Faculty of Maryland, which carried with it membership in that institution.

In 1819 he was invited to lecture on dentistry to medical students at the University of Maryland and gave a series of lectures there in 1823–25. He was awarded an honorary medical degree in 1837 by the Jefferson Medical College of Philadelphia and in 1840 by the University of Maryland—one of only two dentists in America who were so honored.

Chapin A. Harris (fig. 181) was born in the small town of Pompey, New York, in 1806. Nothing further is known of his early life until 1823 when he was in Bainbridge, Ohio, studying medicine under his brother, Dr. John Harris. In 1824, he began to practice in Greenfield, Ohio, and by 1828 records show that he had combined dentistry with the practice of medicine.

Early in the 1830s he left Ohio for Baltimore and became a preceptorial student of Horace Hayden's. After that he moved about the South, practicing for a time in Fredericksburg, Virginia, and finally settling permanently in Baltimore in 1835.

Harris built up an extensive library—literary as well as scientific—and he himself enriched the literature of dentistry with his publication in 1839 of *The Dental Art: A Practical Treatise on Dental Surgery*. This book, one of the most important ever published in the field, was reissued during the next seventy-four years in thirteen editions. No other dental treatise can match this record!

Harris attended Washington Medical College in 1838 as an undergraduate student, but there is no indication that he was ever formally awarded a degree in medicine, though after completing his studies with his brother, he appended an M.D. to his name. Harris did, however, receive an honorary M.A. degree in 1842 from Shurtleff College, Alton, Illinois, because of "attainments in the sciences equal to those of [university] graduates."

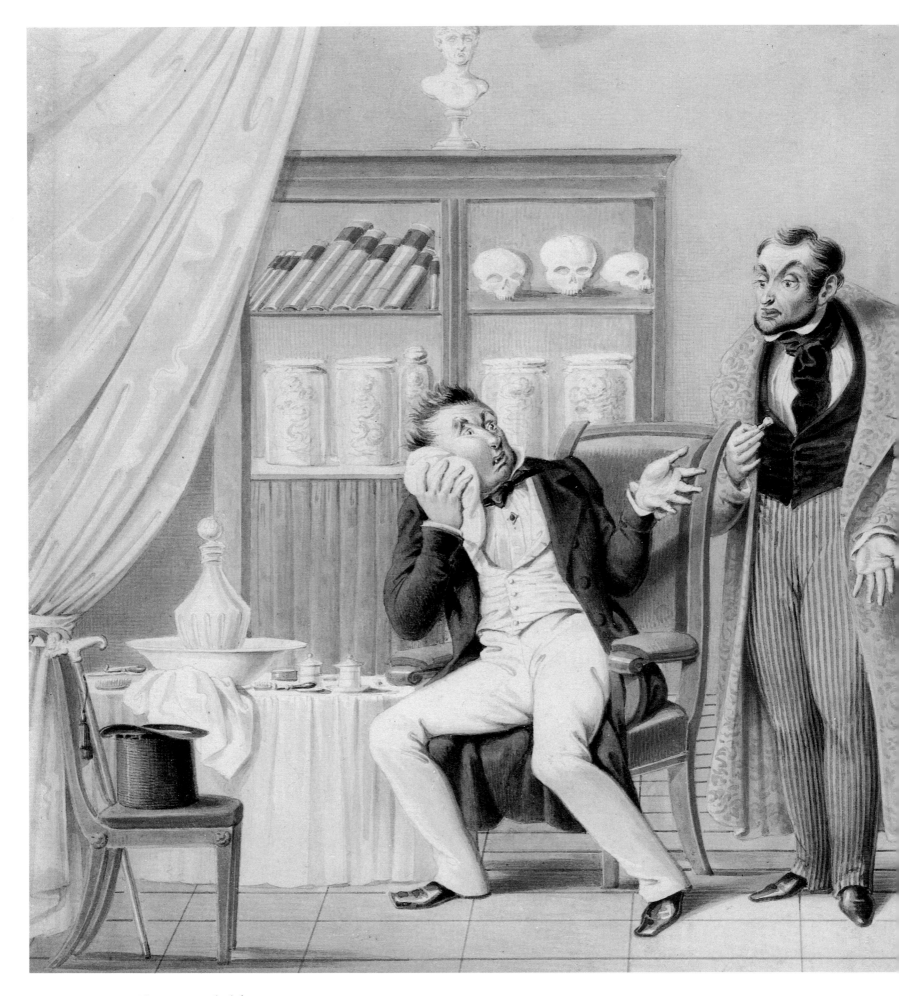

In the ninth century Albucasis remarked that a patient can be misled by pain into thinking a sound tooth is a diseased one. In this colored engraving of 1839 by Johann Christian Schoeller, the shoe is on the other foot. The dentist has made the mistake and extracted the wrong tooth from his patient, who is justifiably annoyed. National Library of Medicine, Bethesda.

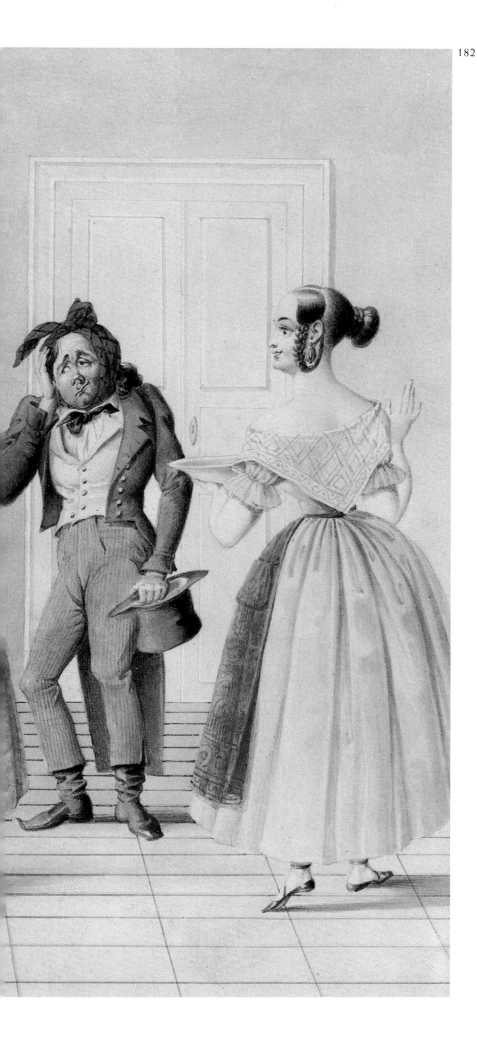

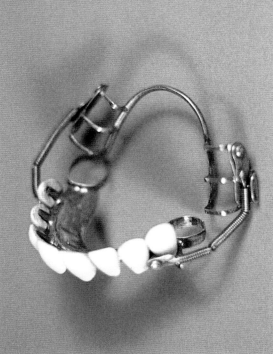

Giuseppangelo Fonzi, an Italian dentist with a fashionable Parisian practice, invented the individual porcelain teeth that revolutionized the construction of dentures in the early nineteenth century. In this partial upper denture of about 1830, porcelain teeth of Fonzi's design have been soldered to a gold backing. The denture was retained by wires surrounding the natural lower teeth. Medicinsk-Historisk Museum, University of Copenhagen.

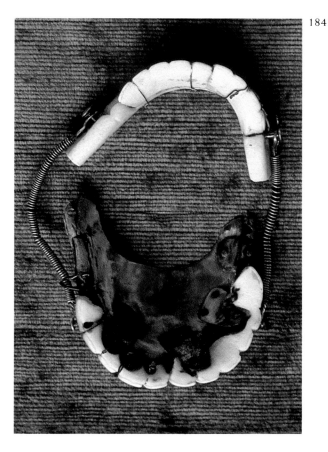

George Washington's last dental prosthesis was made for him by John Greenwood. The palate was swaged from a sheet of gold, and the ivory teeth were riveted to it. The lower denture consists of a single carved block of ivory. The two dentures were held together by steel springs. National Museum of American History, Smithsonian Institution, Washington, D.C.

Education

On March 6, 1840, the first dental college in the world, the Baltimore College of Dental Surgery, was chartered by the state of Maryland, due to the efforts of Hayden and Harris. Under the supervision of a board of visitors consisting of nine physicians, four ministers, and two dentists was a faculty of four. Two were dentists: Hayden, professor of dental physiology and pathology and president of the college, and Harris, professor of practical dentistry and dean. Two were physicians: Thomas E. Bond, Jr., professor of special pathology and therapeutics, and H. Willis Baxley, professor of anatomy and physiology.

Only five students were enrolled in the first class, which began on November 3. The requirements for the newly designated D.D.S. degree were as high as, if not higher than, those for the M.D. degree. The course of study lasted two years, the same amount of time required for a medical degree, with instruction during four months of each year. The remainder of the time was spent receiving practical experience in a dental office. Only two members of the class graduated. One, Robert Arthur of Baltimore, gained renown as the founder, in 1852, of the third American dental college, the Philadelphia College of Dental Surgery, later the Pennsylvania College of Dental Surgery, of which he became dean in 1856.

Organization

Hayden and Harris also collaborated to form the first nationwide association of dentists. The conception was, without question, Hayden's. Close association with other health practitioners at the University of Maryland undoubtedly made him aware of the advantages of a national dentists' organization, but his attempts to establish one in 1817, again in 1829, and again in 1838 had been unsuccessful. Chapin Harris's dynamic drive and force brought the idea to fruition. He instilled a new enthusiasm into the members of a local organization, the Society of Surgeon Dentists of the City and State of New York (SSD), which had been founded in 1834, probably to combat the activities of the notorious Crawcours and other empirics, but which had experienced internal dissension and been dissolved in 1839. The members of the defunct SSD and a number of dentists from other states in 1840 formed the American Society of Dental Surgeons, the first national organization of dentists in the world. The new group chose Hayden as its president. Eleazar Parmly (1797–1874) of New York served as vice-president, Chapin Harris as corresponding secretary, and Solyman Brown (1790–1876) as recording secretary.

Literature

In 1839 Chapin Harris, who long had foreseen the need for an authoritative dental periodical, was instrumental in founding the first in the world, the *American Journal of Dental Science* (*AJDS*). At a meeting held in the home of Solyman Brown in New York City, Harris, Hayden, Parmly, and several other leading dentists agreed that practicing dentists needed to have the latest information published on a regular basis by a reputable journal, though Hayden expressed fears that such a journal would provide the charlatans with a superficial learning that would further entrench them in their practice. Nevertheless, he went along with the proposal.

Parmly, Elisha Baker, and Solyman Brown became the publishing committee, with Harris and Parmly the editors; however, it appears that Brown, as secretary

185

England's first dental school opened in 1859. Before that date, dentistry was often performed by poorly qualified operators such as this jack-of-all-trades, whose sign declares that he also bleeds and makes wigs, sausages, black puddings, powder for the itch, red herrings, and small beer. Satirical drawing by Thomas Rowlandson, 1823. The Francis A. Countway Library of Medicine, Harvard Medical Library/Boston Medical Library, Boston.

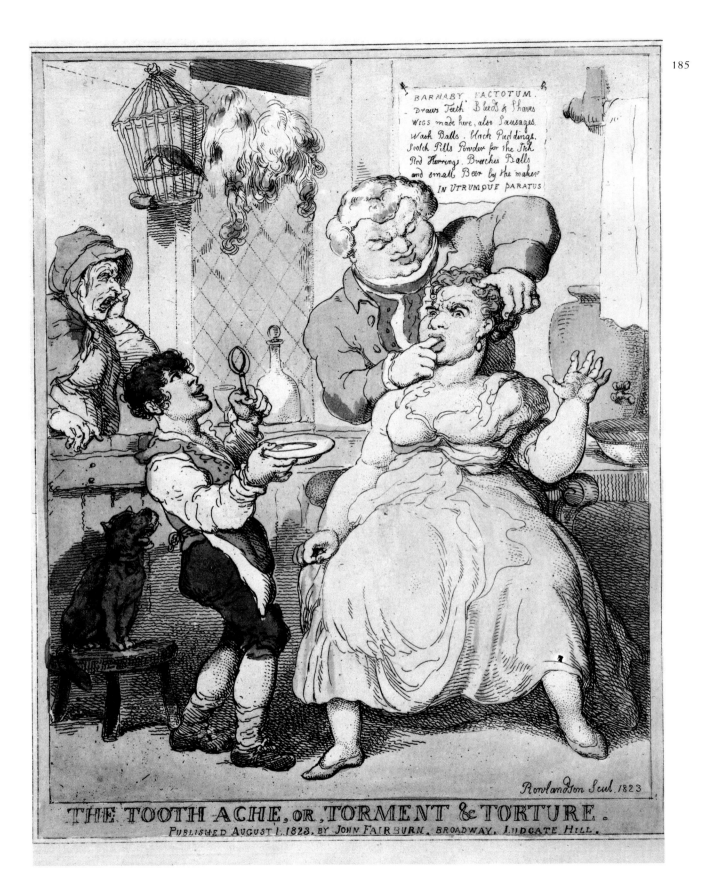

BARNABY FACTOTUM.
Draws Teeth. Bleeds & Shaves
Wigs made here, also Sausages.
Wash Balls. Black Puddings.
Scotch Pills Powder for the Itch
Red Herrings. Breeches Balls
and small Beer by the maker
IN UTRUMQUE PARATUS

Rowlandson Scul. 1823

THE TOOTH ACHE, OR, TORMENT & TORTURE.

PUBLISHED AUGUST 1, 1823, BY JOHN FAIRBURN, BROADWAY, LUDGATE HILL.

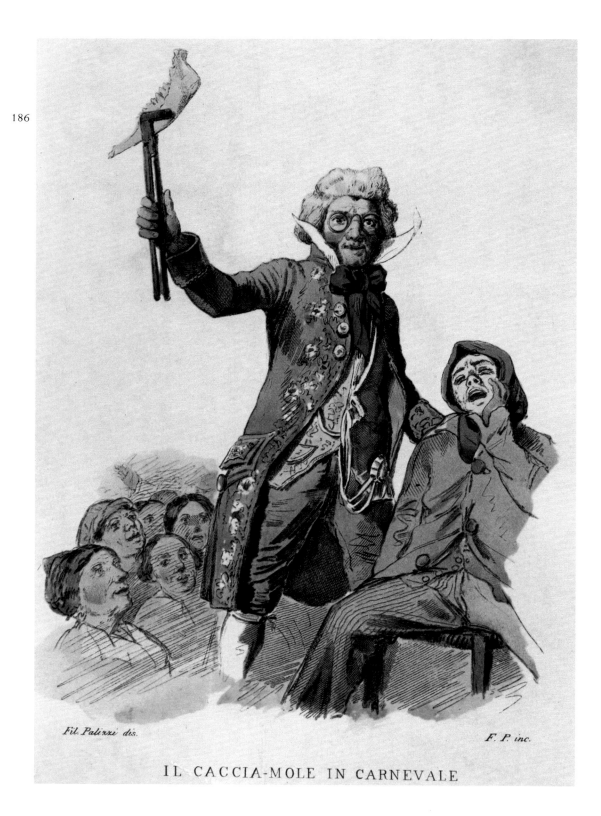

IL CACCIA-MOLE IN CARNEVALE

Fil. Palizzi dis. *F. P. inc.*

During the nineteenth century Europe lagged behind America in dentistry, and quackery was rampant there. In *Il Caccia-Mole in Carnevale*, a painting by Filippo Palizzi, an Italian charlatan attracts a crowd by pretending to extract part of an animal's jaw from a suffering "patient." University of Maryland Health Sciences Library, Baltimore.

This diagrammatic drawing by Christophe François Delabarre shows the action of the key in pulling out a tooth. From *Odontologie; ou, observation sur les dents humaines* (1815).

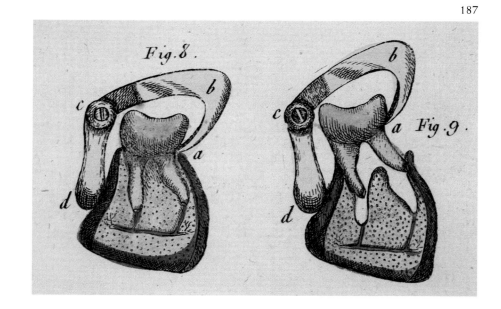

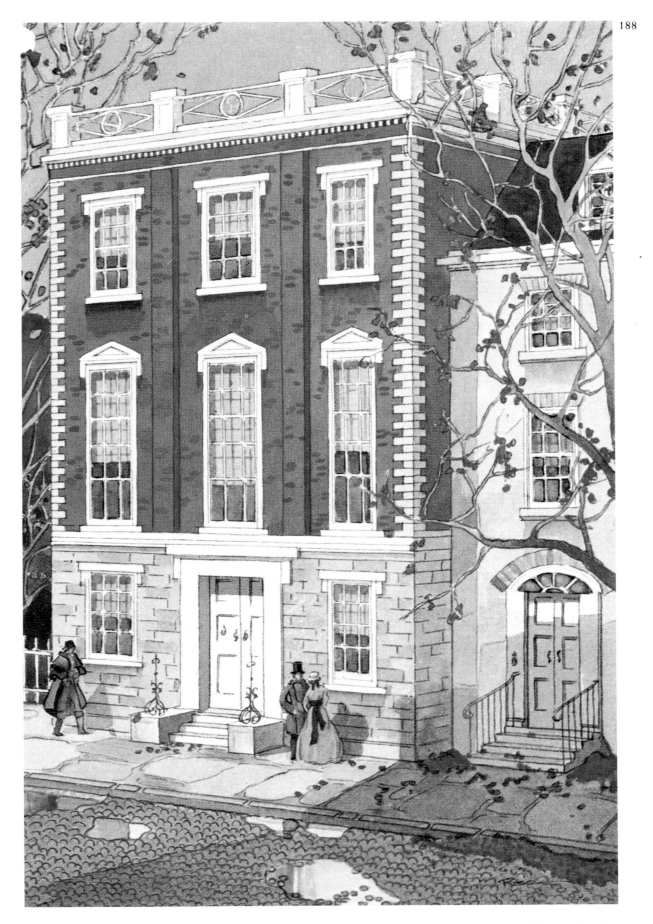

The Baltimore College of Dental Surgery, the first dental college in the world, opened its doors to a class of five students on November 3, 1840.

of the committee, fulfilled the duties of editor for the first volume, and that Harris assumed them for the second. The profession was canvassed for subscriptions (Harris and Parmly contributed $100 each, and Baker, Brown, and nine others put up $50 each). The prospectus was a lengthy one, explaining in some detail why such a journal was needed. "[It] will have the effect of giving dignity and importance to the general subject of practical dentistry, and thus result in a solid advantage to each and all of its professors, as well as to the community at large." "Such a work will have a tendency to expel from dental practice, the quackery which disgraces it, just in proportion as it dissipates ignorance on the subject from the community at large." A list of subscribers was to be published periodically in order to acquaint those professionals "who are not stationary in their labors, to what points their exertions may be most profitably directed," i.e., to help interest dentists in those areas of specialization in which they were most needed, in part also to "check the exuberant influx of half-educated aspirants, who imagine that the field of labor is but partially occupied, and thus expose themselves to ultimate disappointment." On a more idealistic plane the *AJDS* would strive to bring the latest information from every source to the dentist wherever he might be and to unite dentists in "fraternal feeling."

The first issue, published on June 1, 1839, set the tone of the publication. It carried original articles by Elisha Baker, Solyman Brown, Eleazar Parmly, and J.

Electricity was still a novelty in the late 1800s and magical curative properties were ascribed to it. The handle of this toothbrush was purportedly "charged with an electromagnetic current, which acts, without any shock, immediately upon the nerves and tissues of the teeth and gums . . . arresting decay . . . and restoring the natural whiteness of the enamel." This bit of quackery was advertised in *Harper's Weekly* for February 13, 1886.

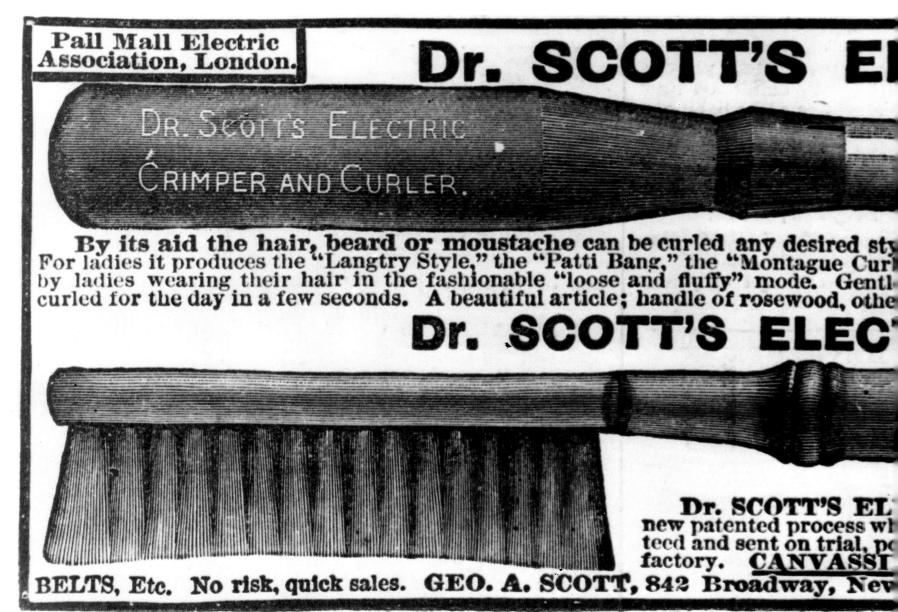

Foster Flagg (a grandson of Josiah Flagg). It also had a review by Solyman Brown of Chapin Harris's new book *The Dental Art;* an extract from Antoine Delabarre's *Second Dentition,* with notes by Chapin Harris; and a catalogue of the library of Elisha Gidney, who had placed his books at the disposal of the publishing committee. And as part of an ongoing endeavor to bring important publications to the attention of its readers, the *AJDS* carried the first installment of John Hunter's *Natural History of the Human Teeth.*

The subscription list for the first issue of the *AJDS* shows where the most informed, enterprising, and dedicated dentists were located in the second quarter of the nineteenth century. They practiced in twenty-three states and the District of Columbia, as well as in England, France, Cuba, Bermuda, and Holland. Most were settled in the major eastern American cities—Boston, New York, Philadelphia, and Baltimore—but a large number, including one from this author's hometown of Batavia, New York, came from small cities and villages farther west and south.

The journal was originally a proprietary one, with the publishing committee as owner, but after a year or two of financial difficulties, the new American Society of Dental Surgeons, recognizing the importance of keeping the publication alive, voted in 1841, at its second annual meeting, to assume ownership of the magazine, declaring it to be its official organ.

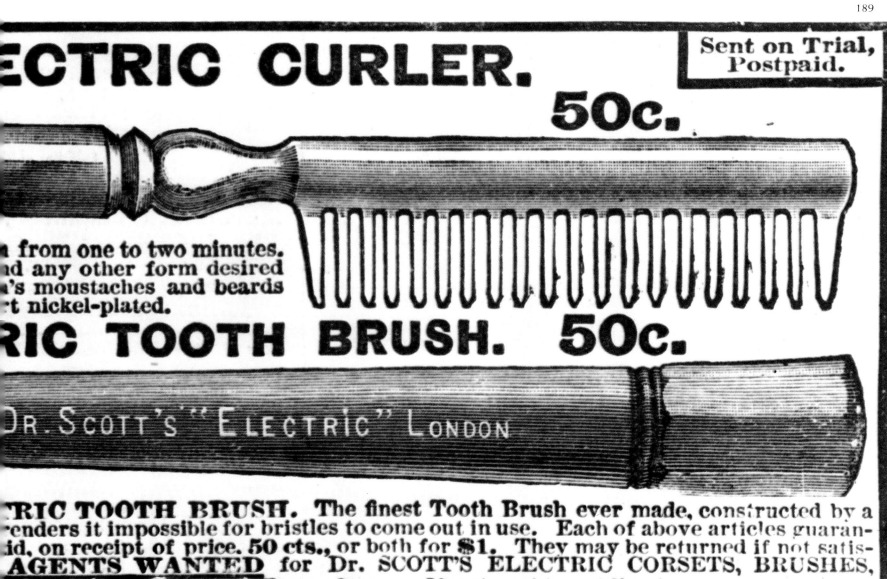

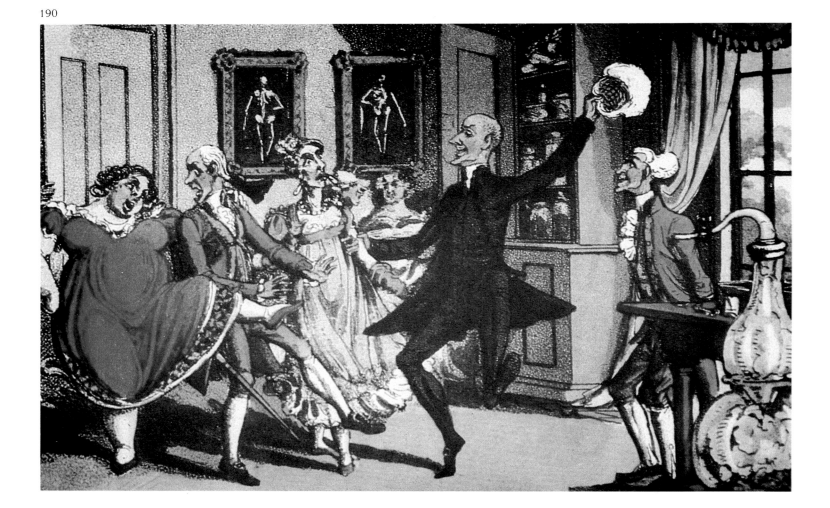

The subject of this satirical English colored drawing of 1820 is the popular story of a Latin tutor named Dr. Syntax, who toured Europe in search of novel experiences. He and his wife have just inhaled nitrous oxide gas from the glass container at right and are showing its effects, to the consternation of others in the room. Nitrous oxide was not used as an anesthetic in dentistry until the 1840s.

Joseph Whiting Stock, a self-taught artist of Springfield, Massachusetts, painted this attractive portrait about 1845. The child holds a teether, a device today usually made of plastic, in earlier times (for the rich) of coral (see figure 199), to expedite the eruption of the first teeth through the gums. Barenholtz Collection.

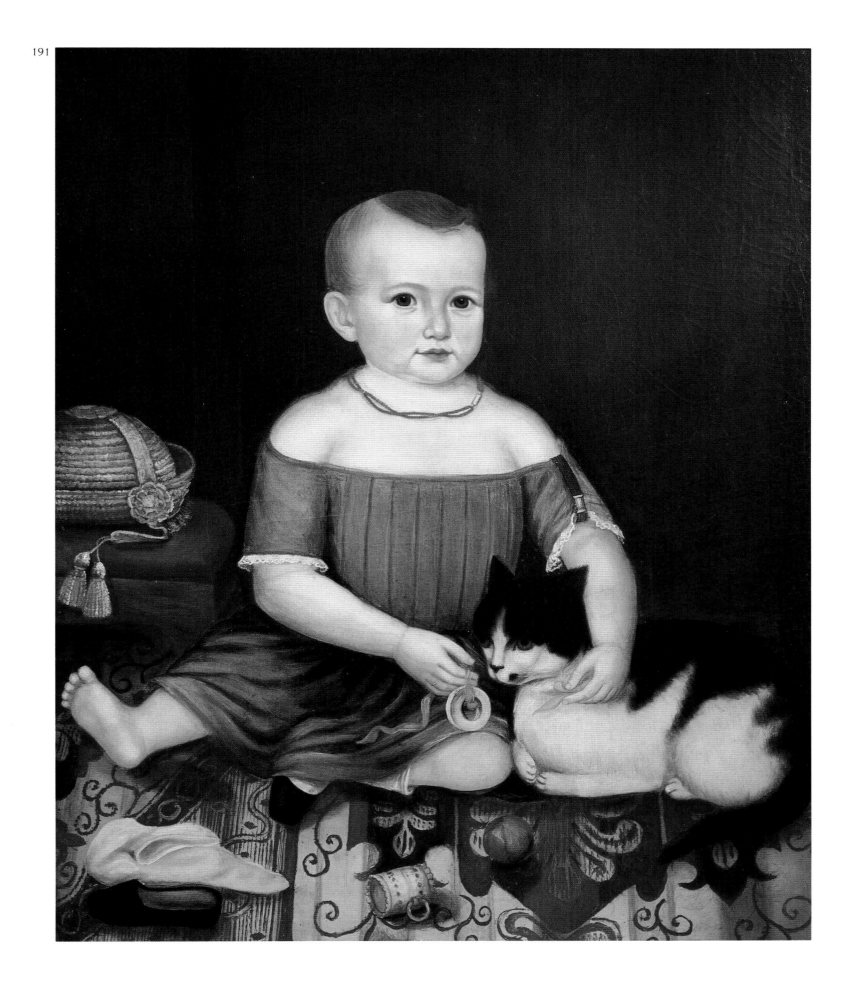

The Amalgam War

Unfortunate it was that the young American Society of Dental Surgeons (ASDS) came into being so soon after the Crawcour brothers had created such a stir with their new amalgam. Their bombastic advertising had posed a threat to more ethical and conscientious dentists. At the same time many other untrained, often unprincipled practitioners in search of easy money seized upon the new material, which was easier to place in a tooth than gold.

Organized dentistry, which at that time represented only a very tiny percentage of practicing dentists, began a campaign against the use of the amalgam, and their drive soon assumed the tone of a religious crusade. Proponents of the amalgam were to be rooted out, and to this end every member of the American Society of Dental Surgeons was required to sign a pledge that it was his "opinion and firm conviction that any amalgam whatever . . . is unfit for the plugging of teeth or fangs [retained roots], and I pledge myself never under any circumstances to make use of it in my practice." Those who refused to sign the pledge were summarily expelled.

But progress, in whatever form it takes, cannot be so easily impeded. Many dentists—including a number of highly reputable ones—soon found in amalgam the answer to certain difficult restorative problems. They also felt compelled to use it to serve the needs of those too poor to pay for gold, and also in order to compete with the quacks, who were using it widely. As a consequence, so many dentists had refused to sign the pledge by 1850 that the ASDS was forced to rescind it. But their conciliatory action came too late, and the annual meeting scheduled for August 1856 had to be canceled for lack of a quorum. Thus came to an end the first national organization of dentists.

In 1850 the ASDS was already too short of money to support the *American Journal of Dental Science*, and so the publication was sold to Chapin Harris, who assumed all its unpaid debts. With rare devotion to his profession, Harris labored valiantly as publisher and editor for ten years until his death in 1860, and he was gradually impoverished by the staggering cost of single-handedly putting out the journal. A pathetic though somewhat ludicrous postscript to Harris's story: his colleagues called a memorial meeting in New York City to raise money to aid his penniless widow, but after $1,000 had been collected by canvassing the profession across the nation, it was discovered that $915 had been expended in raising it! The remaining $85 was turned over to Mrs. Harris, whose first reaction was promptly, and indignantly, to reject the niggardly tribute. On second consideration, she kept the money, as her pressing need was so great.

192

A Familiar Treatise on Dentistry by George Hawes, published in New York in 1846, featured a clever frontispiece. A flap, when lifted, revealed the teeth of the beautiful subject. The Francis A. Countway Library of Medicine, Harvard Medical Library/ Boston Medical Library, Rare Book Collection, Boston.

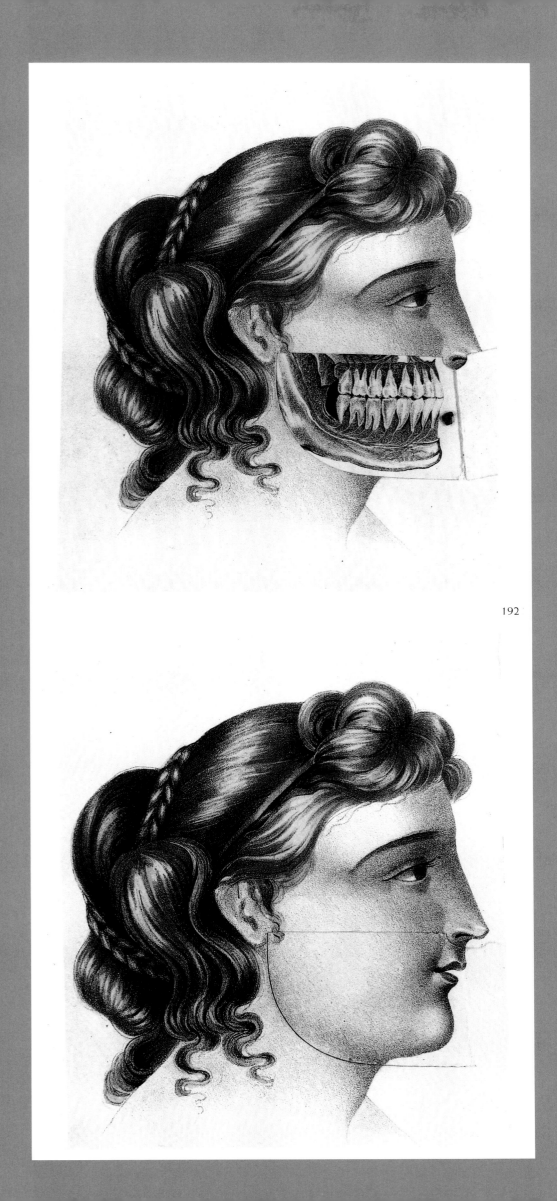

192

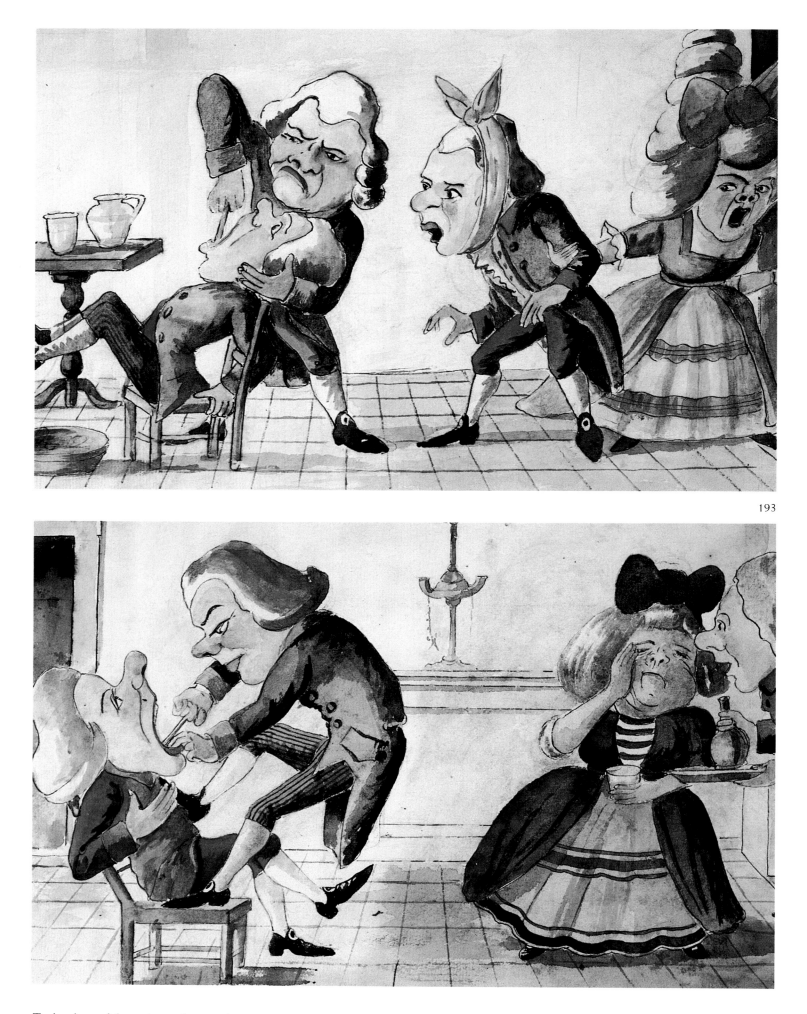

To the alarm of the patients who wait their turn, an athletic Italian dentist draws teeth with energy in these companion drawings of the 1850s. University of Maryland Health Sciences Library, Baltimore.

A Dutch artist of the late nineteenth or early twentieth century designed this poster, published in Berlin, entitled *Tahnuttrecken (Tooth-Drawing)*. The caption describes how important the teeth are, yet how satisfactory it is when aching ones are removed.

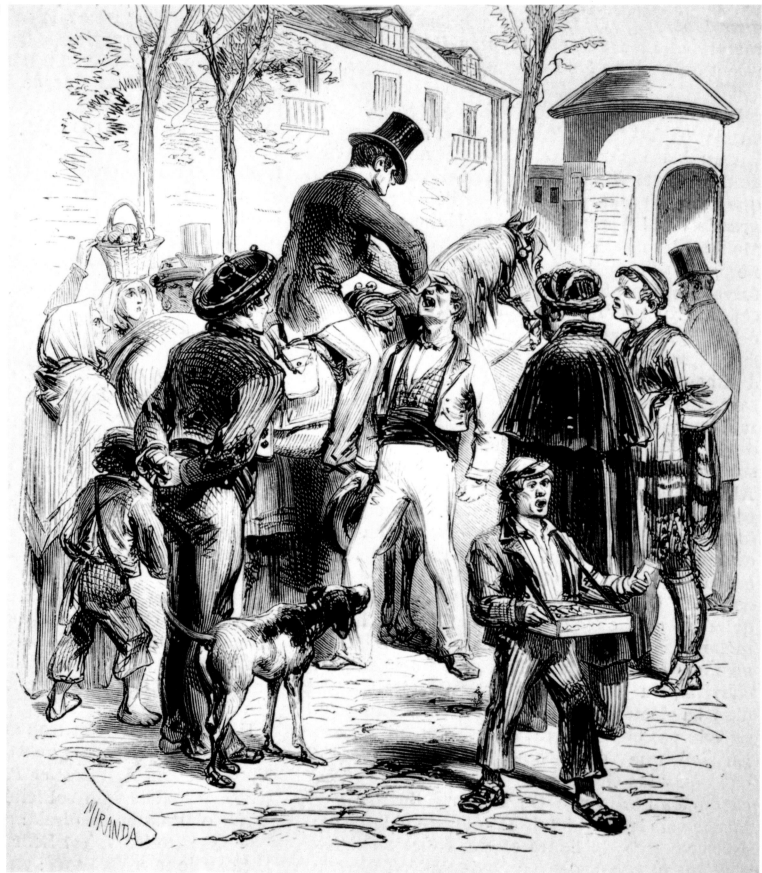

Spain lagged behind the rest of Europe during the nineteenth century, in medicine as in other aspects of culture. This scene in an Iberian town of the 1870s, drawn "from nature" by a Sr. Cuesta, shows a dentist on horseback who, except for his short jacket and high hat, would not have looked out of place in the same street three centuries earlier.

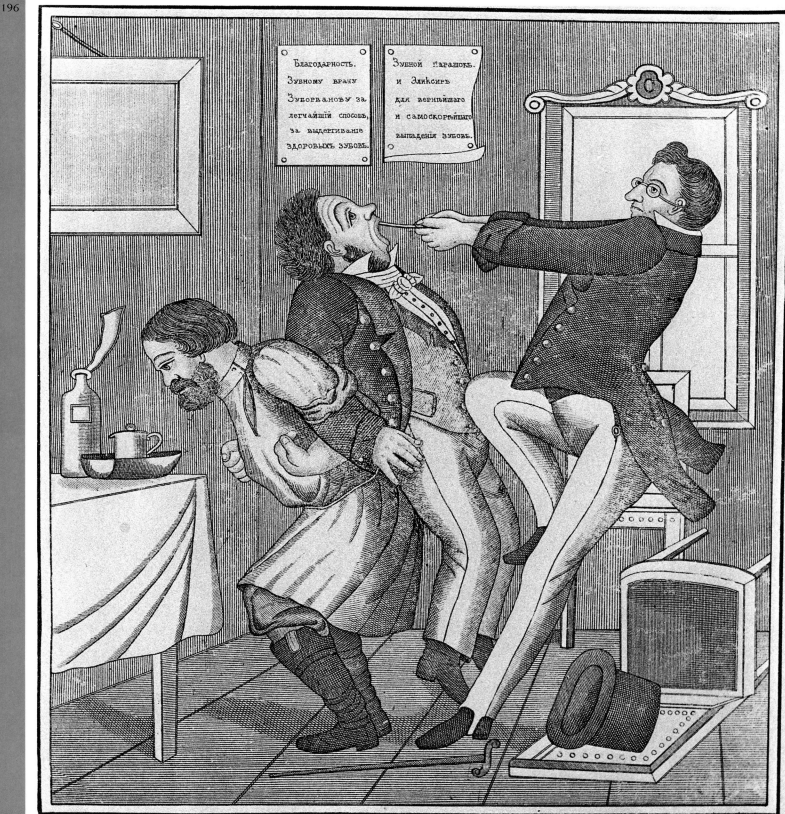

A dentist extracts a tooth with the help of his servant in this Russian cartoon of 1889. The caption below assures the reader that he has done this many times. Collection Dr. F.E.R. DeMaar, The Hague.

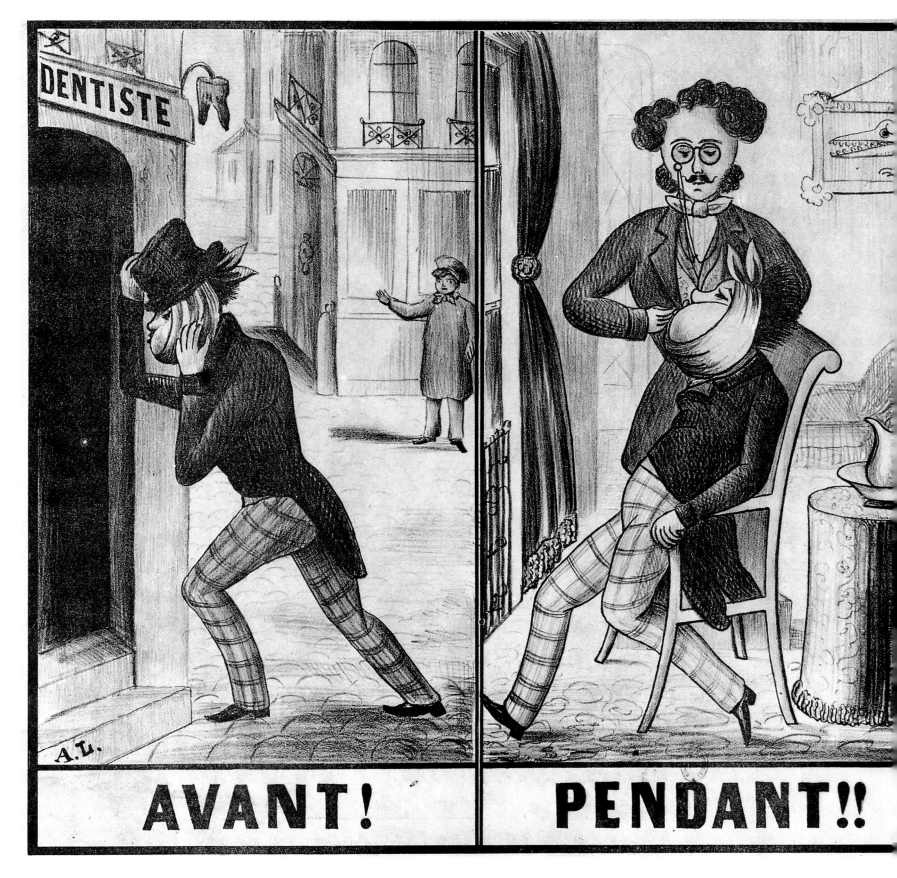

AVANT! PENDANT!!

The apprehension, anguish, and relief that a visit to a dentist inspires are capsulized in this French cartoon of the 1850s by Arthur Lamy. Bibliothèque Nationale, Paris.

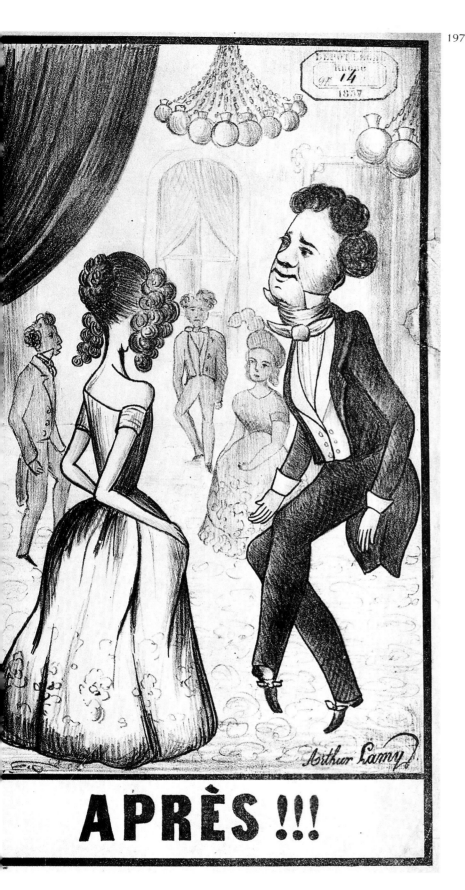

197

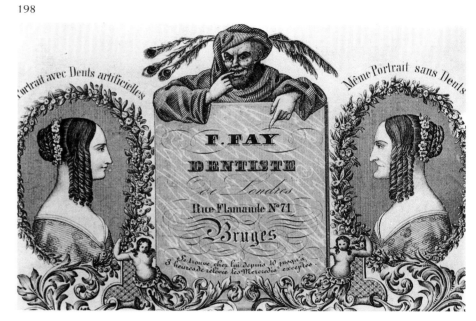

198

The calling card of F. Fay, a dentist of Bruges, Belgium, draws attention to the importance of keeping one's teeth in order to maintain an attractive appearance.

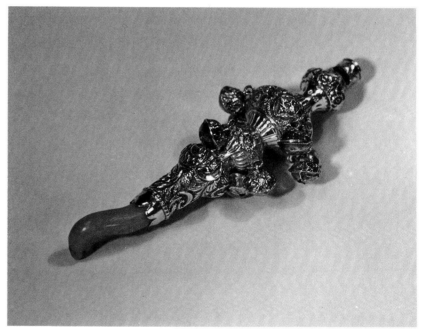

199

This very elegant rattle was made in Birmingham, England, in 1872. The silver handle has two rows of bells and a whistle for a child's entertainment. The teething stick is made of coral. Academy of Medicine, Toronto.

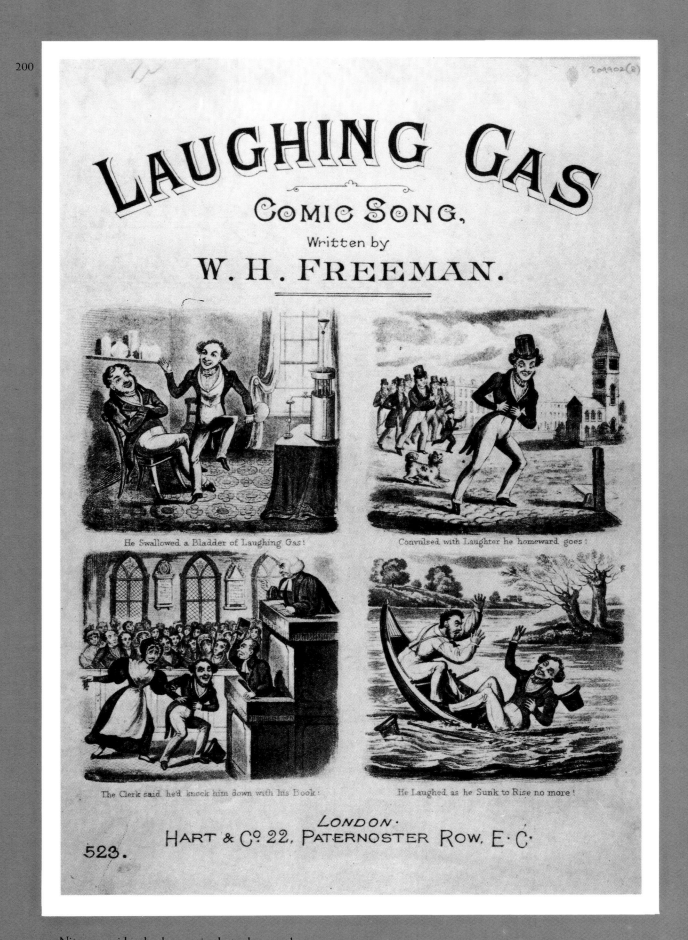

Nitrous oxide deadens pain but also produces pleasant sensations and excitement. During the 1830s and 1840s a vogue developed for inhaling the gas for fun. A young man who tried it, to no good end, was the subject of this comic song of the period entitled "Laughing Gas." Wellcome Institute Library, London.

201

The novel extraction instrument lying in the center of this instrument case is a forceps with detachable ends. Designed to fit any tooth, it was patented in 1876. National Library of Medicine, Bethesda.

XII.
THE LATE NINETEENTH CENTURY IN
THE UNITED STATES AND EUROPE

Anesthesia: Dentistry's Great Contribution to Medicine

Perhaps no advance in medical knowledge has alleviated more human suffering than the discovery of anesthetics. This great gift to mankind was made by an American dentist in 1844.

201

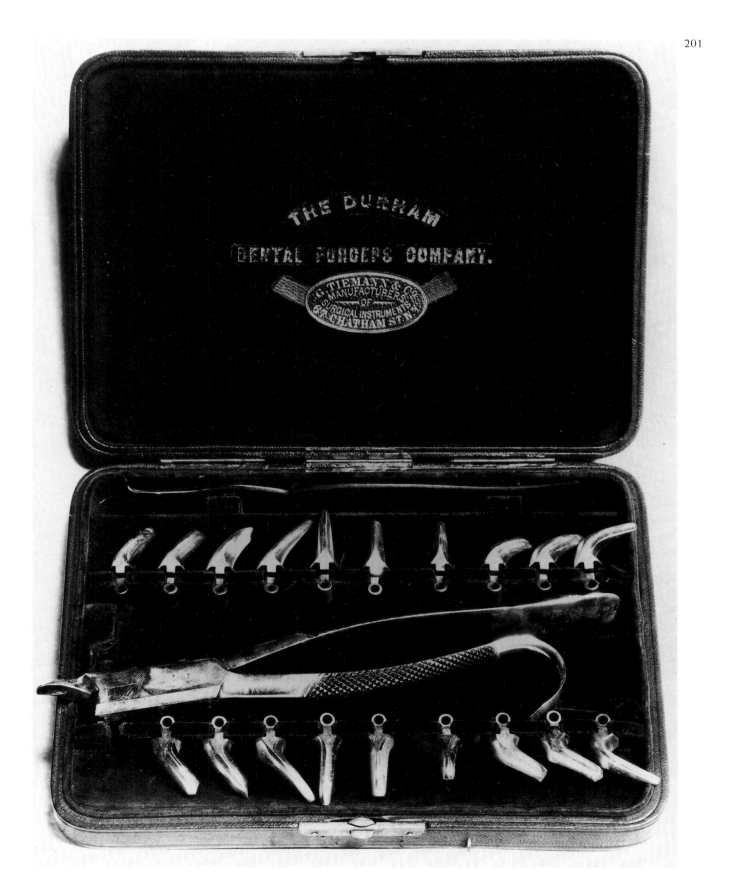

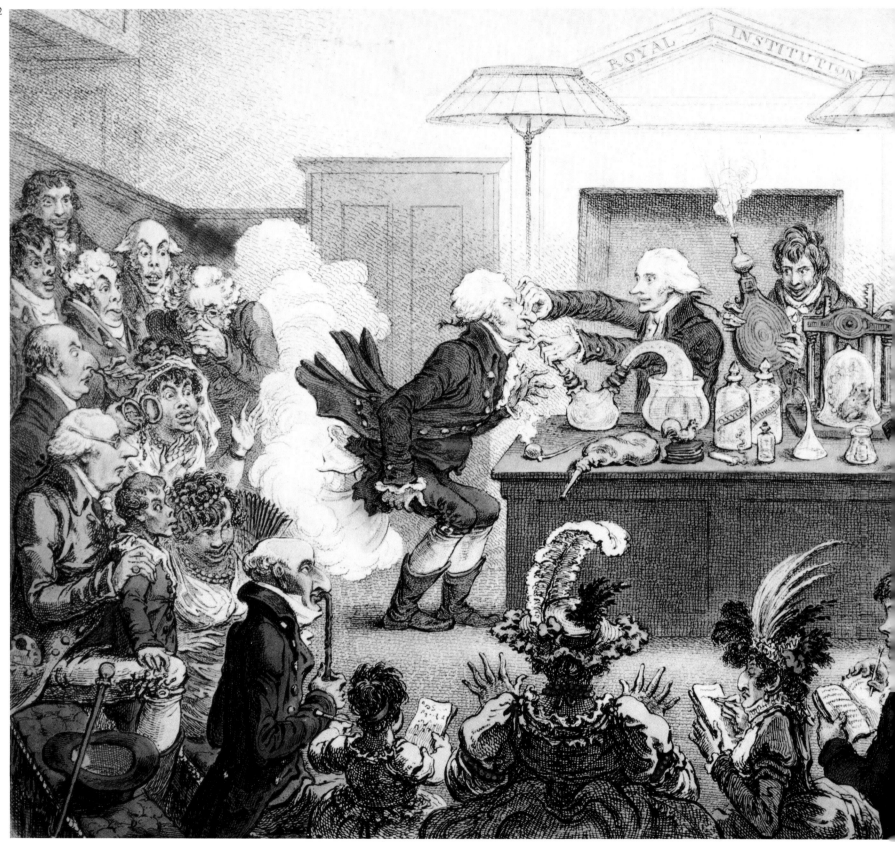

During the late 1700s and early 1800s in England, a great deal of research on the properties of gases, including their effect on human beings, was carried out at "pneumatic institutions." The cartoonists lost no time in lampooning these establishments, and many of their efforts, like this cartoon of about 1800, are genuinely funny. Northwestern University Dental School, Chicago.

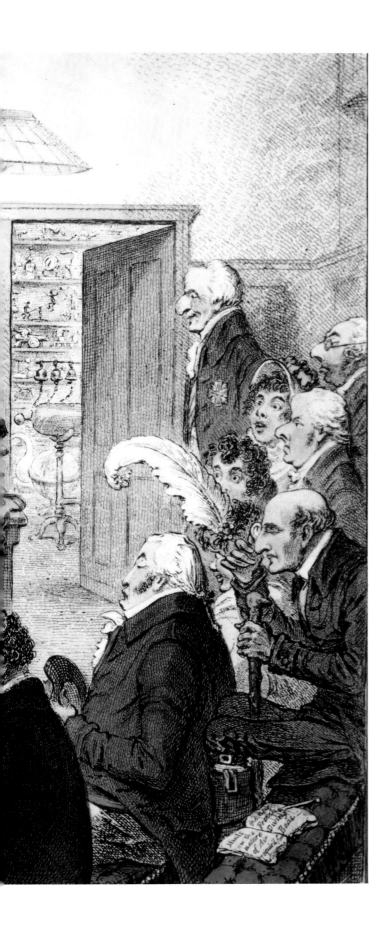

Nitrous Oxide

Chemists were making great strides in the last quarter of the eighteenth century. Many gases were isolated, including nitrogen, by Daniel Rutherford in 1772, and oxygen, in 1774 by the brilliant English cleric Joseph Priestley, who two years earlier had discovered nitrous oxide gas. It was hoped that these new gases might help in conquering disease, and in order to experiment with them, the medical profession set up "pneumatic institutions," where a multitude of gases were administered to patients suffering from illnesses ranging from tuberculosis to diseases of the stomach.

An English chemist and physicist, Humphry Davy (1778–1829), at the age of twenty-one was appointed director of the largest of these institutions, at Clifton. Davy carried out experiments with many gases, but was most intrigued by nitrous oxide. He subjected himself and animals to the gas and made a number of interesting observations, including the fact that inhaling it produced very pleasant sensations and also tended to reduce sensitivity to pain. In 1800 he published his findings in a compendious work, *Researches, Chemical and Philosophical; Chiefly Concerning Nitrous Oxide*, in which he made the prophetic statement, "As nitrous oxide in its extensive operation appears capable of destroying physical pain, it may probably be used with advantage during surgical operations in which no great effusion of blood takes place."

Nitrous oxide, however, first produces excitement and only later sedation and unconsciousness. Though failing to take advantage of the latter attribute of the gas, the medical profession became well aware of the former; indeed, medical students during the thirties and forties often held nitrous oxide "frolics," at which the gas was inhaled for the pleasant effects it produced. A student at Fairfield Medical College near Syracuse, New York, wrote a fellow classmate in November 1838, "Preparations are making to administer pentoxide of nitrogen gas tomorrow. A goodly number of students intend to take it and we expect some sport as usual." During these years, too, itinerant showmen, who often styled themselves professors, traveled about the United States holding popular demonstrations of the effects of nitrous oxide. A wonderful description of such a show put on by Professor Gardner Quincy Colton (1814–1898) in New York City in 1844 appeared in the local *New Mirror* on April 6.

> The candidates for a taste of it [the gas] were many and urgent, crowding up from below like the applicants to St. Peter, and the professor seemed somewhat embarrassed as to selection. A thick-necked and bony youth got possession of the bag, however, and applied his mouth to the stopper. After inhaling its contents for a minute or two he squared away and commenced pummelling the professor in the most approved butcher-boy style.... The "twelve strong men" [appointed to protect the volunteers from injury] rushed to the rescue, the audience applauded vociferously, and the lad returned to his senses, having been out of them perhaps three minutes. A dozen others took their turns, and were variously affected. I was only very much delighted with one young man, who cooly undertook a promenade over the close-packed heads of the audience.... There was one corsair-looking man who rushed up and down the stage, believing himself on the deck of some vessel in pursuit of another, and that was perhaps the best bit of acting. One silly youth went to and fro, smirking and bowing, another did a scene from "Richard the Third," and a tall good-looking young man laughed heartily, and suddenly stopped and demanded of the audience, in indignant rage, what they were laughing at.

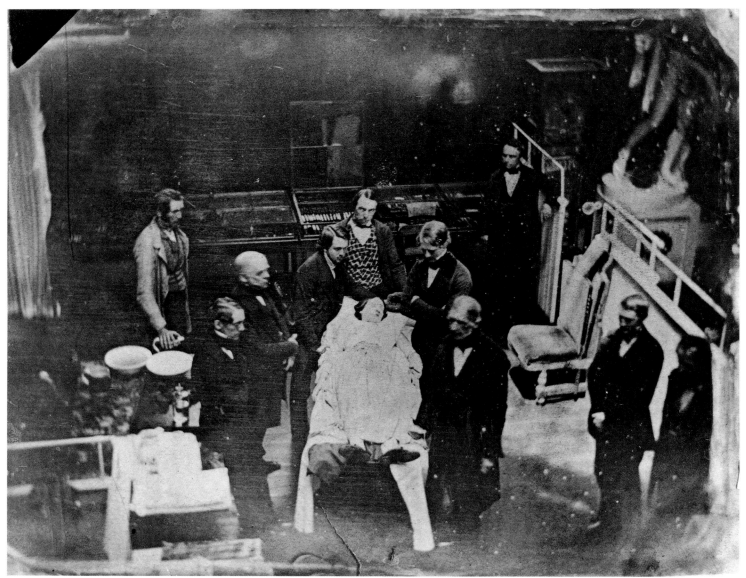

This original daguerreotype was made at the second operation performed under ether anesthesia, on October 17, 1846. The chair in which the patient sat during the demonstration on the previous day is seen at right. At the head of the table, in a checkered waistcoat, is the anesthetist, William T. G. Morton. The surgeon Warren stands in the right foreground. The Francis A. Countway Library of Medicine, Harvard Medical Library/Boston Medical Library, Rare Book Collection, Boston.

On December 11, 1844, a young dentist of Hartford, Connecticut, Horace Wells (1815–1848, fig. 204), attended one of Professor Colton's exhibitions. One of the volunteers from the audience, a man named Cooley who was known to Wells, severely injured his shin while stumbling around the stage. When he returned to his seat, Cooley was totally unaware that he had been hurt. To his great credit, Wells immediately understood the implications of this. He asked Colton to come to his office the next morning with a supply of nitrous oxide gas, and a colleague, Dr. John Riggs, extracted one of Wells's molar teeth after he had inhaled the gas. Upon awaking, he exclaimed, "I didn't feel it so much as the prick of a pin. A new era in tooth-pulling has arrived!"

After using nitrous oxide on a few patients, Wells petitioned the Massachusetts General Hospital, then the nation's leading medical institution, for an opportunity to demonstrate his great discovery. In January 1845 Wells appeared before Dr. John Collins Warren's class and extracted a tooth from one of the students. Unfortunately, he withdrew the gas while the patient was still in the excitement phase, and the student cried out in apparent pain. And although the young man insisted that he had felt nothing, Wells was nevertheless hissed and booed out of the class. Undaunted, he returned to his practice and continued using the gas for extractions. He also discussed his work with a former pupil, a practicing dentist, William T. G. Morton (1819–1868, fig. 205).

Ether

Morton was taking medical courses in Boston and had as one of his instructors a chemist, Charles Jackson (1805–1880), with whom he discussed Wells's new painkiller. Jackson suggested that Morton try ether. Jackson was in the habit of inhaling ether himself, often falling insensible, much as heavy drinkers do, and was aware of ether's ability to bring on unconsciousness.

After experimenting with the drug on small animals as well as on himself, Morton was ready to try extracting teeth with it. His first attempt was a success.

> Toward evening a man residing in Boston came in suffering great pain and wishing to have a tooth extracted. He was afraid of the operation and asked if he could be mesmerized. I told him I had something better, and, saturating my handkerchief, gave it to him to inhale. He became unconscious almost immediately. It was dark and Dr. Hayden held the lamp while I extracted a firmly rooted bicuspid tooth. There was not much alteration in the pulse and no relaxing of the muscles. He recovered in a minute and knew nothing of what had been done for him. He remained for some time talking about the experiment. This was the 30th of September, 1846.

Morton then applied to Dr. Warren for a chance to demonstrate his "new" drug, which, in an attempt at secrecy, he had named Letheon. On October 16, 1846, almost two years after Wells's unsuccessful demonstration, Morton administered ether, after which Dr. Warren excised a tumor from the neck of a young man, Gilbert Abbott (fig. 216). Warren then turned to the hushed audience and exclaimed, "Gentlemen, this is no humbug!"

News of this epochal discovery spread rapidly around the world, and in just over two months the first major operation to be performed under ether was carried out in London by England's greatest surgeon, Robert Liston. On December 21, 1846, he amputated a leg while the patient slept. Afterward, he turned to the audience of physicians and said, "This Yankee dodge, gentlemen, beats mesmerism all hollow!"

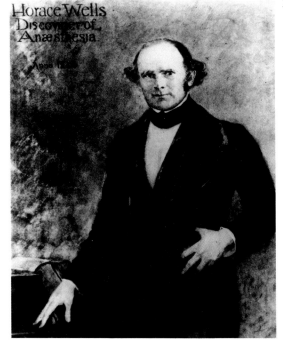

The Connecticut dentist Horace Wells, the first to use nitrous oxide as an anesthetic during surgery, had his likeness painted in 1844, the year of his great breakthrough.

205

William Thomas Green Morton, a Boston dentist, gave the first successful public demonstration of ether anesthesia.

The Claimants Battle for Recognition

When the United States Congress voted to award an honorarium of $10,000 to the discoverer of anesthesia, Horace Wells applied, as did both Morton and Jackson. At this time a new figure entered the picture, Crawford Long (1815–1878), an obscure physician from Jefferson, Georgia. Long claimed that he had used ether for surgical anesthesia in his practice as early as 1842, and he produced affidavits to this effect from his patients. However, his claim cannot be given serious consideration, for he neither introduced anesthesia into his general practice nor wrote or lectured on the subject before any medical group until after Wells and Morton had made their demonstrations. A letter Long wrote to a friend, Robert Goodman, also shows his unawareness of ether's greater importance.

> I am under the necessity of troubling you a little. I am entirely out of ether and wish some by tomorrow night. . . . We have some girls in Jefferson who are anxious to see it taken, and you know nothing would afford more pleasure than to take it in their presence and to get a few sweet kisses. . . . If you cannot send it tomorrow, get Dr. Reese to send it by the stage on Wed'sday, I can persuade the girls to remain until Wednesday night, but would prefer receiving the ether sooner.
>
> Your friend, Crawford Long

The controversy over the discoverer of anesthesia raged unabated for many years until Congress finally withdrew its offer. Horace Wells, after trying vainly to secure the recognition due him, committed suicide. Jackson went insane and was committed to an institution. Morton became impoverished as a result of the protracted legal battles and died a pauper. Long went back to his small-town medical practice. To whom is the credit due? In order for one to be considered the true discoverer of a new technique, one must satisfy three criteria: one must discover something not generally known, must be aware of its significance, and must communicate the discovery to others. Of all the claimants, only the dentist Horace Wells satisfies all three criteria.

Crawford Long was not the only physician who had had the opportunity to make the discovery but had missed it. Among the students who participated in the ether frolics at the Massachusetts General Hospital in 1836 was Morrill Wyman, who in later years was to achieve fame for his use of trocars for the aspiration of pleural exudates. In 1877 he remembered administering ether at a frolic to rats confined to glass globes. "But with all our experiments," he said sadly, "we never thought of trying the sensibility under ether, even by pricking with a pin. It was a great oversight."

The state of Georgia erected a statue of Crawford Long in the Rotunda of the Capitol in Washington, D.C., with the words "Discoverer of Anesthesia" inscribed on it; however, medical historians have rejected this claim prompted by understandable state pride. William Welch of Johns Hopkins University asserted, "We cannot assign to him any influence upon the historical development of our knowledge of surgical anesthesia or any share in its introduction to the world at large." The eminent surgeon Owen Wangensteen also dismissed Long's claim, but was unable to decide whether credit should go to Wells or to Morton.

> There can be little question of the greater influence of Morton's successful demonstration of the efficacy of ether on Oct. 16, 1846, in allaying the pain of operation and speeding the acceptance of anesthesia. Wells had only one scientific publication of Nitrous Oxide (1847). However, survival of the practice continues to be an important determinant in the adjudication of priority. Now, more than 130 years later, it would probably be in the spirit of fairness to cite Wells, with Morton, for division of the honor of discovery. In fact, the use of ether has disappeared in many clinics, while Nitrous Oxide, used in 65 percent of anesthetic procedures, is the more durable legacy.

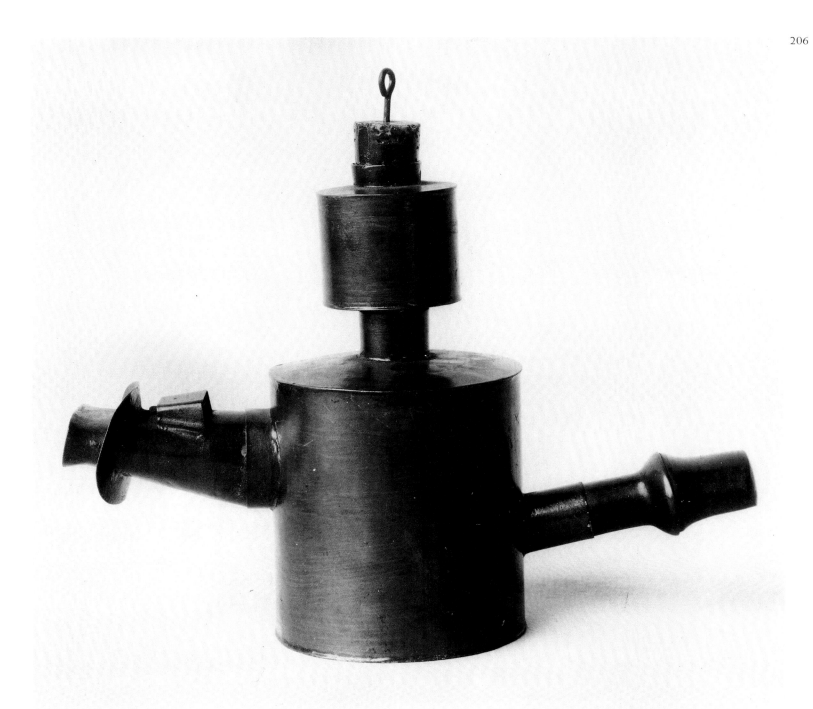

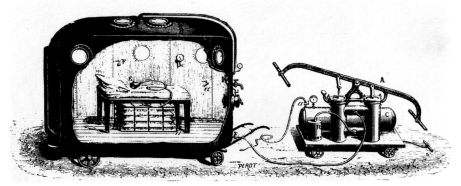

207

This original patent model of the ether inhaler devised by William T. G. Morton is now in the National Museum of American History, Smithsonian Institution, Washington, D.C. Though the inhaler used in the 1846 demonstrations at the Massachusetts General Hospital was made of glass, this model is metal.

During the early days of anesthesia, some doctors decided that smaller (and safer) amounts of nitrous oxide could be administered to a patient if the gas were dispensed under pressure. Complicated hyperbaric chambers were devised—such as this Cloche Mobile, the invention of a Dr. Fontaine of Paris in 1880, which could be moved from hospital to hospital and was large enough to admit ten patients.

Similar conclusions were reached by the major professional organizations. The American Dental Association led the way in 1864 when it passed a resolution that to "Horace Wells of Hartford, Connecticut (now deceased), belongs the credit and honor of the introduction of anesthesia in the United States of America, and we do firmly protest against the injustice done to the truth and to the memory of Dr. Horace Wells, in the effort made during a series of years and especially in the last session of Congress to award the credit to other person or persons."

Six years later, the American Medical Association, at its meeting in Washington, D.C., resolved "that the honor of the discovery of practical anesthesia is due to the late Dr. Horace Wells of Connecticut."

Anesthesia in Dentistry

Just two months after Morton's demonstration and two days before Liston's femoral operation, a prominent young London dentist, James Robinson (1816–1862), performed the first dental extraction under ether anesthesia in England, removing a molar from a young woman. Morton's apparatus consisted of a glass globe into which a sponge saturated with ether had been placed. Both Robinson and Liston devised equipment that differed somewhat from Morton's. And soon investigators were experimenting with different devices for administering the gas in order to control the dosage and render anesthesia safer.

In November 1847, a Scottish physician, James Simpson, introduced chloroform, an easier and more pleasant anesthetic to apply than ether, and countless physicians, dentists, and surgeons on both sides of the Atlantic adopted it enthusiastically. But chloroform is also a very dangerous drug, and soon the early dental journals began to carry accounts of young, vigorous men and women succumbing to chloroform while having their teeth extracted. Consequently, ether again became the anesthetic of choice.

The widespread adoption of nitrous oxide as a dental anesthetic was delayed for too many years—seventeen, to be exact. It was the showman Gardner Quincy Colton who was responsible for its reintroduction. In 1862, at a demonstration in New Britain, Connecticut, a woman in the audience asked Colton if he would give her nitrous oxide so that her dentist, a Dr. Dunham, could extract one of her teeth. Colton did so, and the operation was so successful that Dunham became a staunch advocate of the anesthetic. Within a year he had administered it successfully to more than six hundred patients. Colton, who supplied Dunham with the gas, eventually went into partnership with several reputable dentists and opened a clinic in New York. In less than ten years the Colton Dental Association proudly announced that nitrous oxide gas had been administered successfully on its premises more than twenty-seven thousand times.

Nitrous oxide was used only sporadically by European dentists before 1870. It was through the efforts of an American dentist, Dr. Thomas W. Evans (1823–1897, fig. 208), that it became accepted outside the United States. Evans, Philadelphia-trained, emigrated to France in 1847 to join Dr. Christopher S. Brewster in his successful dental practice in Paris. There Evans introduced two innovative procedures: the use of silver amalgam for fillings and Vulcanite (an inflexible form of vulcanized rubber—cheap, durable, and light in weight) for denture bases. Soon he became dentist not only to the future emperor Louis Napoleon but also to most of the royal families on the Continent.

In 1867 Evans attended the Paris Universal Exposition as U.S. Commissioner to the exhibition. There he met the indefatigable Gardner Colton, who was demonstrating the use of nitrous oxide for dental anesthesia. Evans became an enthusiastic champion of the gas, using it, as he said, "with success in Paris, under my own direction, in the gravest surgical operations." Evans, a careful and responsible doctor, studied the properties of the gas to determine the optimum concentrations to be used and the best methods of administering it, for the procedure was still in its infancy—specialists were not even sure whether the gas should be given with the patient upright in a chair or lying down.

Within a year Evans went to England to acquaint his British colleagues with nitrous oxide. He lectured all around the island and was received in many instances with enthusiasm. The highly conservative British medical establishment, however, made several attempts to discredit the new anesthetic. The medical journal *Lancet* in 1868 offered an extremely negative (and erroneous) evaluation of the drug: "The gas had been treated as an unknown, wonderful, and perfectly harmless agent; whereas in simple fact, it was one of the best known, least wonderful, and most dangerous of all substances that had been applied for the production of general anesthesia."

British dentists were more open-minded and accepted nitrous oxide anesthesia very quickly. It has never been displaced in England as the leading, and safest, general dental anesthetic. In the same year the *Lancet* made its disparaging remarks, the *British Journal of Dental Science* paid glowing tribute to Dr. Evans: "Whatever may be [nitrous oxide's] ultimate fate, the dental profession in England can never forget the liberality of Dr. Evans in devoting his time and money to the introduction among his English brethren of what he believes to be a valuable aid to their labour, and an inestimable boon to suffering humanity."

To measure what the world owes Horace Wells, it is only necessary to imagine the state of mind of a patient anticipating surgery without anesthesia. In 1841 Dr. Alfred Velpeau, France's greatest surgeon of the century, proclaimed, "To escape pain in surgical operations is a chimera which we are not permitted to look for in our days. A cutting instrument and pain in operative medicine are two ideas which never present themselves separately to the mind of the patient, and it is necessary for us surgeons to admit their association." Thanks to Wells, only three years later the sick were no longer, in Wordsworth's words, "doomed to go in company with Pain, and Fear and Bloodshed."

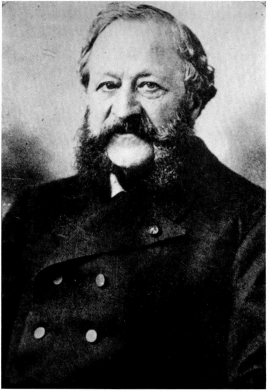

Dr. Thomas W. Evans of Philadelphia, dentist to Louis Napoleon, was responsible for popularizing nitrous oxide as an anesthetic in European operating theaters.

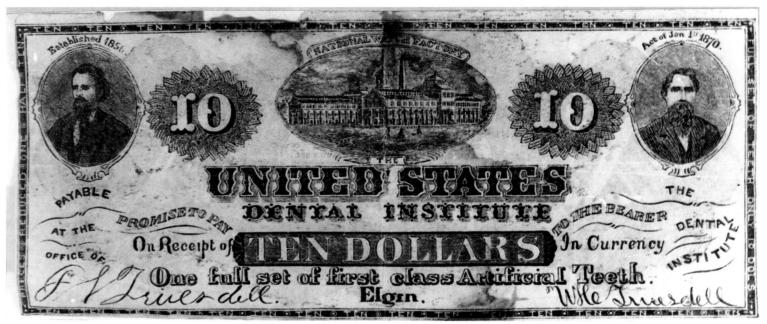

209

Established 1856

Act of Jan 1ˢᵗ 1870

NATIONAL WATCH FACTORY

10   10

THE

UNITED STATES

DENTAL INSTITUTE

PROMISE TO PAY

PAYABLE AT THE OFFICE OF

On Receipt of **TEN DOLLARS** In Currency

TO THE BEARER

DENTAL INSTITUTE

One full set of first class Artificial Teeth.

F S Truesdell.   Elgin.   *WC Truesdell*

1844   79   1875

SIXTY-TWO   S. S. WHITE   PREMIUMS

New York, Jan 3ᵈ 1877

Mess Mayer & Loewenstein

CATALOGUES SENT ON APPLICATION.

Goods sent by Mail will be charged with the Postage.
Goods forwarded with bill for collection on delivery
will be charged with the expense of collection.

☞ All goods are shipped at the risk of the purchaser; therefore, for all
delays or damages, he must look to the transporters of goods, who alone are
legally responsible for their prompt and safe delivery.

BOUGHT OF **SAMUEL S. WHITE,**

Manufacturer of and Wholesale Dealer in

Artificial Teeth and Dentists' Materials,

TERMS: NET CASH.   Nos. 767 and 769 Broadway.

MANUFACTORY AND PRINCIPAL DEPOT: Chestnut Street, corner Twelfth, Philadelphia.
BRANCHES: Nos. 767 and 769 Broadway, cor. Ninth St., New York. Nos. 14 and 16 Tremont Row, Boston. No. 14 and 16 E. Madison St., Chicago.

Please make *Post-Office* Orders payable at Station D, New York.

1 lb # 1 Tooth Powder $ .50

Rcd Paymt
S S White

210

The Establishment of the American Dental Association

During the 1840s and 1850s many new state and regional societies were organized. An association was formed in Virginia in 1842, in Pennsylvania in 1845, and in New York in 1847. By 1859 more than a dozen had been established in various parts of the nation. Organized in Cincinnati in 1844, the Mississippi Valley Association of Dental Surgeons became one of the most influential dental associations in the nation, and its official organ, *The Dental Register of the West*, was soon considered one of America's outstanding dental journals.

In 1855, the year before the American Society of Dental Surgeons was disbanded, several dentists who had not taken strong positions in the Amalgam War formed a new national organization, the American Dental Convention. Although the group continued in existence until 1883, it never had a major impact upon the profession for several reasons. It had no fixed set of bylaws and it admitted to membership even those who were unqualified to practice. In addition, the governing board of the ADC was inflexible and insensitive to the wishes and practice of the majority of the membership.

In 1859, twenty-five delegates representing eight different dental groups gathered in Niagara Falls, New York, and organized the American Dental Association (ADA). An important early act of the ADA was the promulgation of a very advanced code of ethics, which served as a model for the codes adopted subsequently by many state and local societies. The ADA was intended to be a truly national organization, but the outbreak of the Civil War made this objective impossible, and even after the defeat of the Confederacy, bitterness between the northern and southern states prevented dentists nationwide from joining forces. In 1869, forty-eight dentists from the former Confederate states established a Southern Dental Association (SDA). This organization grew rapidly, and its influence extended beyond the borders of the South. By 1897 a number of its members were residents of northern states, including Pennsylvania, New York, New Jersey, and Connecticut, and also California. Indeed, at the century's turn the SDA had a larger membership and more influence than the ADA.

After repeated attempts on the part of the SDA to join forces with the ADA, finally in 1897, at a meeting in Old Point Comfort, Virginia, the ADA voted in favor of a merger, and the expanded organization took a new name, the National Dental Association (NDA).

The combined membership of the two associations remained pitifully small by comparison with the number of practicing dentists in the country. In 1905 Dr. Arthur D. Black of Illinois proposed a bold plan, first implemented in his home state: All the local societies in each state would be combined into a single organization, and membership in any local society would carry with it membership not only in the state society but also in the NDA. Membership in the Illinois state society jumped overnight from 274 to more than 1,200.

During the next eight years, local societies in fifteen additional states regrouped under the Black Plan, which was formally adopted by the NDA at its meeting in 1913. In 1922, when the NDA numbered 33,000, the organization's name was changed back to the American Dental Association. (In 1923 the name National Dental Organization was freely given by the ADA to a group of black dentists who wished to form an organization of their own.)

209

Any person producing this advertising certificate of about 1870, plus ten dollars, would receive a set of artificial teeth from the United States Dental Institute, Elgin, Ohio. National Museum of American History, Smithsonian Institution, Washington, D.C.

210

In 1877 the Samuel S. White Company, then established in Philadelphia, New York, Boston, and Chicago, sold Drs. Mayer and Lowenstein one pound of their number one variety of tooth powder. The bill amounted to $1.50. New-York Historical Society, New York City. Bella Landauer Collection.

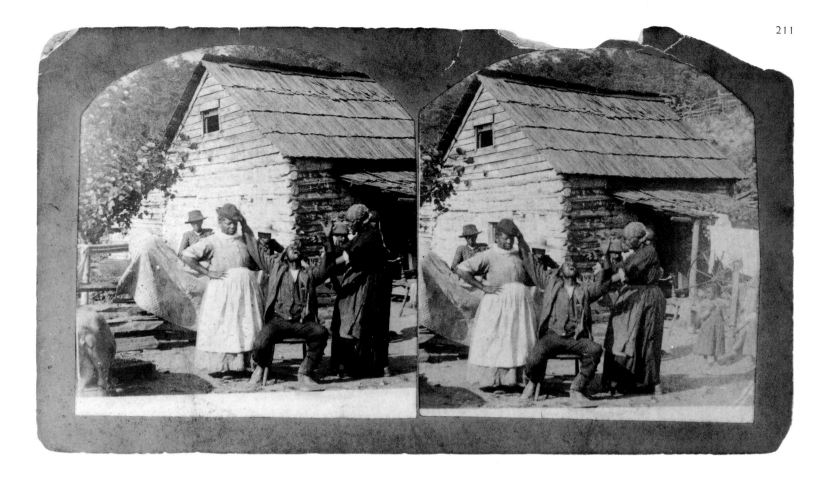

"Aunt Sophia," an untrained practitioner in the Rorer Iron Mines in Virginia did necessary dental work, principally extractions, for the black miners. In this stereopticon slide of the 1890s she appears engaged in an operation while her daughter steadies the patient. Library of Congress, Washington, D.C.

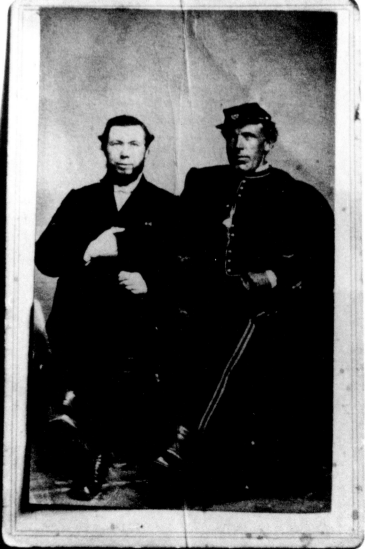

A contract dentist with the Union Army during the Civil War poses here for the camera with his commanding officer.

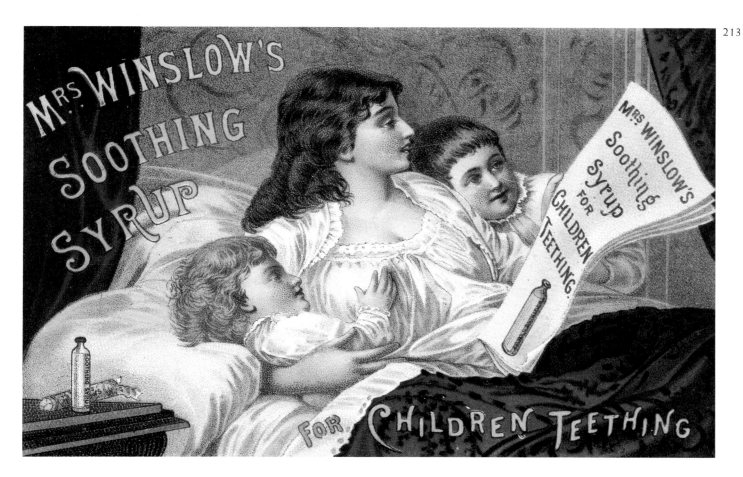

Nineteenth-century Americans were great believers in self-dosage. Mrs. Winslow's Soothing Syrup, a popular nostrum intended to quiet fretful children during teething, contained a high percentage of alcohol. Antique postcard in the author's collection.

This advertisement by a Dr. Shiffman appeared in 1898. Library of Congress, Washington, D.C.

214

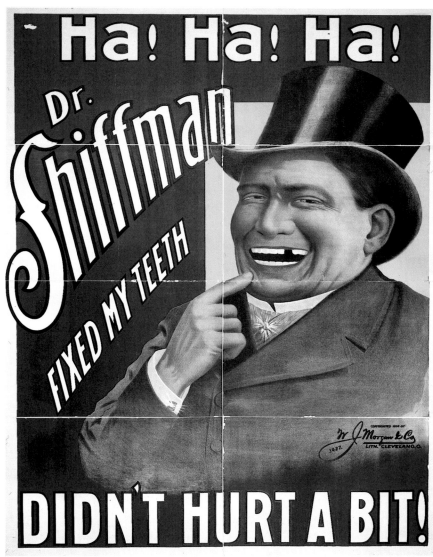

Inventions and Patent Wars

Denture Base Construction

A great breakthrough in the construction of dentures came in 1851, when Nelson Goodyear, brother of Charles Goodyear, the rubber magnate and the inventor of vulcanization, learned how to change flexible rubber into a hard, unyielding substance that he named Vulcanite. It was used to manufacture a variety of products but found its most important application as a material for artificial denture bases. Sold through dental depots, or supply houses, Vulcanite revolutionized the field, and within a very short time supplanted gold as the material of choice in the construction of denture bases. Ease of manipulation was reflected in a marked reduction of dental fees, for rubber dentures cost only about one-third as much as gold dentures.

In 1864 an obscure dentist, Dr. John A. Cummings, succeeded in securing a patent covering the entire process of making rubber dentures, from taking impressions and pouring models, through placing the teeth and fabricating the denture itself. Why Cummings got the patent is a mystery since the Patent Office for twelve years had rejected his repeated applications on the grounds that most of the procedures involved had been in common use for more than a hundred years. Nevertheless, the patent was granted, and Cummings immediately sold it to the Goodyear Dental Vulcanite Company (GDVC), which thereafter insisted that a dentist could henceforth make rubber dentures only after receiving a license from the rubber company for a substantial fee, ranging from twenty-five to one hundred dollars per year, depending on the size of his practice. In addition, a fee was exacted for each denture made, the amount to be determined by the number of teeth set in the denture.

The dental profession reacted in various ways. About five thousand dentists purchased licenses; others went back to using gold; some tried inferior substitutes; and many others continued using Vulcanite surreptitiously. The job of enforcing collection of fees and prosecuting cases of patent infringement fell to Josiah Bacon, treasurer of the rubber company. He blanketed the nation with newspaper notices advising not only dentists but patients as well that they were liable to prosecution for patent violation if they made or purchased dentures of Vulcanite without a proper license.

The organized dental profession formed groups to fight Goodyear's patents in the courts—the United States Dental Union in Boston, the Dental Protective Union in New York, and a number of others—and found a leader in Samuel S. White, head of the important dental manufactory that bore his name and publisher of *Dental Cosmos*, the most influential dental journal in the world (see below). White devoted much time and money and many of the pages of his journal to the fight. Unfortunately, a ruling in 1877 by the Supreme Court against the dentists seemed to spell the end of the struggle. Meanwhile, Josiah Bacon continued to savage the profession, bringing suit across America against dentists who had infringed the patents. By and large he was successful, backing off only in cases in which a vigorous plea proved the defendant had not used Vulcanite at all. Eventually, however, he went too far, pursuing a respectable dentist named Samuel Chalfant, who refused to pay GDVC's fee, from Wilmington, Delaware, to St. Louis, to San Francisco. In each city Bacon secured injunctions against Chalfant, and at the trial in San Francisco he treated Chalfant so cruelly that the dentist was reduced to tears. In 1879, driven to desperation by Bacon's vows to destroy him, Chalfant killed Bacon, a murder that made headlines in newspapers from coast to coast.

215

The struggle against the rubber company's patents resulted in the introduction of a number of substitutes for rubber in denture base construction, but most of them had none of the excellent qualities of Vulcanite; some were soon discarded, others had a longer vogue. As early as 1851, the year Goodyear perfected vulcanization, Dr. Edwin Truman brought out dentures made of gutta-percha, but the material was too unstable and to work with it required complicated equipment. Chapin Harris's son-in-law, Dr. Alfred A. Blandy, in 1856 introduced into his London practice what he called cheoplastic dentures, made of a compound of silver, bismuth, and antimony that has a low fusing point. He imbedded a wax model of the denture in plaster of paris, and after melting the wax he poured in the metal compound. Although his metal denture was never accepted, Blandy's molding and pouring technique was adapted for the manufacture of Vulcanite dentures.

Collodion, a solution of gun cotton in ether, was tried in 1859 as was cast tin (as early as 1820), with little success. In 1866 aluminum was introduced by Dr. J. B. Bean, but he could not eliminate inaccuracies in the cast and found it difficult to attach teeth to the metal. Celluloid looked to be a most promising material, when, in 1870, two dentist brothers, I. S. and J. W. Hyatt, introduced it to the profession; indeed, many predicted it would soon replace Vulcanite because of its translucency and light weight. But within a short time it was proved very unsatisfactory. Dr. Alfred P. Southwick, a leading Buffalo dentist (whose fate, incidentally, it was to be remembered as father of the electric chair, since he headed the commission that recommended this method of execution in New York State), reported of the celluloid dentures he had made: "One by one they came back on my hands; until today the last, I believe, has come, for which I thank Heaven. Some turned black as ink directly; others well fitting and satisfactory at first, gradually warped out of shape or fit; others . . . began to shed the teeth." Happily for the dental profession, GDVC's Vulcanite patents expired in 1881 and the company made no further efforts to press licensing upon dentists.

In 1872 the Eighth District Dental Society, located in western New York State, raised money from its members to carry on a legal fight against the Goodyear Dental Vulcanite Company's patents on the process of making hard rubber dentures. A Dr. Danforth of Jamestown pledged fifty dollars to the struggle. Receipt in the author's collection.

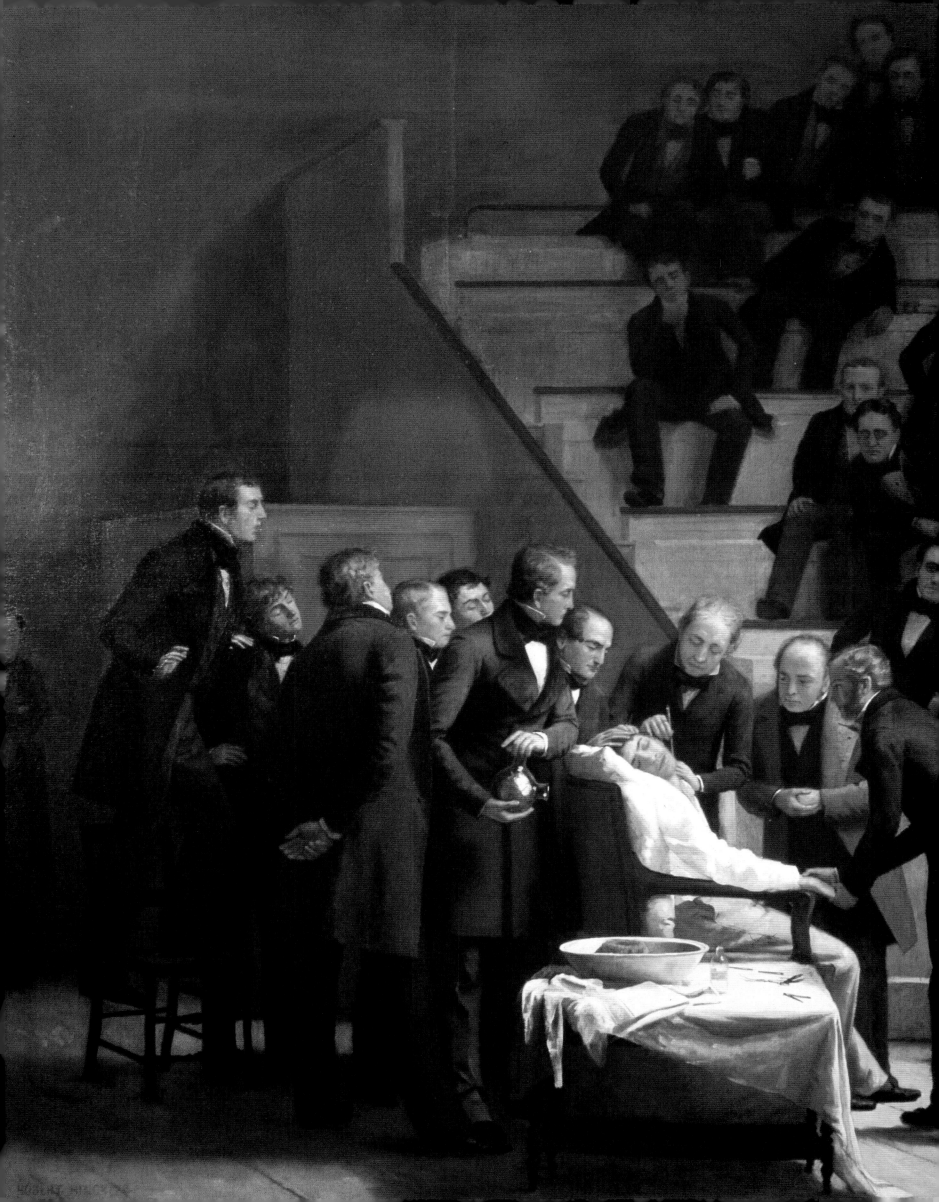

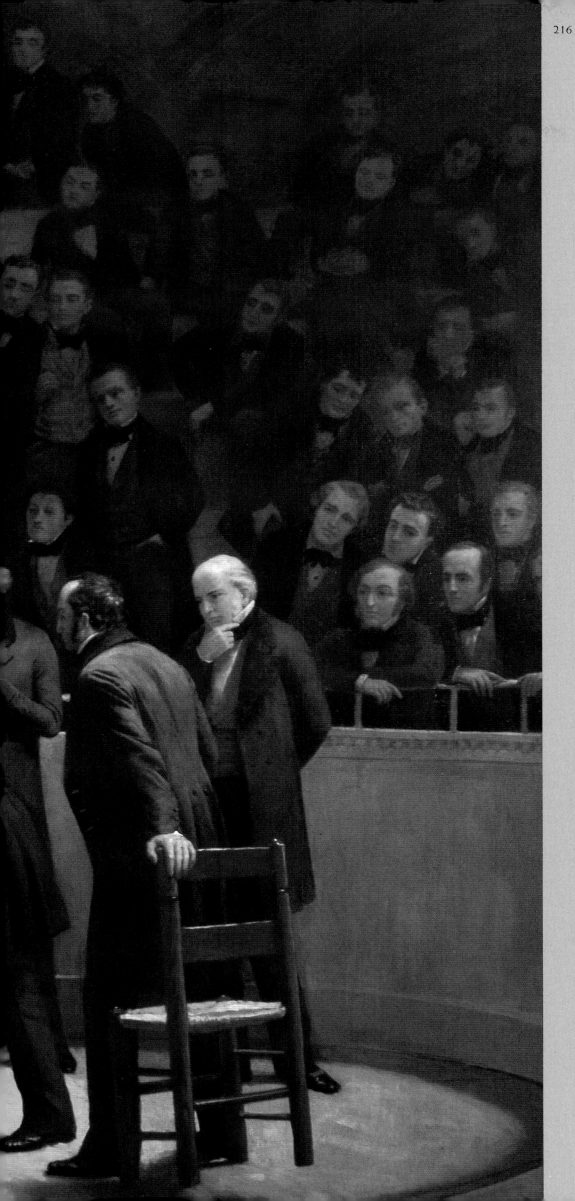

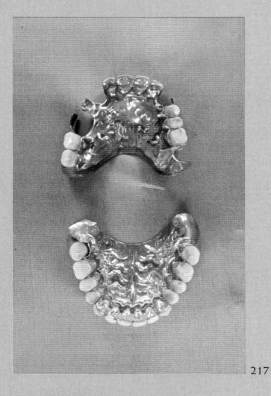

217

By the 1880s most denture bases were constructed
entirely of Vulcanite; however, this full set has a
palate of swaged gold and porcelain teeth set in
Vulcanite. Musée de la Chirurgie Dentaire, Lyons.

In *Ether Day*, a painting of 1882, Robert Hinckley
shows William T. G. Morton's successful demonstration of ether anesthesia at the Massachusetts
General Hospital on October 16, 1846. Morton is
in the center of the picture holding the glass inhaler he devised. The surgeon, Dr. John Collins
Warren, scalpel in hand, is bending over the sleeping patient while an awestruck audience looks on.
The Francis A. Countway Library of Medicine,
Harvard Medical Library/Boston Medical Library,
Boston.

Other entrepreneurs, following Goodyear Dental Vulcanite Company's example, soon attempted to profit from the host of new inventions that were made in the United States during the last quarter of the nineteenth century. For American dentists had by then taken the world lead in introducing new techniques. Some of the most notable improvements were made in bridges and crowns, which, as we have seen, had first been constructed by the Etruscans as long ago as the fifth century B.C. In 1880, Dr. Cassius M. Richmond patented a porcelain tooth soldered to a gold backing. Four years later, Dr. Marshall Logan, a Pennsylvania dentist, patented a crown constructed entirely of porcelain, except for a metal dowel incorporated inside before firing. Though neither the Richmond nor the Logan crowns could be put in place without killing the natural tooth and removing the natural crown, nevertheless they represented a major breakthrough, porcelain being a significantly more esthetic material than metal.

Within a short time more than twenty-five similar patents had been granted. A group of clever manipulators bought them from the inventors and announced the formation of the International Tooth Crown Company (ITCC). Newspaper announcements appeared nationwide, and dentists found themselves threatened with prosecution for making *any* crowns or bridges without paying a fee ranging between one hundred and five hundred dollars to the ITCC. Furthermore, the company immediately brought suit against some of the most prominent dentists in the country.

Desperate situations call forth men of courage, and in this case it was Dr. J. N. Crouse of Chicago who refused to be intimidated. In 1887, at his own expense, he began traveling across the land, urging his colleagues to support his newly launched United States Dental Protective Association. A great number of dentists rallied to his support, and in 1900, after lawsuits were filed by Crouse's organization, the ITCC's patents were declared invalid. When three years later Land's truly revolutionary full-porcelain crown came on the market, dentists and their patients were able freely to reap the benefit.

Charles Henry Land (fig. 219), a dentist in Detroit who had been experimenting with porcelain, in 1888 had devised and patented a method of fashioning porcelain inlays on a matrix of thin sheet platinum. Moderately successful, their application was limited and their fit not ideal because porcelain remained difficult to fuse. With the invention in 1894 of the electric furnace and in 1898 of low-fusing porcelain, Land was at last able to make a major contribution by constructing a full-porcelain crown built up on a platinum matrix. By 1901 a method of fusing porcelain at higher temperatures had been perfected, and in 1903 Land introduced his strong, esthetic porcelain-jacket crown to the profession.

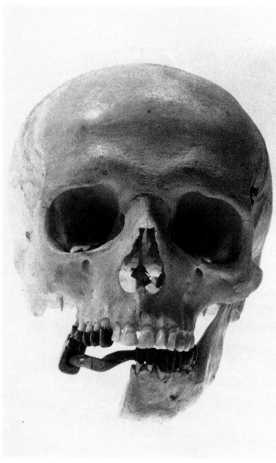

218

In 1890 a unique dental restoration was made for a Massachusetts minister who had had the right half of his lower jaw surgically removed along with a tumor. It consisted of an extensive system of gold crowns soldered together and attached to a hinge device. After the prosthesis was inserted, the patient was able to resume chewing as well as preaching. Harvard University Medical Museum, Boston.

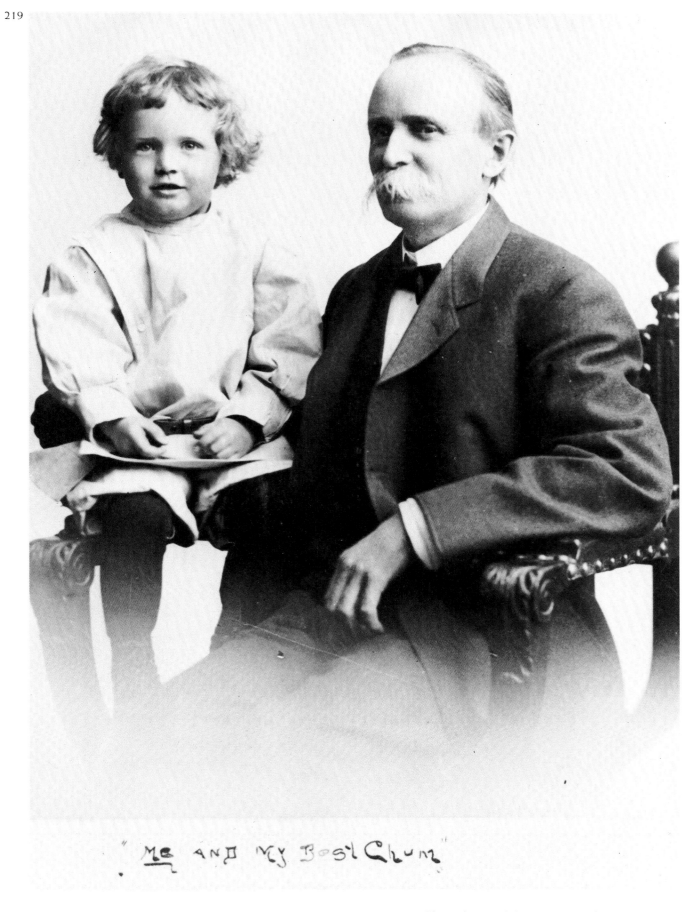

" ME AND MY BEST CHUM "

Shown here with his soon-to-be-famous grandson, Charles A. Lindbergh, is Charles Henry Land (1847–1919), inventor of the porcelain jacket crown. Lindbergh later related that his grandfather used to fire small toys for him in his kiln. National Museum of American History, Smithsonian Institution, Washington, D.C.

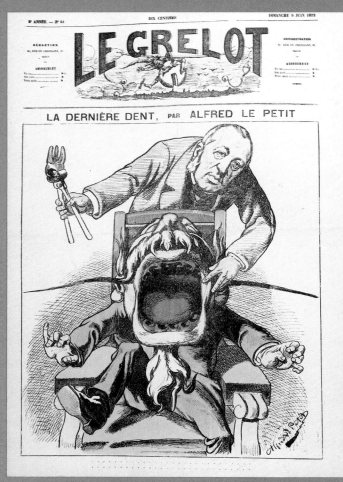

LA DERNIÈRE DENT, PAR ALFRED LE PETIT

220

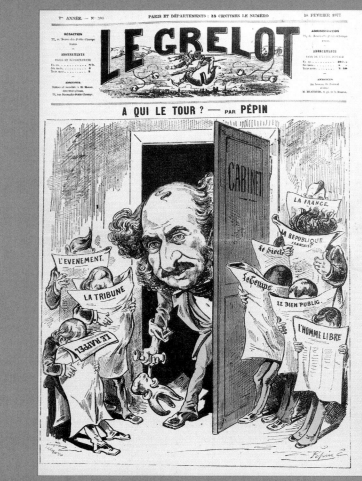

A QUI LE TOUR ? — PAR PÉPIN

221

222

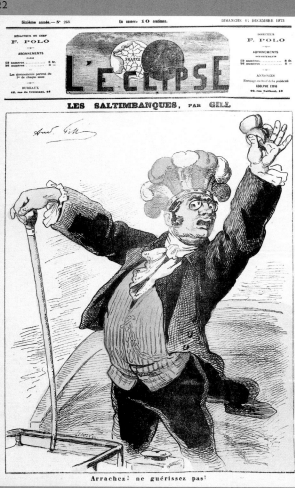

LES SALTIMBANQUES, PAR GILL.

Arrachez! ne guérissez pas!

220

Alfred Le Petit's illustration for the cover of the June 9, 1872, issue of *Le Grelot* is entitled *The Last Tooth*. Collection William Helfand, New York.

221

"Whose turn is it?" asks the dentist, and his patients hide behind their newspapers. Like many nineteenth-century cartoonists, Pépin delighted in wry analogies between dentistry and politics. From *Le Grelot*, February 18, 1877. Collection William Helfand, New York.

222

"Pull! Don't cure!" was the prescription of many dentists before the twentieth century. This cartoon by Gill entitled *Les Saltimbanques (Mountebanks)* appeared in the December 14, 1873, issue of *L'Eclipse*. Collection William Helfand, New York.

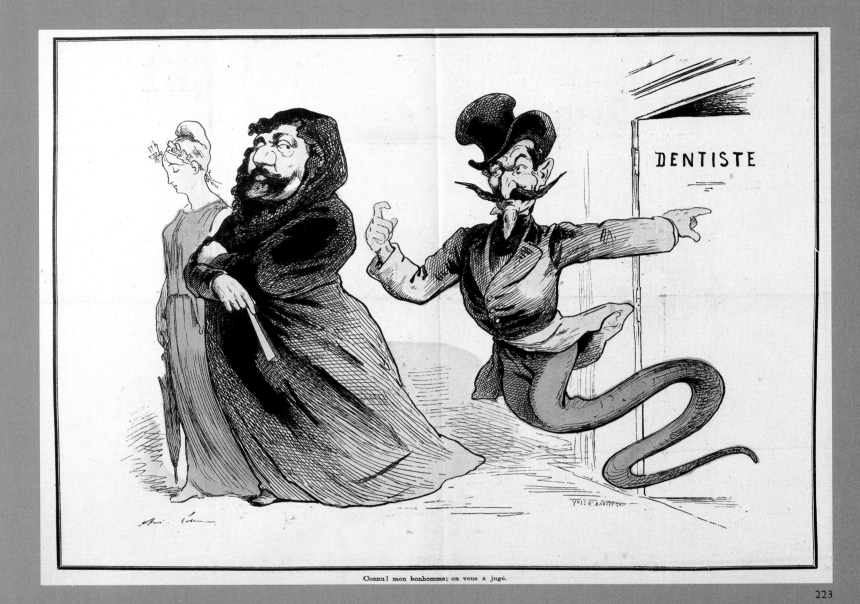

Connu! mon bonhomme; on vous a jugé.

223

As late as 1878, when this cartoon by Gill appeared in *La Lune Rousse*, the dentist's office still had sinister connotations. Collection William Helfand, New York.

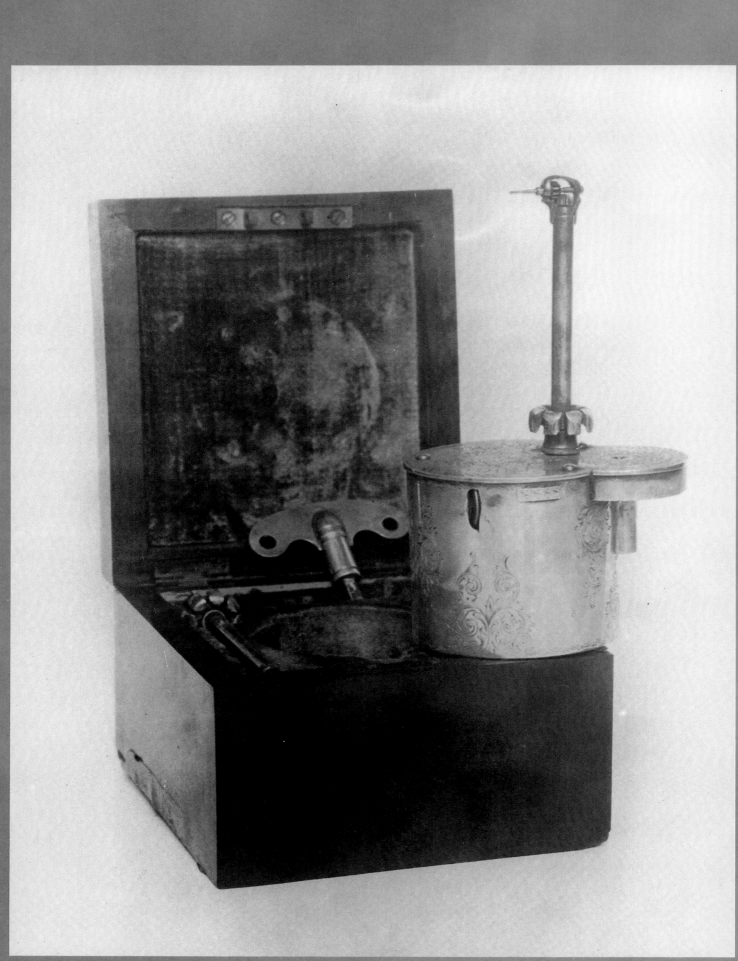

This clockwork dental drill was patented in 1864 by George F. Harrington of England. National Library of Medicine, Bethesda.

With the introduction of anesthesia and Vulcanite, tooth extraction became the alternative of choice in the dentist's office. Tooth restoration remained exceptionally difficult. Preventive and restorative dentistry waited upon the development of equipment that would enable an operator to cut teeth precisely. Since Fauchard's day, different types of drills had been introduced, ranging from the simple ring drill of Amos Westcott, which was spun between the thumb and forefinger, to such elaborate but essentially ineffective mechanical contrivances as the heavy and clumsy clockwork mechanism brought out in England in the 1860s that is shown in figure 224.

Isaac Singer's treadle-driven sewing machine gave the impetus for a breakthrough. Charles Merry of St. Louis had brought out in 1858 a simple hand-held drill that consisted of a short spiral cable that rotated a bur. By driving a variant of this cable with a foot treadle and a series of pulleys, the inventive James Beall Morrison was able to deliver sufficient speed to a bur so that it could cut smoothly through enamel and dentine. He received his patent in February 1871 (fig. 225). Soon thereafter, the S. S. White Company improved on Morrison's design by introducing a flexible cable in which the strands of wire were woven from both directions, thus eliminating the chance of dangerous backlash.

In 1872 the S. S. White Company put on the market the first electric-powered drill, which had been invented by George F. Green (fig. 226). The motor was incorporated directly into the handpiece of the instrument, which was extremely heavy and awkward, and though many improvements were made in the electric drill over the next decade, the majority of dentists continued to use the foot-driven drill because most offices in the country were not electrified. Only in the late 1880s did the illustrious Dr. C. Edmund Kells become the first to bring electricity to his office.

The foot-treadle drill shown here in a patent drawing revolutionized the practice of dentistry in the 1870s. James Beall Morrison, son of a carriage builder and nephew of a watchmaker of East Springfield, Ohio, was the inventor.

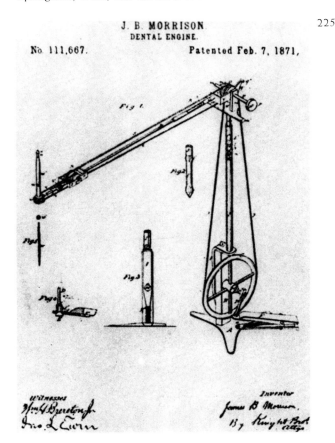

225

J. B. MORRISON.
DENTAL ENGINE.

No. 111,667.   Patented Feb. 7, 1871,

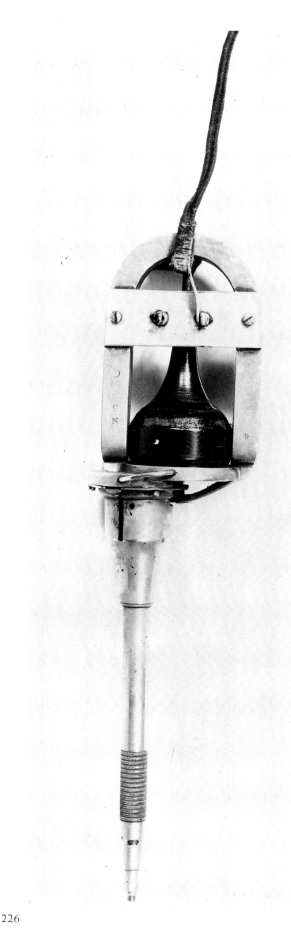

226

The first electric dental drill, shown here in an early photograph, was invented in 1868 by George F. Green, a mechanic of the S. S. White Company. National Library of Medicine, Bethesda.

Dr. Twister's device for retaining timorous patients was a metal door that slammed shut behind them. F. M. Howarth's cartoon appeared in *Puck* in 1874. Collection William Helfand, New York.

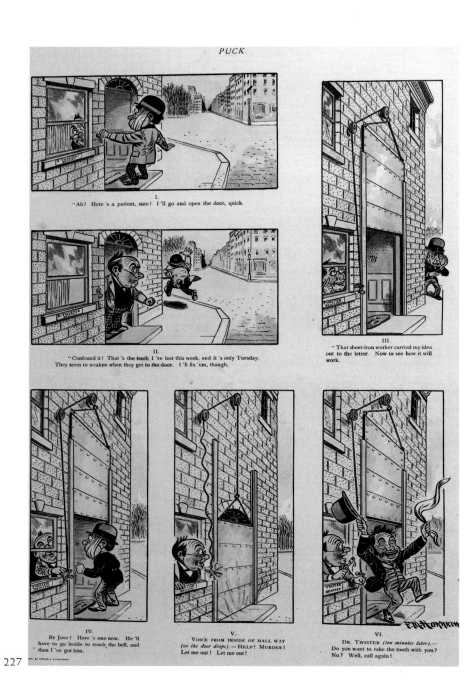

This richly upholstered and decorated German dental chair of the 1890s could be raised and lowered by means of a foot pedal. Library, University of Pennsylvania, School of Dental Medicine.

229

On view in the National Museum of American History, Smithsonian Institution, Washington, D.C., is this replica of Dr. G. V. Black's operating room in Jacksonville, Illinois, about 1885.

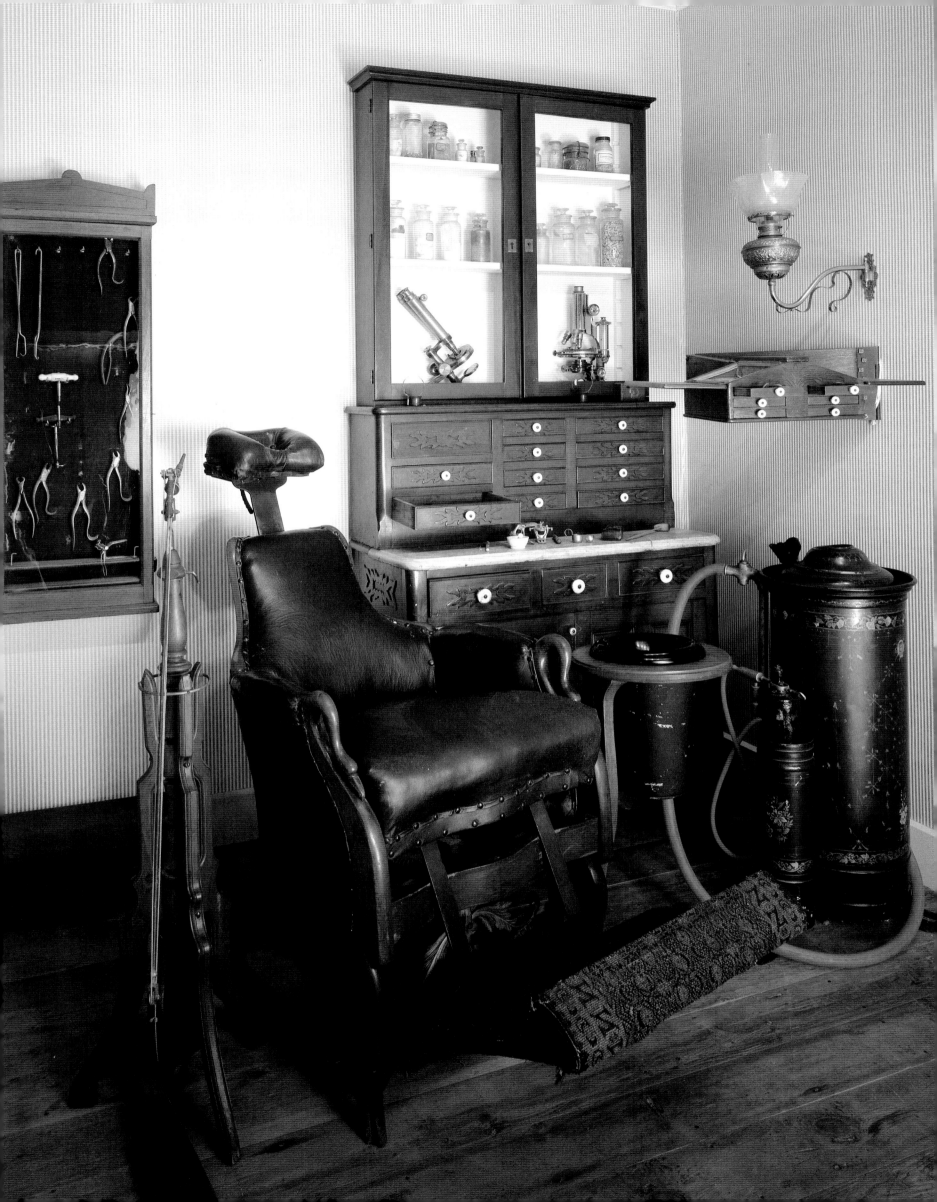

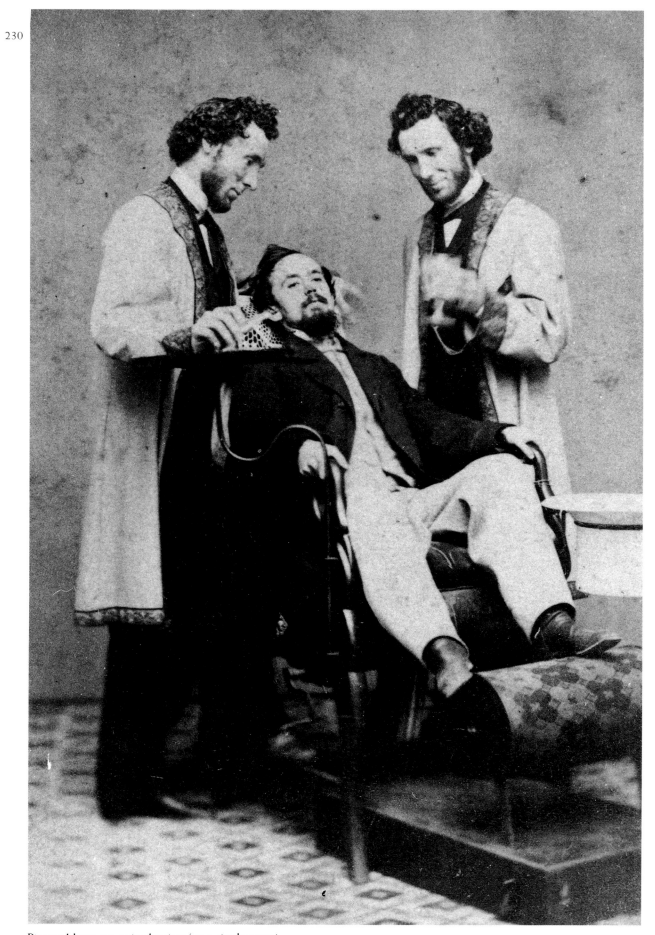

Pictured here are twin dentists (or a single practitioner replicated through trick photography)
about to draw a tooth with an extraction key. The
patient, seated in an Archer's Swan Chair, readies
himself for the operation, which was probably performed about 1870. Edward G. Miner Library,
University of Rochester, School of Medicine and
Dentistry, History of Medicine Collection.

Office Equipment

The first reclining dental chair was made by James Snell in 1832. This was well upholstered and had a spirit lamp and mirror ingeniously arranged to cast and reflect light into the mouth. For many years, however, most dentists continued to use ordinary kitchen chairs, to which they attached a type of portable headrest that was introduced in 1847 by Jones, White and Company, who advertised it as "well-suited to traveling dentists."

Full dental chairs were manufactured by a number of companies in the 1850s and 1860s (generally of walnut, rosewood, or mahogany, these recliners were upholstered in plush, including the footrest). One of the best known was the Swan Chair (Archer's Number 2) because the arms were carved to resemble a swan's neck (fig. 230).

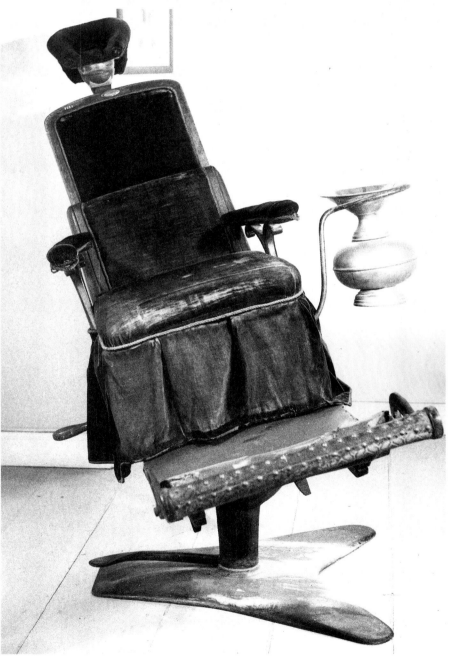

231   James Beall Morrison's dental chair of 1868 had a unique mechanism which allowed the dentist to tilt it in any direction. Despite its obvious advantages, only four examples of this chair were manufactured. Medicinsk-Historisk Museum, University of Copenhagen.

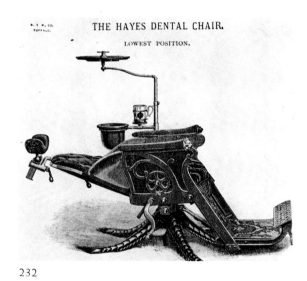

232

The Hayes Dental Chair, introduced by the Buffalo Dental Manufacturing Company in 1875, could, according to the promotional literature, be tilted far enough back to allow a dentist to work sitting down. But most dentists chose to stand at their tasks until about 1950.

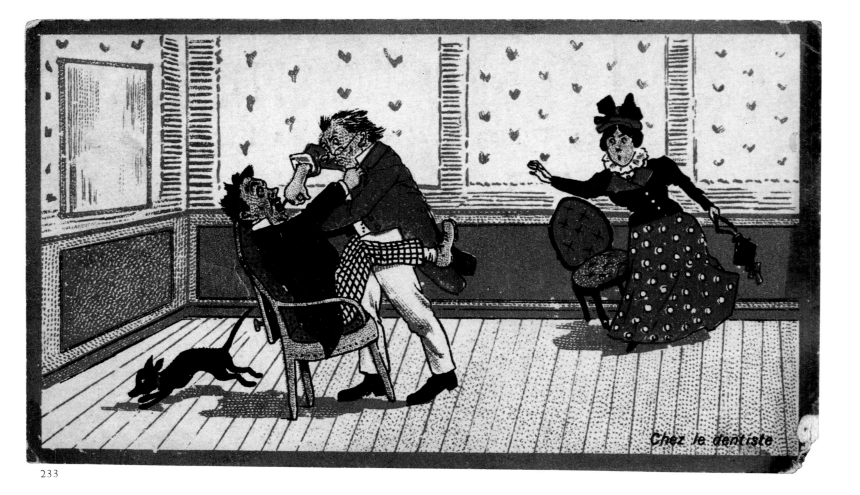

233

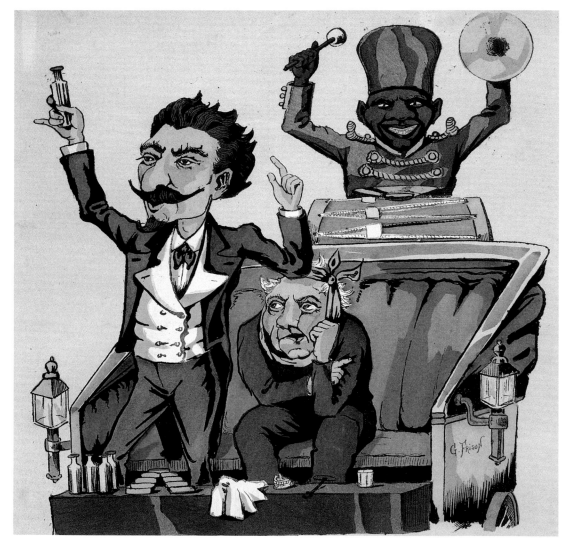

Chez le dentiste

256

234

233

This lighthearted drawing appears on the front of a nineteenth-century advertising card that announces the many and various bargains to be found at branches of the French department store Au Gaspillage. Collection William Helfand, New York.

234

Cartoonist G. Frison lampooned itinerant medicos in this early twentieth-century print. Standing in his carriage, the charlatan makes his pitch, ignored by a pair of assistants who have heard it all before. Not only does he promise to cure constipation and baldness, he will doctor your chickens and cows, paint signs, and attend to your teeth. Collection William Helfand, New York.

235, 236

From 1835 to 1848, the great French caricaturist Honoré Daumier produced thousands of humorous cartoons for *Le Charivari*. Some of these lithographs gently poke fun at dentists and their clienteles. In figure 235, a patient cries, "Ouch! Ouch!" but is reassured that the pain means the tooth is loose at last. In figure 236, a dentist who has pulled two good teeth by mistake thinks quickly and declares that they would have rotted anyway; furthermore, "false teeth never hurt, and everyone's wearing them now." Collection William Helfand, New York.

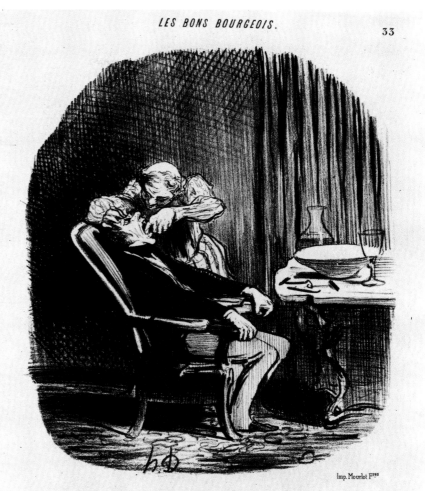

— Oh! la....la....*la......la !*

— *Tant mieux.....tant mieux........ça prouve qu'elle vient!....*

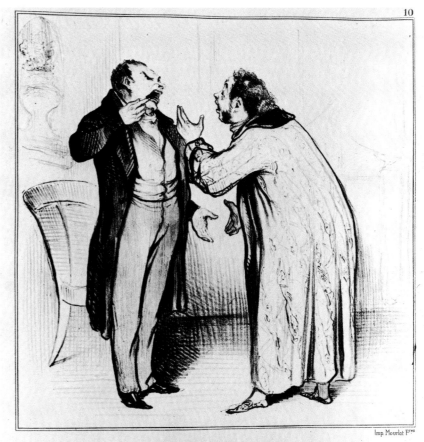

10   236

Robert Macaire Dentiste.

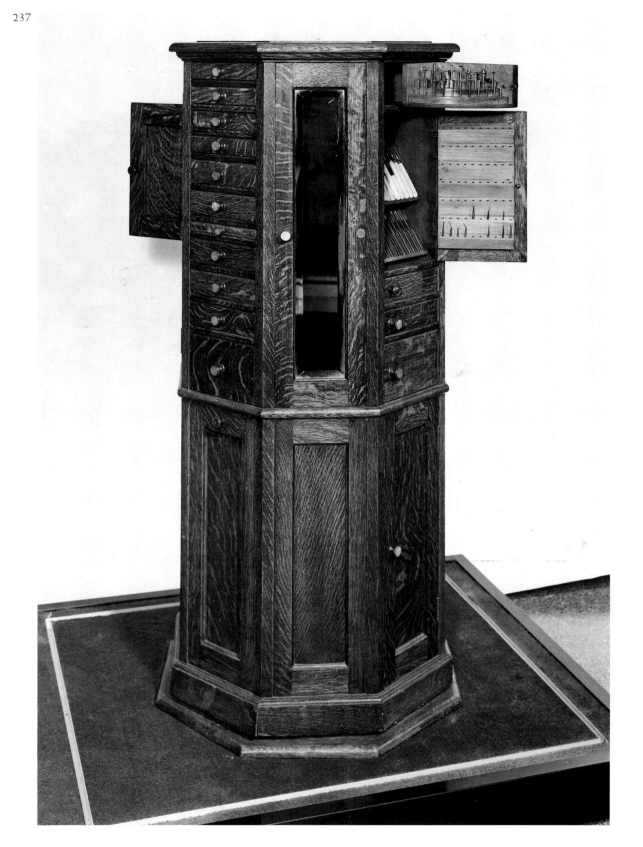

This rotating dental cabinet was patented in 1905. It has twelve drawers, five cupboards, two medicine cases, six swinging drawers, and two forceps compartments. National Museum of American History, Smithsonian Institution, Washington, D.C.

In 1871, the same year that Morrison invented his treadle-driven drill, the S. S. White Company brought out the first all-metal dentist's chair, which could be raised or lowered by turning a crank attached to a central screw. The first pump-type hydraulic chair (the Wilkerson chair) was brought out in 1877, and as an added innovation, it offered a compensating backrest (one that moves to maintain the same position relative to the patient's back).

In the 1860s most dental offices lacked not only electricity but plumbing as well. Patients rinsed their mouths and spat into an old-fashioned brass contrivance attached to the chair arm. Even when the spittoon was enclosed in an attractive cabinet, it still had to be emptied by hand. The first self-cleaning cuspidor, which of course required modern plumbing, the Whitcomb Fountain Spittoon, was introduced in 1867 (fig. 239). Water was supplied through numerous perforations in a pipe surrounding the bowl, and drinking water flowed from the beak of a miniature swan perched daintily on a rod over the basin.

Until the invention of the fountain spittoon, which made the modern saliva ejector a possibility (it was finally introduced in 1882), dentists struggled with the problem of keeping the teeth dry while they were being filled or otherwise restored. Many devices were tried: stoppers that clamped over the openings of the salivary ducts; cotton napkins that were folded and stuffed into the mouth; "bibulous paper"; wax cofferdams; and even an ingenious patient-operated suction bulb that drew out saliva and deposited it in a reservoir on the floor. The big leap forward came in 1864 when, frustrated by the seepage of saliva that made his work well nigh impossible, Dr. Sanford C. Barnum, a dentist practicing in the Catskill Mountain area of New York, invented the rubber dam. Years later he recalled that "on the 15th of March, 1864, a case presented itself of a cavity in a lower molar...in a mouth as wet as—well, as water gushing from every duct could make it." After stuffing absorbent paper around the molar, "in a sort of half-desperate way" Barnum cut a hole in his napkin protector, a thin sheet of oilskin, and tucked it over the paper. Then he pushed a little rubber ring down over the neck of the tooth. To his jubilation, "Over the tooth it went. There I found I had the ring of rubber and an apron combined! There was the rubber dam!" Two months later Barnum demonstrated his great invention before the New York Dental Society, which was meeting at Cooper Union Institute in New York City. Although there were those who scoffed, by 1867 Barnum's dam was being widely used both in America and abroad.

An item frequently found in dental offices of the late nineteenth century was the container in which nitrous oxide was stored. The gas was generally prepared by the dentist himself in retorts purchased from a supply house and then stored over water in an often elaborately decorated nickel-plated tank called a gasometer.

Cabinets underwent many changes, and some very beautiful models were manufactured. Most featured a myriad of small drawers that popped up or pivoted out of the most unexpected places. A finely constructed oak or mahogany example might sell for as much as one hundred dollars. They were made in a variety of sizes so that they could be placed in different areas of an office. One ingeniously constructed octagonal model rotated on a stationary base, occupying a minimum of space, yet offering enough drawers for all the instruments, materials, and medicines that were by then available to the profession (fig. 237).

The dental unit as we know it today did not yet exist, and the dentist of the late nineteenth century used instead a bracket table fastened to a wall by an extendable arm for his instruments. This table, too, was often fitted with tiny drawers for burs and other small pieces of equipment. Until electricity became common in offices, dental treatment was performed only during the day, with the patient seated facing a window. These pieces of equipment and furniture, including a desk, since a separate business office had not yet become standard, plus a washbasin of sorts, constituted all that would be found in the average dental office of the period.

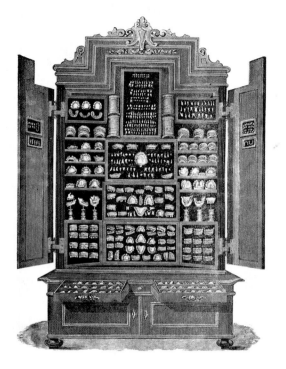

This commodious dental cabinet designed in Italy in 1876 is shown here filled with teeth, dentures, and models for the instruction of students. The Francis A. Countway Library of Medicine, Harvard Medical Library/Boston Medical Library, Rare Book Collection, Boston.

239

WHITCOMB'S DENTAL "FOUNTAIN SPITTOON."

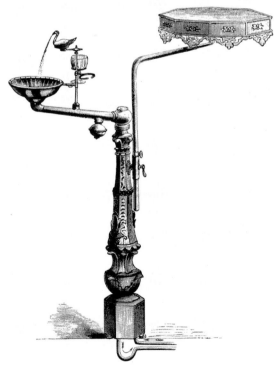

The Whitcomb Fountain Spittoon, introduced by the S. S. White Company in 1867, was the first to feature running water. The Francis A. Countway Library of Medicine, Harvard Medical Library/Boston Medical Library, Rare Book Collection, Boston.

In the 1870s a group of dentists led by the prominent J. Foster Flagg, initiating what they called a New Departure, effectively brought to an end the last hostilities of the great Amalgam War. The basic tenet of the movement was that no single filling material could serve equally well in every case. Gold had its uses, as did silver amalgam (which, in fact, was claimed by the group to be the more versatile material of the two).

A number of attempts to improve the resistance of the amalgam to shrinkage had been made since the Crawcours' day. Thomas W. Evans, who was chiefly responsible for popularizing the use of silver amalgam in Europe, experimented with a mixture of tin, cadmium, and mercury. Though he eventually found it necessary to reintroduce silver into the mixture, tin, which reduces shrinkage, has remained an essential ingredient to this day. At this time innovations to enhance the utility of amalgam were brought out: retentive pins that screwed into the dentine (fig. 240), patented in 1871, and matrix retainers and matrices, which came on the scene in that same year.

To carry the story forward to its conclusion, in 1895 the great G. V. Black, often called the father of scientific dentistry, announced his formula for a truly satisfactory amalgam. After years of experimentation, using instruments of his own design to measure hardness, flow, and other characteristics, Black hit upon a mixture of metals that has remained essentially unchanged: 68 percent silver, with small amounts of copper, tin, and zinc. With this new alloy expansion and contraction could be precisely controlled.

Meanwhile, gold remained popular—indeed, gained some ground when in 1855 Dr. Robert Arthur introduced cohesive gold foil. Since the days of Giovanni d'Arcoli, gold in thin, beaten sheets had been compressed into place in the cavities of teeth with four strong walls against which pressure could be exerted. Weak or damaged teeth could not be repaired with gold. Arthur, who, it will be recalled, was one of the first dentists to receive a dental degree when he was graduated from the Baltimore College of Dental Surgery in 1841, discovered that by annealing gold and increasing its cohesiveness by passing it through the flame of an alcohol lamp, he could insert it with little pressure into a tooth cavity, and, using tiny pluggers with serrated points, could construct elaborate and extensive fillings.

It was in this period, too, that modern dental cements were introduced. Adapted from a substance containing zinc chloride used for cementing mosaic tiles to walls and floors, the first mixtures were later modified because zinc chloride is harmful to dental pulp. The zinc compound was replaced with a weak phosphoric acid, and the forerunner of modern zinc-oxyphosphate cements was introduced in 1879.

The search for a suitable tooth-colored filling material continued, led by the prominent artist-dentist Adelbert J. Volck, who brought out a somewhat unsatisfactory product as early as 1857. Though a superlative product was not available until the next century—the modern synthetic porcelains, or silicate cements— porcelain inlays fashioned to fit prepared cavities precisely were first marketed about 1880. These, however, were of limited application.

240

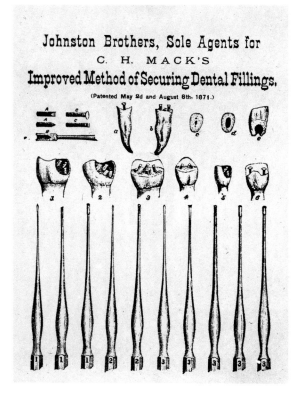

About 1871 Johnston Brothers advertised what was, as they said, an "improved method of securing dental fillings"—pins that could be screwed into the dentine to help retain amalgam inserted into badly broken-down teeth.

241

About 1900 a photographer, perhaps the practitioner himself, took this snapshot of a dental office in Baltimore, Maryland. The all-metal chair is of James Beall Morrison's design. Introduced in 1872, it was the first to feature a compensating backrest. There is no dental unit; a movable bracket table holds the instruments. Although there was running cold water in this office, there was no electricity. A gas lamp fastened to the wall illuminated the room. University of Maryland Health Sciences Library, Baltimore.

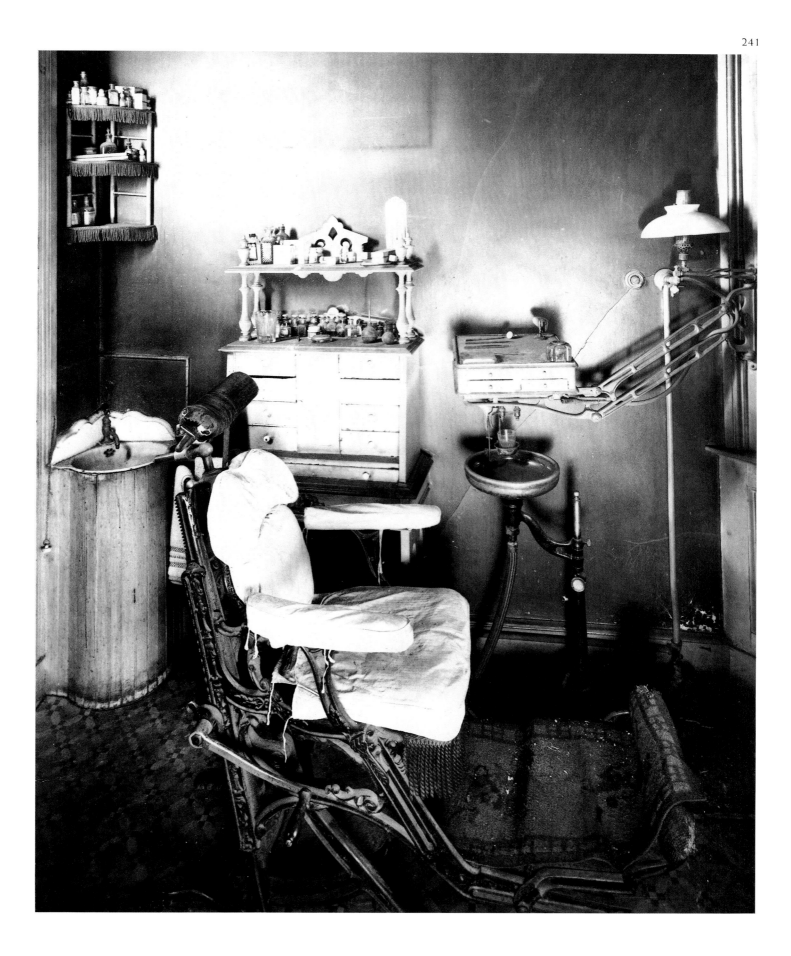

Figures 243–47 show a variety of dentures in different materials manufactured between 1840 and 1880. The Francis A. Countway Library of Medicine, Harvard Medical Library/Boston Medical Library, Rare Book Collection, Boston.

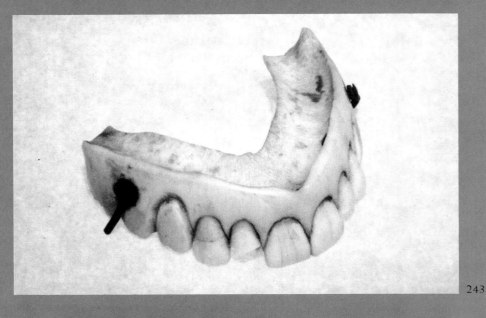

243

Carved ivory upper denture retained in the mouth by springs, with natural human teeth cut off at the neck and riveted to the base, c. 1840.

242

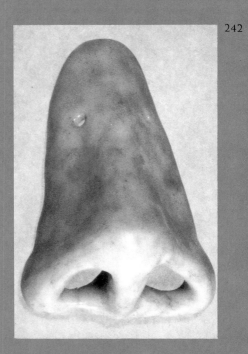

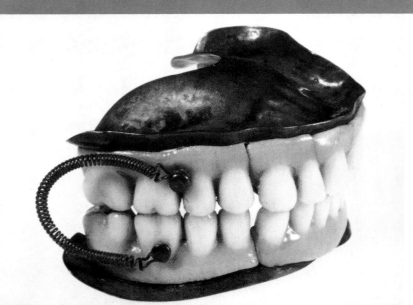

244

By the nineteenth century dentists had become expert in creating many different kinds of porcelain prostheses. Dr. Willard Codman of Massachusetts made this porcelain nose in 1840. A cord could be drawn through the holes on either side of the bridge and tied behind the head. The Francis A. Countway Library of Medicine, Harvard Medical Library/Boston Medical Library, Boston.

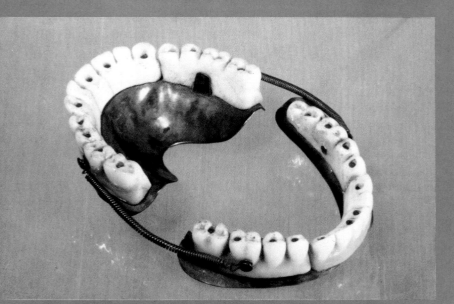

Full denture (closed and open) with porcelain teeth carved in blocks attached to swaged bases of soft silver, retained in the mouth by springs, c. 1850.

245

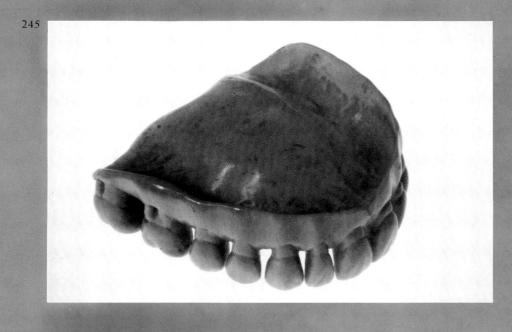

One-piece porcelain upper denture crafted by Dr. John Scarborough, Lambertville, New Jersey, 1868.

246

Partial upper denture with silver base and porcelain teeth made by Dr. P. B. Lasky of Massachusetts, 1869.

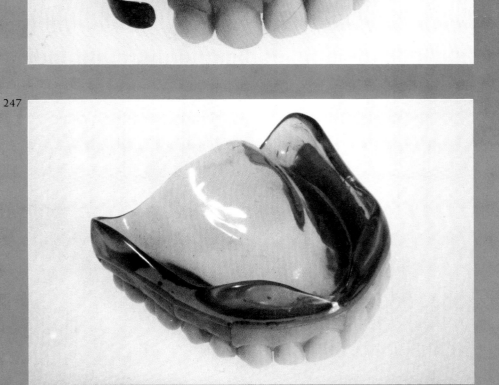

247

Full celluloid upper denture, c. 1880. Celluloid as a substitute for Vulcanite was unsuccessful, as it absorbed stains and odors in the mouth, gradually turned black, and was flammable.

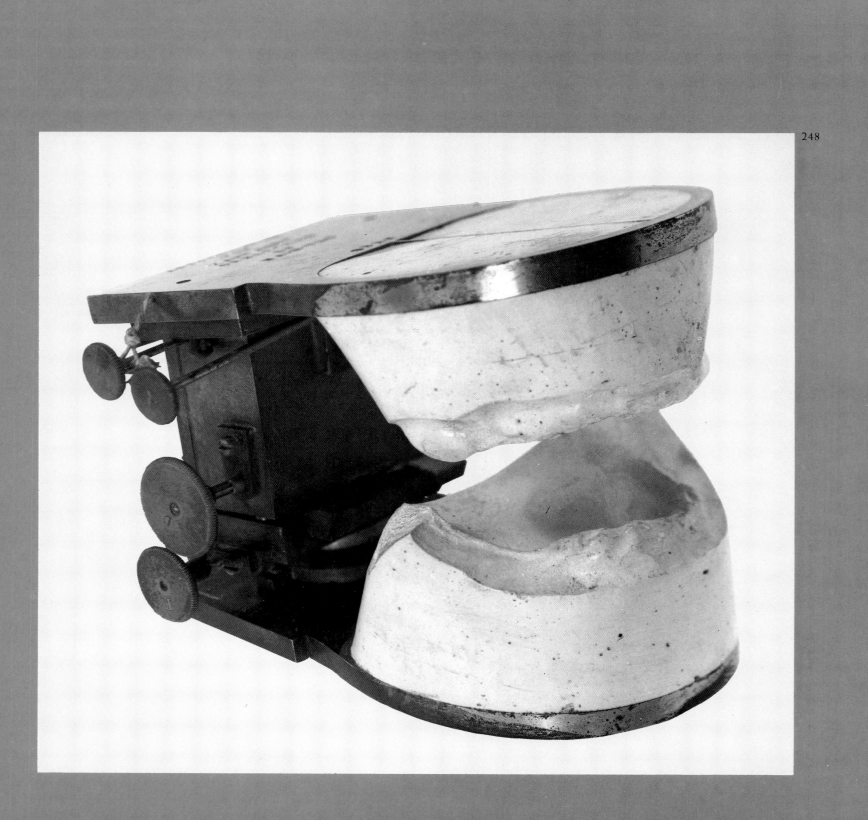

Denture Construction

The metal impression tray, which is used to hold the substance pushed against the gums when taking an impression, had been introduced in France about 1820 by Christophe François Delabarre, and its design had been steadily improved upon in the United States when in 1857 a London dentist, Charles Stent, introduced the first impression compound, a substance that can be softened in hot water and that hardens when removed from the mouth. Some American dentists had used plaster of paris for impressions in the 1840s, and the technique was presented to the profession at large by Chapin Harris in 1853.

The necessity of establishing the correct relationship between the upper and lower jaw in denture construction had been recognized as early as 1756 by Philip Pfaff. A nineteenth-century French dentist, J.-B. Gariot, is credited with having invented a simple "barn-door hinge" articulator. The first articulator that approximated movement in three dimensions, the forerunner of the modern ones that can accurately reproduce mandibular movements, came out in 1840, patented by an American, Dr. Daniel Evans. The first truly superior articulator was demonstrated in 1864 by a dentist who was also a mechanical genius, Dr. William A. G. Bonwill of Philadelphia. His articulator, the first to allow "the condyles [to] move away from the position they occupy during hinge closure," won quick acceptance by the advanced members of the profession and set a standard for the many articulators introduced in the succeeding half century. It was Bonwill who coined the term "articulation" to describe the relative positions of maxilla and mandible during jaw movement (it has replaced the older "occlusion") and developed what became classic rules for positioning teeth in dentures. Unfortunately, much of the new information regarding articulation and news of the many new devices did not spread among the profession at large, and the majority of dentures were constructed by the trial and error method. In many cases, only a protracted period of adjustments and the patient's perseverance resulted in a satisfactory denture.

Bonwill made numerous other contributions to dentistry, including an electromagnetic mallet of advanced design for condensing gold foil; a superior drill-driving mechanism (dental engine); rubber-corundum discs for polishing (corundum separating discs had been invented by Robert Arthur in 1872); cervical matrix forms for holding filling material in place while setting; a diamond-tipped reamer for root canal work; and a specially designed crown.

248

During the nineteenth century several devices for imitating and measuring the movement of the jaws came on the market. Oehlecker's articulator of 1878 was the first in a long line of instruments with an array of knobs and dials that permitted sophisticated control of the movements of upper and lower casts. National Museum of American History, Smithsonian Institution, Washington, D.C.

Dental Literature

When the *American Journal of Dental Science* went out of existence in 1860 with the death of Chapin Harris, the dental profession lost a truly great resource. As Dr. William H. Trueman, a noted dental historian of the 1920s, has rightly observed, the *AJDS* had "a stateliness and dignity, a professional tone and a scholarship that has not been excelled. The twenty volumes published by dentists for dentists, apart, uncontrolled, and unaided by trade or business concerns, have a place of honor among dental journals. It is not to the credit of the profession that from first to last it was published at a financial loss."

From the mid-nineteenth century until the first quarter of the twentieth century, almost all dental periodicals were published under the auspices of dental-supply houses or firms manufacturing dental equipment. Some of these journals were of high quality, edited by responsible and ethical dentists. Some, however, were merely vehicles for advertising dental products. The first dental journal sponsored by a supply company was *Stockton's Dental Intelligencer*, launched in 1843 by Samuel W. Stockton who, as we have learned, was proprietor of a dental depot in Philadelphia. In 1847, following suit, Jones, White and Company of the same city brought out a *Dental News Letter*. Though not a dentist, John R. McCurdy, business manager of the firm, was appointed first editor of the periodical and, happily, he had a keen appreciation and understanding of the problems dentists face. The *Dental News Letter*, which sold for fifty cents a year, soon achieved a secure place in dental literature. By the time the seventh volume appeared, Dr. James D. White, a respected dentist, had joined McCurdy as coeditor. The journal went out of existence about 1860, upon McCurdy's retirement. Shortly thereafter, Jones, White announced the publication of a monthly called *Dental Cosmos*. Three outstanding individuals would produce it: Dr. James D. White, in charge of "original communications"; Dr. John H. McQuillen, responsible for "reporting and dental literature"; and Dr. G. J. Zeigler, covering aspects of "medical and general science in their relation to dentistry." Under their able direction, *Dental Cosmos* became the most influential dental periodical of all time. In its pages were announced almost every major advance in dentistry made throughout the world during the second half of the nineteenth century.

In 1871, Dr. James W. White, brother of the publisher, S. S. White, became editor and held that post until his death in 1891, when the exceptionally well qualified Dr. Edward Cameron Kirk took it over. (After S. S. White's death in 1879, the S. S. White Dental Manufacturing Company assumed the role of publisher.) *Dental Cosmos* remained a force in the profession until 1920, when it merged with the *Journal of the American Dental Association*.

A host of other proprietary journals sprang up in the late nineteenth century, among them the *Dental Quarterly*, of Philadelphia; the *New York Dental Journal*; the *Southern Dental Examiner*, of Marietta, Georgia; the *Dental Advertiser*, of Buffalo; and the especially popular *Johnston's Dental Miscellany*, founded in 1874, discontinued in 1881, when Johnston Brothers merged with S. S. White Company.

Though they were far outnumbered by the commercial organs, a few journals published by dental organizations also came into existence: the *Dental Register of the West*, published by the Mississippi Valley Association of Dental Surgeons, and the *Dental Times*, issued by the faculty of the Pennsylvania College of Dental Surgery in Philadelphia between 1863 and 1873, were the most outstanding. In addition, a few dentists launched journals, some of which were very fine. The notable *New York Dental Recorder* was established as early as 1846, but was sold to a dealer in dental equipment about ten years later because of the financial difficulty associated with individual ownership and publication of a journal.

By 1900 many dental periodicals had been brought out—and had, often in a short time, gone under: *Merit's Dental Messenger*, of Bridgeport, Connecticut; *The Family Dentist*, of Portsmouth, New Hampshire; *The Forceps*, established in New York City by the eminent Solyman Brown; *The Dental Monitor*, of New York; the *Dental Enterprise*, of Baltimore; and the *Cincinnati Dental Lamp*. The ground had been prepared for the introduction of professional literature in the next century.

Women Enter the Profession

In the eighteenth century and the early nineteenth century, it was universally accepted that none of the newly established dental schools would admit women as students. Preliminary schooling as a requisite for admission effectively screened out most would-be applicants since very few educational institutions in America or Europe offered a higher education to women. As late as 1873 the *American Journal of Dental Science* published an article by Dr. Emilie Foeking of Danzig, Prussia, entitled "Is Woman Adapted to the Dental Profession?" Foeking pointed out that only two universities in Europe admitted female students for undergraduate study: Geneva and Zurich. In Germany, she noted, a woman seeking higher education faced even more formidable obstacles: while there were 407 high schools for boys supported by the Prussian state, there was none for girls. Thus, a woman seeking a career in dentistry had immense obstacles to overcome.

America's first woman dentist was Emeline Roberts, who, in 1854, at the age of seventeen, married Dr. Daniel Albion Jones, of Danielson, Connecticut. Within a year she was assisting her husband in his dental practice and studying, at night by herself, the basic sciences. In 1859 she became her husband's partner, and when he died in 1864, leaving her with small children to support, Jones took over the practice and carried it on by herself for sixty years. She was elected to membership in the Connecticut State Dental Society only in 1893, after she had been in practice for thirty-four years!

About the same time Dr. Jones became her husband's partner, Lucy Beaman Hobbs (fig. 249), of upstate New York, decided on dentistry as a career. After graduating at the age of sixteen from a teacher's school, she found employment in a small town in Michigan. There she tried to secure admittance to the newly organized Ohio College of Dental Surgery (OCDS), but even though Dean Jonathan Taft sympathized, he regretted that "women are not admitted as students." Undaunted, Hobbs canvassed all the dentists in the Cincinnati area and finally found one who agreed to take her on as a preceptorial student, Dr. Samuel Wardle, himself a recent graduate. In 1861 she opened her own Cincinnati office, but soon moved to Iowa and established a flourishing practice. Hobbs persisted in her crusade, securing the backing of the entire Iowa delegation to the American Dental Association, who threatened to withdraw from the ADA if she were not admitted as a full-fledged student at OCDS, and Taft at last allowed her to enroll in 1865. Granted the D.D.S. degree on February 21, 1866, she became the first woman in the world to graduate from a dental school.

In 1865, in an unprecedented move, the Iowa State Dental Society amended its bylaws to permit women as members. Hobbs was unanimously elected and was immediately named a delegate to the American Dental Association convention held later that year in Chicago. (There was opposition, however. In the *Dental Times* for April 1866, Dr. George T. Baker deplored the entrance of women into the profession and proposed "to offer an amendment to the constitution of the American Dental Association at its next meeting in Boston, to allow none but males to be eligible as delegates from local societies.")

Other pioneers included Henriette Hirschfeld of Germany, who struggled long and hard for admission to the Pennsylvania College of Dental Surgery (one professor asserting that he "would not teach anatomy to a woman"), and she received her dental degree in the school's first graduating class. She returned to Germany and became the first woman to practice in Berlin. According to her sister-in-law, the Berliners were incredulous because Hirschfeld "was not in man's clothing, she did not smoke, and she was not what the world called an 'emancipated' woman." She was a true ground-breaker, soon taking another woman into partnership. Within a few years many other European women entered the profession.

OCDS can boast another early female graduate of distinction. Dr. Marie Grubert, the second woman to receive a dental degree from OCDS, was elected vice president of the Mississippi Valley Association of Dental Surgeons in 1872, becoming the first woman to hold office in a dental society.

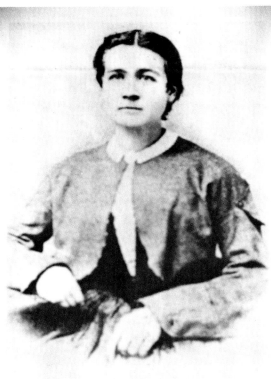

Lucy Beaman Hobbs graduated from the Ohio College of Dental Surgery in 1866, becoming the first woman in the world to receive a dental degree. That year, at the age of thirty-three, she sat for her portrait, shown here.

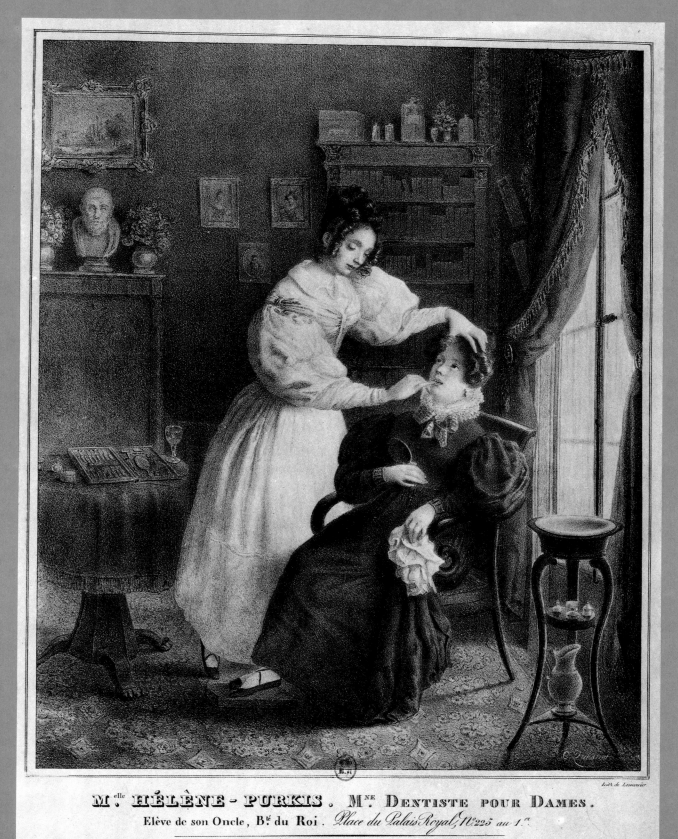

Lith. de Lemercier

M.ᵉˡˡᵉ HÉLÈNE-PURKIS. Mᵐᵉ DENTISTE POUR DAMES.

Elève de son Oncle, Bᵗᵉ du Roi. Place du Palais Royal, N.²²⁵ au 1.ᵉʳ

Cette Artiste, mentionnée honorablement, prévient les personnes qui ont eu le malheur de perdre leurs dents en partie ou en totalité, qu'elle les remplace sans douleur, à peu de frais, avec l'imitation parfaite de la nature.

Elle soigne les dents, les nettoie, les cautérise, les orifie et cherche toujours à conserver celles qui restent : ses conseils sont gratuits. On trouve chez-elle tout ce qui est relatif aux soins, à la propreté et à l'ornement de la bouche.

Son Elixir Diaphénix, qui guérit incontestablement les maux de dents, se distingue de tout ce qui se débite abusivement par la seule raison qu'il est d'une efficacité reconnue et qu'il n'est livré qu'à l'essai et sous condition.

250

Advances in Education, Regulation, and Supply

At the end of the Civil War, only three dental schools existed: the Baltimore College of Dental Surgery, the Ohio College of Dental Surgery (organized in 1845 by Dr. James Taylor, a close friend of Chapin Harris), and the Pennsylvania College of Dental Surgery. Several short-lived schools had come and gone: the Dental Department of Transylvania University, Lexington, Kentucky (1850–52), and the New York College of Dental Surgery, founded in Syracuse by Amos Westcott (1852–55).

The need for another school was keenly felt in the East and several prominent dentists, including George E. Hawes, Norman Kingsley, and William Dwinelle, were successful in setting up, in 1865, the New York College of Dentistry in New York City (today, the College of Dentistry of New York University, one of three dental schools in the world that have continued in existence uninterruptedly from the nineteenth century to the present). The following year, the Missouri Dental College (later the dental school of Washington University) was established in St. Louis.

A step forward of profound significance was made in 1867 when Harvard University established a dental school, the first dental college to be affiliated with a university. Harvard's lead was followed in 1875 by the University of Michigan and in 1878 by the University of Pennsylvania. But progress of this nature was very slow, for although by 1884 twenty-eight dental colleges existed, most of them were privately owned.

Requirements for admission remained minimal. In the beginning there had been none at all. In 1865, at the first meeting of the newly organized National Association of Dental Faculties, "a good English education" was suggested as a requirement for admission, but the level of achievement was not specified, and not until the turn of the century was a minimum of one year of high school required for admittance to dental colleges in the United States.

The length of the period of instruction varied among the individual schools during the nineteenth century, increasing from the sixteen weeks of formal instruction (in addition to preceptorial training in a dental office) required by the Baltimore College of Dental Surgery in 1840, to twenty-two and later twenty-eight weeks at other schools. Harvard introduced stringent requirements characteristic of a university discipline: three years of apprenticeship; classes for two academic years; defense of a thesis; examinations in various subjects; and demonstration of technical skill. By the late 1870s all American dental schools required two years of attendance at classes lasting at least twenty weeks each (strangely, the second year was a mere repetition of the first).

Along with improvements in dental education came efforts to regulate the profession by licensure. New York took the lead in 1868, empowering the state dental society to establish a Board of Censors to examine candidates. In time this body became the present State Board of Dental Examiners. Other states followed suit, and laws regulating licensure were passed in most other states by the end of the century.

Although commercial dental laboratories of a sort had been in operation since the middle of the nineteenth century, they either offered only a very specialized or limited service—vulcanizing, for example—or were merely manufacturers of dental materials. The few that offered diversified services were for various reasons unsuccessful and quickly went out of business. The first major commercial dental laboratory to thrive and prosper was organized in Boston by two enterprising men in partnership: Dr. William H. Stowe, a practicing dentist, and Frank F. Eddy, a toolmaker and machinist. Stowe had developed a reputation in prosthetics, and his fellow dentists often asked his help in difficult cases. In the attic of his home he fitted up a simple laboratory where he worked on jobs for his colleagues on evenings and Sundays. He was eventually approached by Eddy, who suggested a partnership and offered to supply the capital to build a properly equipped dental laboratory to serve the dental profession alone. Stowe agreed,

250

Mlle Hélène-Purkis, a woman dentist who treated female patients, had her offices in the chic first *arrondissement* of Paris during the 1880s. Her advertisement tells us that she did all kinds of dentistry and offered free consultations. A glass containing what may be her special Elixir Diaphénix stands on the table behind her. Bibliothèque Nationale, Paris.

Willoughby D. Miller, American dentist and bacteriologist, first proposed the acid-dissolution theory of caries in 1890.

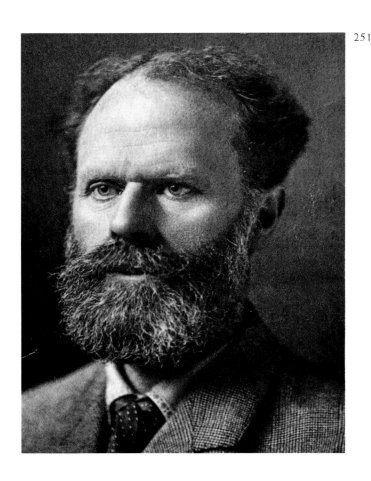

and W. H. Stowe and Company Dental Laboratory opened for business in 1887, having issued a prospectus that read, in part:

> There is a large and ever-increasing number of dentists ... who desire to have their artificial work, more particularly the metal plates, etc., made outside their offices. There are others who would do so, could they be assured of first-class work, which we will endeavor to do. This, as you are doubtless aware, is practically a "new departure" in dentistry, for none have attempted to make a business in itself as we propose doing and we claim that having every convenience and appliance with the best workmen that can be procured, under the personal supervision of a Mechanical Dentist of many years experience, we can do this work—the mechanical portion of it—better than those whose time is principally occupied with other branches of the profession.... You will be convinced that you can better afford to send us whatever work ... your practice may demand, than to wear yourself out in trying to do it before and after office hours, thus depriving yourself of the rest and recreation you need to enable you to do your best work for your patients.

Theirs was an ambitious undertaking, and not the least of the difficulties to be overcome was the absence of "workmen" promised in the prospectus (Stowe gave up his practice and devoted the next twenty years to the training of technicians, which he did with great success). Within fifteen years W. H. Stowe and Company had to build a new and larger laboratory, the finest anywhere, and opened a branch in New York City—so well had it prospered. By the turn of the century several other similar enterprises were flourishing, notably Samuel Supplee's in New York City and A. O. Eberhart's in Atlanta, and the commercial dental laboratory had become firmly established as a valuable partner to the profession, assuming much of the dentist's burden of tedium and drudgery.

Two Revolutionary Developments

During the last two decades of the nineteenth century two major discoveries revolutionized the profession of dentistry and pointed the way to new paths, their effects extending into every aspect of research, teaching, and practice.

Preventive Dentistry: The Work of Willoughby D. Miller

Dentists had for centuries confronted what was a presumably unalterable circumstance. Teeth decayed, and it was the task of the dentist to repair them. Preventive dentistry was an impossibility until some basic knowledge of the nature of decay was secured. It was an American scientist, Willoughby D. Miller (fig. 251), who opened the door to a solution with his classic work on the microbiology of the mouth.

Armed with a B.A. degree in chemistry, physics, and applied mathematics granted by the University of Michigan in 1875, Miller went to Europe to continue his studies in chemistry and physics. In Berlin he met an American dentist who practiced there, Dr. Frank P. Abbott, who advised him to enter the field of dentistry because the profession needed men with scientific training such as he possessed. Miller entered Dr. Abbott's office as a preceptorial student, but within a short time returned to the United States and, in 1879, received a D.D.S. degree from the University of Pennsylvania. Thereupon, he returned to Berlin and entered practice with Dr. Abbott, whose daughter he married. In 1884 he became professor of operative dentistry at the University of Berlin, the first foreigner ever to receive a professorial appointment in a German university. While practicing he continued his studies and earned the M.D. degree. During the 1880s he did a vast amount of original research on all aspects of dentistry, stimulated by study of bacteriology under the renowned Robert Koch, discoverer of the cause of tuberculosis. Miller's work culminated in the publication of a major opus, *Microorganisms of the Human Mouth*, in 1890.

The book's revolutionary thesis was that carbohydrates trapped around the teeth were fermented by bacterial components of the normal oral flora and the resulting acids decalcified the tooth enamel; other bacteria then entered the tooth through the initial defect and destroyed the underlying dentine. Dentists eagerly accepted Miller's theory. Taking up the battle against tooth decay along the lines Miller had suggested, and armed with the somewhat simplistic slogan "A clean tooth never decays," they launched a campaign to teach oral hygiene to the public. Because he lacked clinical experience, Miller had not fully appreciated the role plaque plays in both caries and periodontal disease, and it eventually became clear that toothbrushing alone will fail to stop the ravages of decay. Then other researchers took steps to develop dentifrices and medicinal washes that might counter the destructive acids. In fact, all future work in the field of caries prevention was based on Miller's initial research.

Miller's discovery led to many improvements in the general practice of dentistry: more stringent exercise of oral prophylaxis by both dentist and patient; greater care in sterilization; and eventually the development of modern cavity-preparation techniques, by the great G. V. Black (see below). It also furthered immeasurably the study of pulp disease (endodontics) and oral pathology and provided a solid incentive for research in all the other areas of dental science.

Miller, the outstanding dental scientist of his generation, received many professional honors, and in 1885 his alma mater conferred on him an honorary Ph.D. As he was extremely interested in the organization of the profession, he was appointed the leader of many such groups, and served them with distinction. He was president of the Central Association of German Dentists for six years, and at the important Fourth International Dental Meeting in St. Louis in 1904 was elected president of the Fédération Dentaire Internationale. At this meeting he was offered the deanship of the School of Dentistry of the University of

Michigan. He accepted, and in July 1907, returned with his family to America, but before he could take up his new duties he died suddenly at the age of fifty-four, of peritonitis contracted after his appendix ruptured.

His death shocked and saddened the entire scientific community. But his legacy was an enduring one, for he had put dental research on a sound biological basis.

252

This last photograph of Wilhelm Roentgen, the discoverer of X rays, was taken shortly before his death in 1923. Collection Museum of Medical History, Stockholm.

Radiography: The Work of Wilhelm Conrad Roentgen and C. Edmund Kells

The development of X-ray photography, or radiography, ranks only slightly less in importance than the discovery of anesthesia in the progress of the healing arts. A great deal of experimentation with the effects of electric currents as they passed through vacuum tubes was being done in Germany in the 1880s. Heinrich Ruhmkorff had invented the induction coil, Heinrich Geissler had succeeded in evacuating all air from a glass globe, and Johann Hittorf had discovered the cathode ray, which was created when electricity generated by Ruhmkorff's coil passed through Geissler's tube.

The investigation of these cathode rays was a particular interest of Wilhelm Conrad Roentgen's. One day in 1895, while experimenting in the Würzburg Physical Institute, he noticed that a sheet of paper coated with barium platino-cyanide lit up every time the electric current surged through a tube. Even more mysterious: this happened even when the tube was inside a black box. Roentgen (fig. 252) reasoned that this effect could not have been due solely to cathode rays but must derive from a hitherto unknown ray of much greater penetrating power.

Roentgen pursued his investigation in a precise and scientific manner. By putting a hand between the paper and the tube and intermittently switching the tube on and off, he found he could make the paper glow at will. He was puzzled, though, to discover that when he reached for the paper a peculiar black line moved along it in the same way he moved his hand. He asked a physiologist working in a neighboring laboratory to take a look and the latter identified the image as the bones in Roentgen's arm!

Working for weeks in solitude, Roentgen exposed numerous photographic plates to the rays, having first covered portions of his plates with different objects: a platinum disc, a compass, a box with weights, even a double-barreled shotgun. In each case, a shadow picture of the object appeared on the film. Roentgen published his discovery in the last ten pages of the December 1895 issue of the *Proceedings of the Physical-Medical Society* (of Würzburg) and he sent reprints to about a hundred colleagues around the world. Reaction was instantaneous. The scientific world wanted to learn more about the mysterious emanations that Roentgen had named X rays, and soon the popular press filled pages with stories about the photographs Roentgen had taken and the ability of the rays to penetrate solid substances. A prophetic note was sounded by the *Frankfurter Zeitung* on January 7, 1896, only ten days after the initial publication of Roentgen's paper: "Biologists and physicians, especially surgeons, will be very much interested in the practical uses of these rays, because they offer prospects of constituting a new and very valuable aid in diagnosis."

Honors and awards were heaped upon Roentgen and in 1901 he received the first Nobel prize in physics. In typically generous manner he willed the prize money to the University of Würzburg to use in the interest of science. Roentgen's fortunes ebbed, however, with that of the German nation in the aftermath of World War I. Intestinal illness aggravated by poor nutrition in those lean years ravaged his health, and he died on February 10, 1923 at the age of seventy-eight.

The application of the X ray to diagnosis in dentistry was made possible by the pioneering work of C. Edmund Kells (fig. 253), a New Orleans dentist, one of the profession's most innovative geniuses. The son of a prominent dentist, Kells was born in 1856. After spending several years in his father's office learning laboratory techniques, he enrolled in the New York College of Dentistry, from which he was graduated in 1878. Returning to New Orleans to practice with his father, he soon developed a reputation as an outstanding clinician.

Kells also possessed an insatiable curiosity and a genius for invention; more than thirty patents were granted to him for devices with a wide range of applications: a fire extinguisher, an automobile jack, and the starter and brake that are still used today in every building elevator. In dentistry he was also a trailblazer. Not satisfied with the storage batteries that powered some of his equipment, he was the first in the United States to connect his dental office electrically to a central power station, and he also built the first dental engine to run on commercially produced current (fig. 254). He introduced compressed air into the dental office and found many uses for it. One of his most notable inventions was a suction pump that found use not only in dentistry but in every field of surgery where rapid aspiration of fluids was required to clear the operating field. "This invention alone," said one grateful surgeon, "is sufficient to immortalize the name of Dr. Kells, and has won for him the eternal gratitude of every working surgeon in the land." Always progressive, Kells hired a young woman as a chair assistant—a new departure frowned upon by his more conservative father. It was in the field of radiology, however, that Kells made his greatest contribution to dentistry. Upon learning of Roentgen's discovery, he immediately ordered equipment to build his own X-ray machine, the first in America. He fitted out a room in his home as a laboratory and with his assistant as subject, took the first dental X ray in America. With no guide as to the correct exposure time, he seated the patient "in a chair with the film holder in position. With the teeth held together and the mouth closed, she could swallow without causing any movement of the film. With the face leaning against a firmly fixed thin board in order to steady her, the tube was placed on the other side of the board. Thus, I unknowingly used a filter, which possibly prevented my patient from being burned during the long exposure." Kells cut his film himself from large sheets, and wrapped them in black paper and placed them in a rubber dam to keep them dry while in the mouth. He also devised a simple film holder made from modeling compound.

In July 1896, only eight months after Roentgen's discovery was published, Kells demonstrated the use of X rays in dentistry before a meeting of the Southern Dental Association in Asheville, North Carolina, transporting his own delicate but heavy equipment from New Orleans to Asheville.*

Unfortunately, Kells learned too late the dangers inherent in the remarkable rays and as a result of having often held the film in place with his own fingers, he developed cancer in his right hand. Twenty agonizing years followed, during which time Kells underwent forty-two operations, progressively losing hand, arm, and shoulder. Nevertheless, he continued to serve the profession he loved, devising instruments that could be used with one hand, lecturing widely (preventive dentistry and the conservation of teeth had become major interests), contributing more than one hundred fifty articles to leading dental publications, and writing several books.

But the intense suffering proved too much even for a man of Kells's determination, and to spare his family further distress, he took his own life on May 7, 1928, at the age of seventy-two.

Although Kells had laid a substantial foundation, dentists were very slow in adopting the remarkable new tool. Popular opinion had it that X-raying was too difficult for anyone but a specialist and that its application to dentistry was limited to rare and extraordinary cases. Thus, by the time another pioneer dental radiologist, Dr. Howard W. Raper, took up its study in 1909, fewer than a dozen American dentists had followed Kells's lead, and the situation was no different in Europe. At that time, and for several years thereafter, no commercial dental X-ray machine existed on the market.

*The first public demonstration of the potential of X rays in dental analysis had been made some three months earlier in America by Dr. William J. Morton, at a meeting of the New York Odontological Society on April 24, 1896. Morton, however, radiographed skeletal teeth, not the teeth of a living person; moreover, as a physician who was not a dentist, he chose teeth as his subject simply because they were available and easy to photograph, not out of any professional interest.

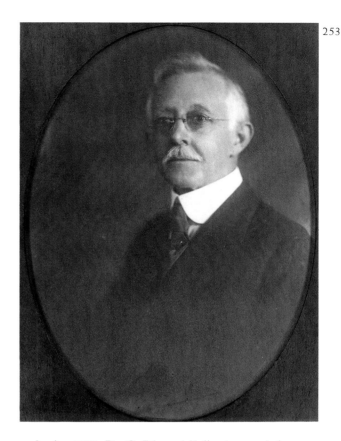

In the 1890s Dr. C. Edmund Kells pioneered the infant field of dental radiography. He was innovative in many other areas, being the first to electrify his office from a central power station and to employ a female assistant. National Museum of American History, Smithsonian Institution, Washington, D.C.

In 1887 Dr. C. Edmund Kells patented this electrical control panel, to which a motor-driven handpiece as well as a mallet to insert gold-foil fillings could be attached.

254

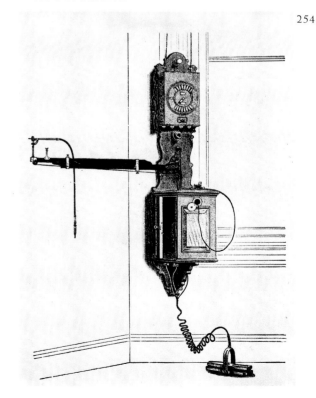

A Dentist Famous to All Ages: Greene Vardiman Black

Surrounding the top of the Illinois State Building in Springfield is a frieze containing the names of sixty-one prominent sons of the state. Beside the names of Abraham Lincoln, Stephen Douglas, and Ulysses S. Grant is the name of Greene Vardiman Black. It was Black (fig. 256) who truly brought dentistry into the modern world and put it on the solid, scientific foundation it now occupies. The impact of Black's work and teaching was concentrated at the end of the nineteenth century, and it is fitting that this chapter end with an account of the life and accomplishments of this remarkable individual.

He was born in Scott County, Illinois, in 1836, one of eight children of a farmer and cabinetmaker. As a youngster he had an aversion to study and rarely attended school. At seventeen, he was sent to Clayton, Illinois, where his older brother, Thomas, was a practicing physician. For four years he "read and rode" with his brother, learning as much medicine as he could.

At the age of twenty-one he moved to Mt. Sterling, Illinois, and became associated with the dentist J. C. Speer, because he found that dentistry appealed more to his mechanical abilities than did medicine. He watched Speer and did some minor work; then, after only four months, he moved to Winchester, Illinois, where he hung out his shingle as a dentist. There, he became friendly with the local gunsmith and watchmaker, and from them he acquired many skills that he later put to use in designing and constructing instruments for his practice and research.

In 1862 Black entered the Union Army as a scout, but an injury to his knee led to his discharge in 1864. While he was in the army, his infant son died and his wife also succumbed to the dreaded "consumption." With no domestic ties, he moved to Jacksonville, Illinois, where he was to remain until 1897.

Jacksonville, the Athens of the West, was the site of the first college in the state and had a reputation as an intellectual center. It boasted three dentists and a dozen physicians, and association with them was fruitful and stimulating for Black. He married for the second time and had three children, among them Arthur D. Black, who like his illustrious father became a renowned teacher.

In Jacksonville Black became acquainted with David Prince, a progressive physician who introduced him to the writings of Darwin, Virchow, and other leading thinkers of the day. Black aided Prince in his practice, helping to quell a typhoid epidemic. When a medical society was established in Morgan County, Black participated in its activities. In 1878 was passed the first Illinois Medical Practice Act, requiring every physician to register. Black could have received a license by virtue of his training with his older brother, but he elected to stand examination, which he passed with an excellent score. He thus became a licensed physician on January 15, 1878. (Incidentally, Black helped Thomas, who was a member of the state legislature, to write the first Illinois Dental Practice Act, which became law in 1881, and from 1881 to 1887 G. V. Black served as president of the State Board of Dental Examiners.) Black's operating room in Jacksonville is on view in the National Museum of American History, in Washington, D.C. (fig. 229).

Black was accustomed to travel to St. Louis, about one hundred and seventy-five miles away, to attend meetings of the Missouri Dental Society, and there he became acquainted with some of the leaders of the dental profession and read voluminously in the books he borrowed from their private libraries. He attended meetings of the Illinois Dental Society in Springfield beginning in 1868, presenting papers there for more than thirty years. The subject of his first address, given in 1869, was "Gold Foil," a particular interest, for Black had become aware that gold fillings, in time, lost their cohesiveness and had decided to find out why. To do so he taught himself chemistry and fitted up a laboratory. So proficient did he become that he was asked to teach a course in chemistry for the high-school teachers of Jacksonville.

During the last quarter of the nineteenth century, much work of scientific importance was being done in Germany. But Black knew no German, so he set himself the task of studying the language with a local German-Jewish merchant.

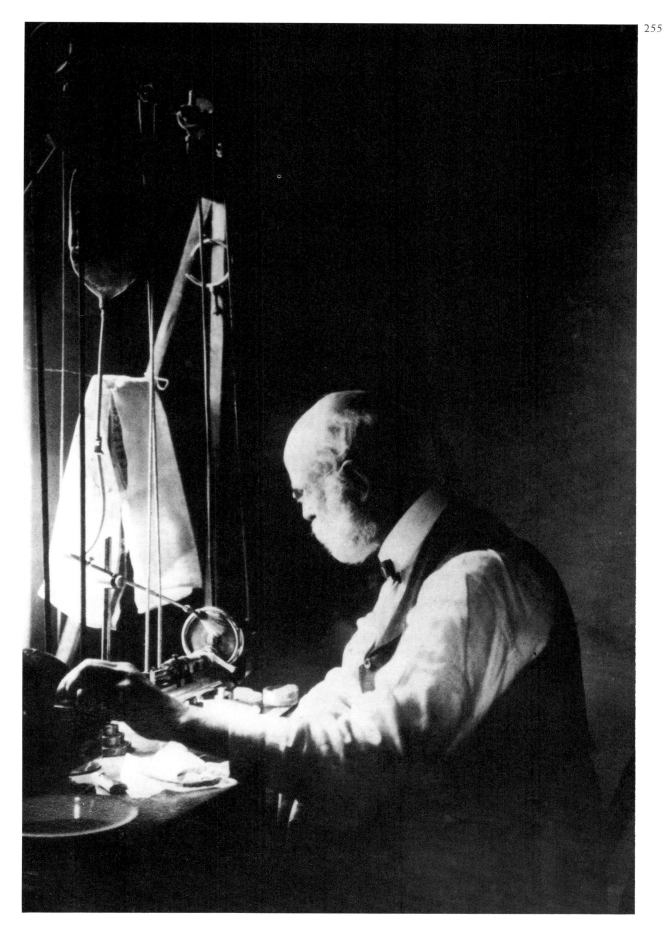

Dr. G. V. Black in his laboratory, grinding tooth sections.

After reading Virchow, Black became deeply interested in cellular pathology. He acquired a microscope and soon was the only pathologist in the county serving the medical profession. Admirers circulated the story that a local ophthalmologist brought Black a mysterious foreign body he had removed from the eye of a patient, and Black was promptly able to identify it as the first joint of the third leg of a potato bug.

In 1870 Black was invited to teach at the Missouri Dental College (MDC) in St. Louis, and the first formal lecture he ever heard was his own (in all, he had received only twenty months of elementary-school education). His first years at MDC were spent as lecturer on histology and microscopy; later he became lecturer on pathology and operative dentistry. After he had been eight years on the faculty, the school awarded him an honorary D.D.S. But Black believed that dentistry should stand as a profession independent from and equal to that of medicine, and because the Missouri school was strongly dominated by medical men Black severed his connection with MDC.

By 1883 Black was teaching again, this time in Chicago: first at the Chicago Dental Infirmary, then, from 1885, at the Chicago College of Dental Surgery, commuting from his home in Jacksonville, a tedious trip indeed. For one year he also taught at the dental department of the University of Iowa, but resigned in 1891 after being appointed to the faculty of the newly organized Northwestern University Dental School as professor of pathology and bacteriology. In 1897 he was made dean of the college and in that year relocated in Chicago. As dean, he assembled the finest specialists for his faculty, making Northwestern the outstanding dental educational institution of its day. Under his aegis the library's holdings also increased by thousands of volumes.

Black continued to write and publish. He authored more than five hundred articles and several outstanding books, which became recognized classics in the field. His *Dental Anatomy* appeared in 1890, and in 1908 his great two-volume *Operative Dentistry* was issued.

An indefatigable researcher, Black invented numerous machines for testing alloys. He also did more to standardize operative procedures than any dentist before or since. Two major contributions were his principle "extension for prevention," bringing the margins of a filling out to the point where they can be readily reached by a toothbrush, and his standardized rules of cavity preparation. In that day, photographic slides were nonexistent, and Black devised oversize models of teeth and mammoth hand instruments to demonstrate to his students exactly how teeth should be prepared for filling (fig. 258).

Honors and awards were generously bestowed upon Black. He received honorary degrees from Illinois College and Northwestern University, and in 1915 the University of Pennsylvania granted him an honorary Sc.D.

Still at work on the mottling of tooth enamel associated with fluorosis, Black died on August 31, 1915, at the age of seventy-nine, having immeasurably enriched the field of dentistry. Nineteen years earlier, in 1896, he made a prophetic statement to some of the students he so markedly influenced: "The day is surely coming, and perhaps within the lifetime of you young men before me, when we will be engaged in practicing preventive, rather than reparative, dentistry. When we will so understand the etiology and pathology of dental caries that we will be able to combat its destructive effects by systemic medication."

256

This photograph of the faculty of Northwestern University Dental School in Chicago, was made at the turn of the century. Dr. G. V. Black, then dean of the institution, is seated at the center of the table before the door. National Museum of American History, Smithsonian Institution, Washington, D.C.

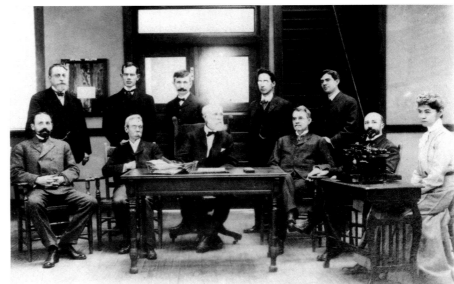

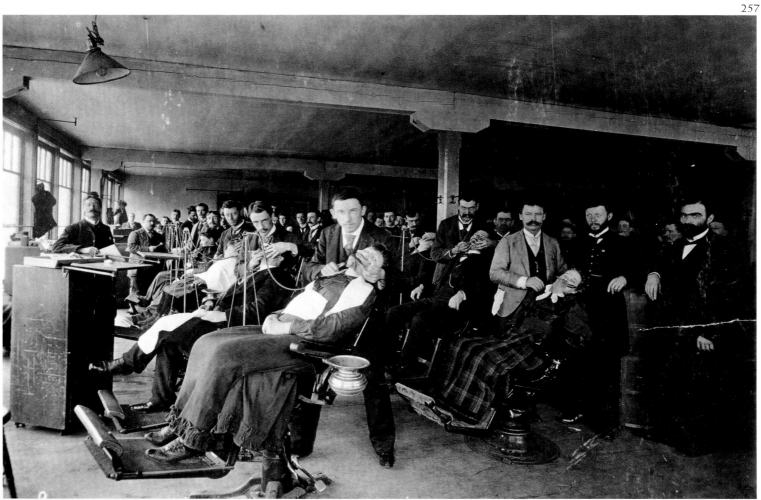

258

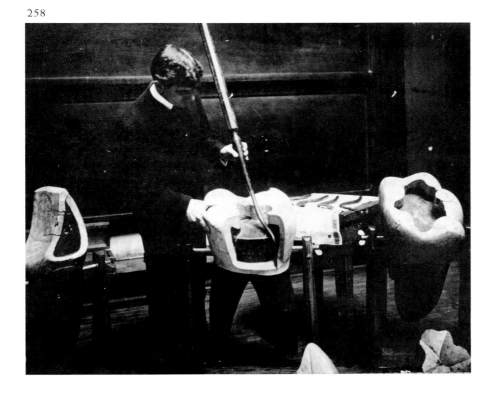

Shown here in 1900 is the dental clinic at the University of Illinois, Chicago, filled to capacity. The patients closest to the camera have rubber dams over their mouths. These sheets of rubber, the invention of Dr. Sanford C. Barnum, were used to isolate teeth and keep them dry during a dental procedure.

Probably during the 1890s, a student at Northwestern University Dental School was photographed as he demonstrated the correct way to prepare a tooth cavity for filling using the oversized models and instruments designed by Dr. G. V. Black.

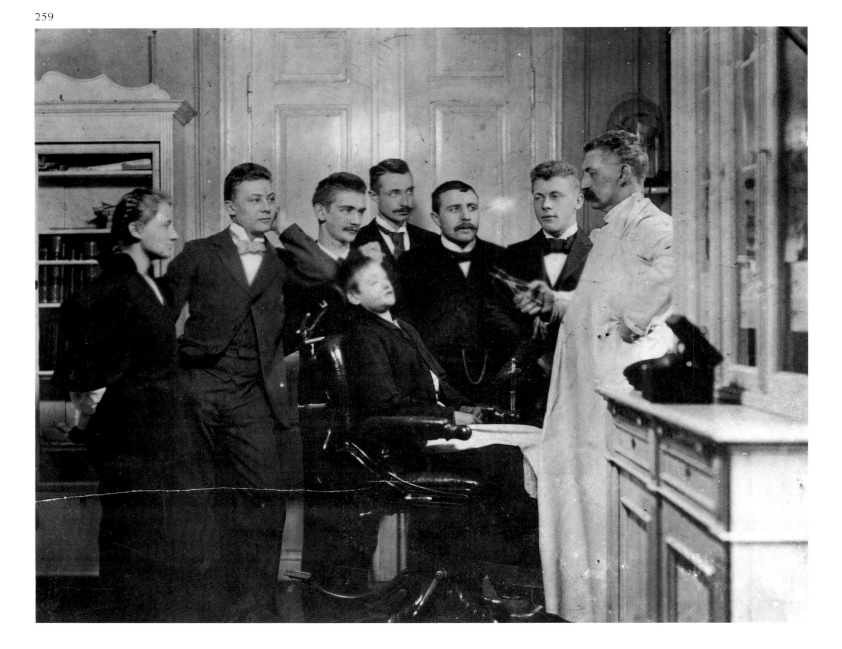

A Danish professor of dentistry demonstrates a
point to a class of students about 1904. Shortly
after this photograph was taken, the students
staged a successful strike against dress requirements and were thereafter allowed to dress as casu-
ally as the professor.

260

Dental students at the School of Dentistry, University of Buffalo, posed for the camera in the gross
anatomy laboratory about 1904.

XIII
THE TWENTIETH CENTURY

By 1900 the profession of dentistry had become well established and respected in both Europe and the United States. The basic systems of education and practice were functioning smoothly, and dental organizations were flourishing. During the twentieth century, changes in all these areas would take place, dental equipment would see marvelous transformations, and truly revolutionary steps would be taken in the fields of preventive dentistry, public-health dentistry, and prosthetic dentistry.

In 1904 operative clinics like this one at the Dental School, University of Pennsylvania, were housed in large auditorium-like rooms. Since World War II the trend has been to simulate as closely as possible within the clinic the conditions of a private office. Today each student-dentist usually works in a private cubicle. Library of Congress, Washington, D.C.

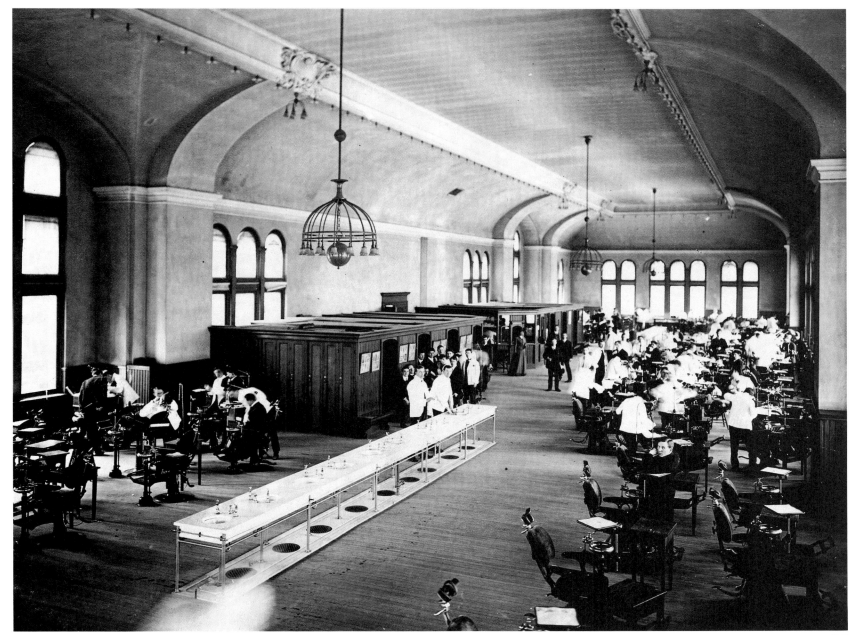

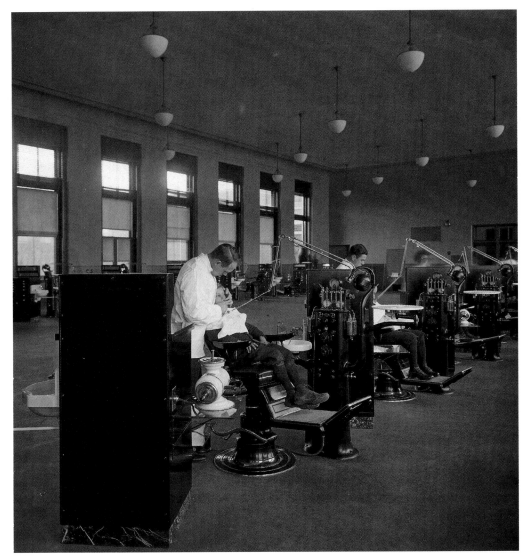

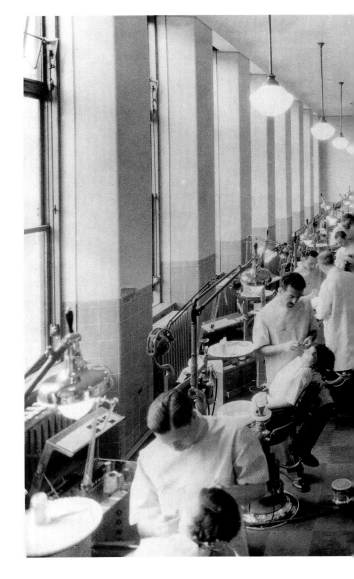

262

The main clinic at the Eastman Dental Dispensary in Rochester, New York, is seen here on opening day in 1917. The dentists, all recent graduates of dental schools, were interested in receiving postgraduate training.

263, 264

The Guggenheim Clinic in New York City is one of the principal dental facilities in the United States not only for the treatment of children but also for the training of intern dentists. These photographs date from the 1940s. 263: Library of Congress, Washington, D.C. 264: Museum of the City of New York.

265

Student dental hygienists from the Eastman Dental Dispensary treat workers of the Eastman Kodak Company at the Rochester, New York, factory in 1926.

266

The main operative clinic of the Baltimore College of Dental Surgery was electrified by about 1905, as this photograph shows; however, the students were still using foot-treadle drills. The instructor in the right foreground is checking a student's articulator to see if the artificial teeth have been properly arranged. Baltimore College of Dental Surgery, University of Maryland.

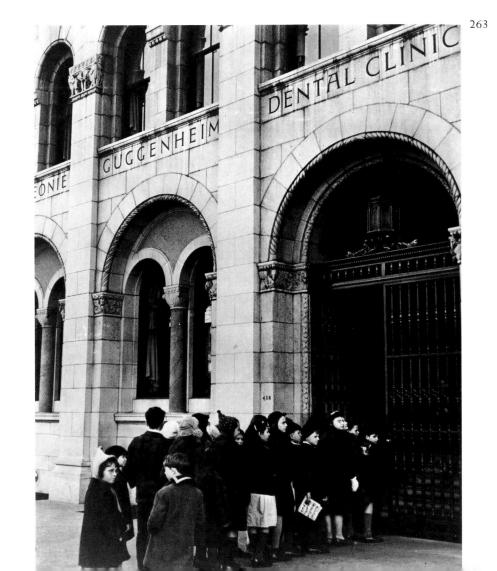

263

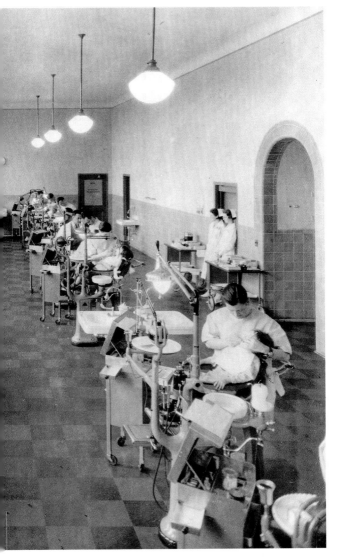

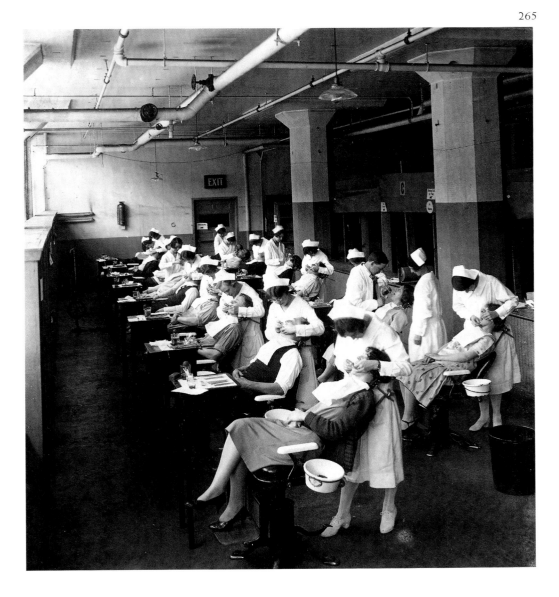

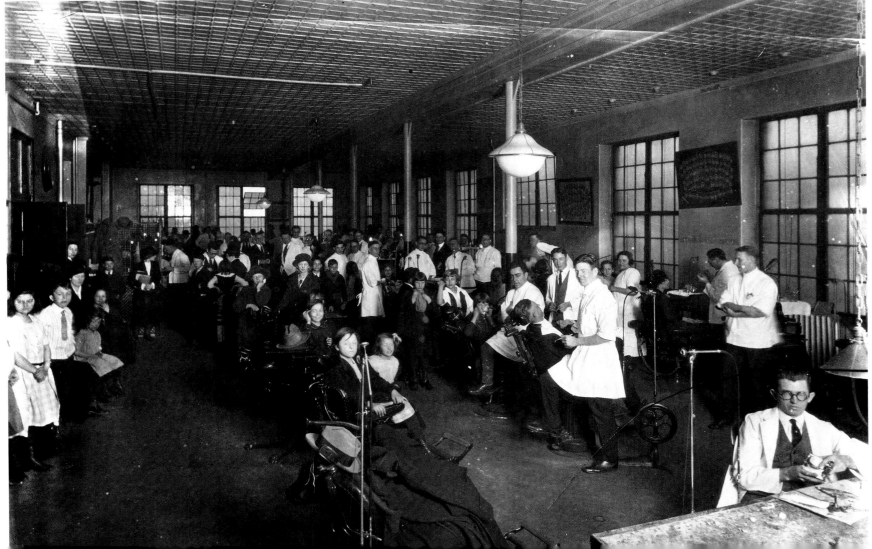

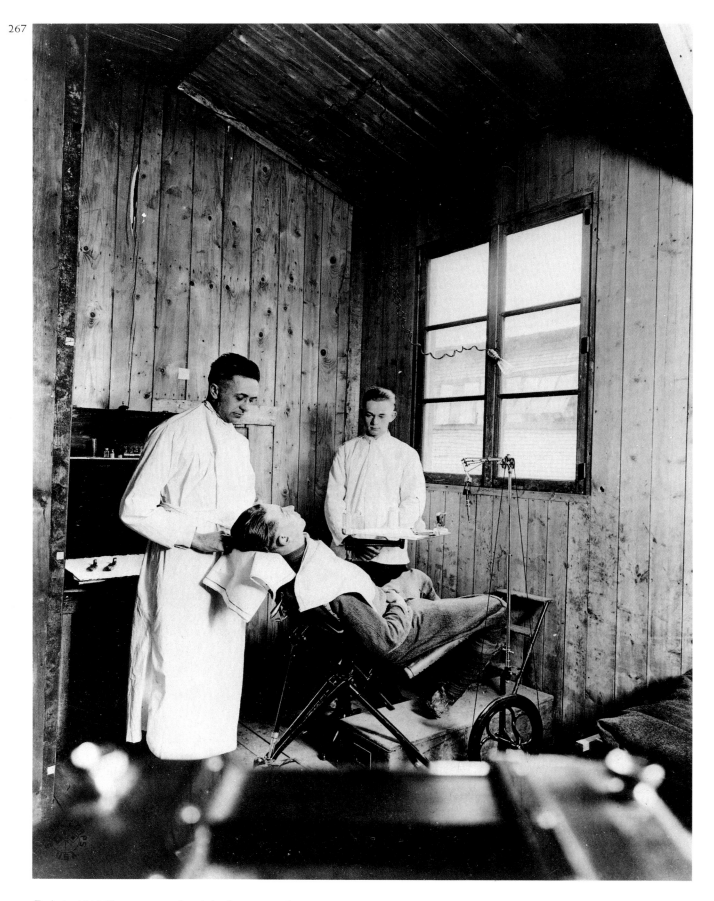

Early in 1918 Congress mandated the formation of
a Dental Reserve Corps composed of graduates of
"recognized dental colleges." In this photograph
made in 1918, an American Dental Corps officer
treats a soldier at Camp Hospital 9, Châteauvillain
(Haut-Marne), France. National Library of Medicine, Bethesda.

Advances in Education

Before 1925, American dental schools were of varying degrees of quality. In addition to the university-affiliated schools such as Harvard, Michigan, and Buffalo, there existed a host of independent institutions. Some of the latter were excellent, offering adequate preparation for professional life; those operated strictly for profit, however, were deplorable (one such establishment with an enrollment of 650 employed only a single instructor!). The standards for admission in all these institutions were very low. By 1905 an attempt was being made to establish two years of high school as a minimum requirement for matriculation, but virtually nullifying this was an escape clause written into the resolution permitting students to enter dental school with an education "equivalent" to ten years of schooling but nowhere spelling out what this meant. Although university-affiliated dental schools were in the minority, they nevertheless had sufficient prestige to take the lead in elevating the level of dental education. In 1908 these institutions organized the Dental Faculties Association of American Universities, which took up the fight to establish two years of high school and four years of dental school as a requirement for an accredited diploma, against the bitter opposition of the proprietary schools.

An attack by the prominent London doctor Sir William Hunter on American dentistry spurred on those who sought to improve dental education in the United States. In 1910 Hunter delivered a lecture to the medical faculty of McGill University in Montreal on the role of sepsis and antisepsis in medicine. A medical lecture for an audience of M.D.s, Hunter's address surprisingly contained a biting condemnation of American dentistry. He claimed that he had treated many obscure complaints that disappeared only after he had ordered to have removed from the patients' mouths prostheses inserted, he claimed, by American-trained dentists. He said he had found crowns and bridges in septic oral environments and full dentures placed over retained roots. He condemned *all* root-canal therapy, tarring good and bad dentists, Europeans as well as Americans, with one brush. In one striking phrase he characterized American dental prostheses as "mausoleums of gold over a mass of sepsis," a metaphor that was immediately picked up by the newspapers. Naturally, a multitude of Americans suffering from stubborn illnesses clamored to have teeth and prostheses removed and a rash of extractions followed—many of which were unnecessary. American dentists responded vigorously to Hunter's challenge. Edward Cameron Kirk, the respected editor of *Dental Cosmos*, asserted that, as a result of the work of G. V. Black, American dentistry had become exemplary. Furthermore, he pointed out, unscrupulous European dentists were known to have added an undeserved D.D.S. after their names; it was probable, he said, that Hunter had seen the work of these dentists, not of accredited American professionals. Nevertheless, Hunter's attack continued to rankle—to beneficial effect. It caused American dentistry to examine itself and discard some unsound techniques, such as incomplete filling of canals in root-canal therapy. A crusade for better techniques ensued, led by Charles Rosenow, who performed his research at the Mayo Clinic, in Rochester, Minnesota, and Frank Billings, who worked at both Rush Medical College in Philadelphia and Presbyterian Hospital in Chicago. They stated what was the most salutary consequence of the Hunter episode: "The prevention of oral sepsis in the future, with a view to lessening the incidence of systemic diseases, should henceforth take precedence in dental practice over preservation of the teeth almost wholly for mechanical or cosmetic purposes, as has been so largely the case in the past."*

The big impetus for change in dental education came with World War I. Early in 1918 as a war measure Congress mandated the formation of a Dental Reserve Corps composed of graduates of "recognized dental colleges." A Dental Educational Council (DEC) was also set up and charged with the task of establishing acceptance standards for the colleges. In August, the DEC announced that "a

---

*A proper balance between the interests of disease prevention and of tooth preservation eventually came about with the widespread use of radiology, which allowed dentists to determine accurately the presence or absence of infection at the apex of a nonvital tooth. With the introduction of the precision-casting technique, the policy of devitalizing teeth before reconstructive work was done became outmoded.

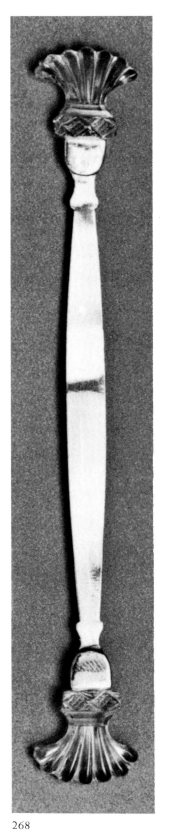

268

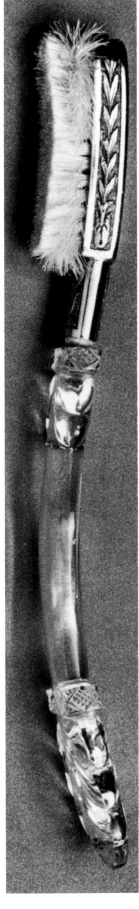

The handsome bronze and crystal toothbrush and tongue-scraper shown here belonged to a member of the Swedish royal family about 1900. Hakan Lind, Royal Collections, Stockholm.

dental school conducted for a profit to individuals or a corporation does not meet the standards of fair educational ideals and [is] excluded from 'A' classification." Private schools fought back bitterly and forced some short-term reverses, but in 1923 the DEC announced that after a three-year period of grace no school would receive an A-rating unless it established as an entrance requirement one year of college plus four years of high school. By 1937 the achievement level had been raised to two years of college study that included courses in chemistry, physics, and biology. Today, most American schools require two years or more of college preparation and one and a half years of chemistry, one year of biology or another science, and two years of a modern foreign language. In Europe the training is quite different: in Portugal, Italy, Spain, and Austria, for example, five to seven years of medical-school education are required before any training in dentistry is begun.

Since the 1800s dentistry had suffered from a severe case of schizophrenia. By some of its practitioners it was regarded as a branch of medicine, by others as a separate and independent field. In Europe stomatology (as dentistry was known) was taught in medical schools after the student earned an M.D. degree; in the United States dentistry was taught in completely separate schools. Thus, in Europe, the practical skills of dentistry were somewhat underrated, and in a majority of American schools the emphasis was on the mechanical aspects of dentistry, to the neglect of the biological sciences.

The Carnegie Foundation for the Advancement of Teaching, which had issued the Flexner Report of 1910 evaluating medical education in the United States, twelve years later chose William J. Gies to head a similar commission to study dental education. Gies, who was not a dentist, taught biochemistry at Columbia University. He had developed a keen interest in dentistry, however, and since 1909 had been doing research on dental problems. In 1919 he founded the prestigious *Journal of Dental Research* and served as editor, with no compensation, for the next seventeen years. In 1920 he and a number of colleagues organized the International Association for Dental Research to promote, on an international level, all aspects of dental research. Aware of the importance of dental education to the profession, he was instrumental in helping to form in 1923 the American Association of Dental Schools.

Gies was thus the logical choice of the Carnegie Foundation, and his report, which appeared in 1926, entitled *Dental Education in the United States and Canada*, resulted in the complete reorganization of dental education in those countries. The four years of investigation spent in preparing the report led him to conclude that dentistry as a health profession ought to remain separate from conventional medicine; nevertheless, he predicted correctly that dentistry must and would develop into a health service equal to medicine.

> I am hopeful and confident that the day is not far distant when dentistry, freed from the demoralizing trade dominance that has held it back from its highest professional attainments, will be universally accorded the full degree of respect and regard that is due to every branch of the arts and science of medicine.

Progress in Organization

In 1900 Dr. Charles Godon (1854–1913), dean of L'Ecole Dentaire de Paris, attended the Third International Dental Congress then being held in the French capital. Having long wanted to see the establishment of an international organization of dentists, he discussed the idea with his colleagues and succeeded in interesting eight leading dentists from different countries. They met on August 15, constituting themselves the first executive council of a new Fédération Dentaire Internationale (FDI). Godon was chosen as its first president.

The Third International Congress had pointed out some paths this new group should explore. The congress had determined that in every nation schoolchil-

269

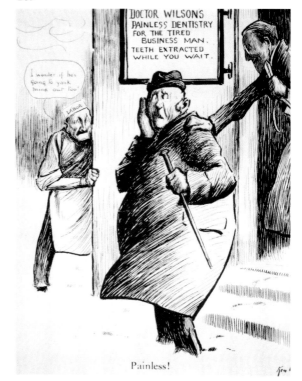

Painless!

President Woodrow Wilson, who in 1913 and 1914 had signed into law the Federal Reserve and Clayton Antitrust acts, was regarded with dislike and suspicion on Wall Street. This cartoon of about 1915 suggests that Wilson has drawn the teeth of American business and may have designs on American labor as well.

dren should have regular dental examinations and free treatment if necessary; that if a state provided medical services to its citizens it should also provide dental services; that dentists should be included in the armed forces of all nations; that the amount of preliminary education required for matriculation in dental schools should be increased; and that the course of study in dental schools should be set at a minimum of four years. These were lofty goals, but the new FDI faced up to the task squarely. The executive committee agreed the new organization should organize task forces on public hygiene and education, for example, to carry out the recommendations of the body as a whole and work with energy and imagination to improve the profession of dentistry.

The first official meeting of the FDI was held in Cambridge, England, on August 7, 1901. Although not many dentists yet knew of the new group, word soon spread around the world, and the 1902 meeting in Stockholm was well attended. The Fourth International Dental Congress, held in St. Louis in 1904 to coincide with the Louisiana Purchase Exposition, is felt by many to have been the greatest and most important international dental meeting ever held. The chairman was Harvey J. Burkhart, a dentist practicing in Batavia, New York, who would later achieve international renown as director of all the Eastman Dental Centers in the world. At that meeting the FDI's constitution was amended to provide for constituent memberships by national societies as well as individual memberships— the form it holds today. Chosen as president of the reorganized federation was the greatest dental scientist of his day, Willoughby D. Miller.

Meetings were held for many years by the FDI, interrupted only by the two world wars. At the conclusion of hostilities in 1945 there was universal feeling among dentists, as among so many other groups, that national hatreds ought to be put aside in the interest of professional unity. Chosen for the task of revitalizing the federation was Harvey J. Burkhart, the only original FDI founder still alive. Although he suffered failing health, Burkhart was successful in bringing the federation back to life and function. Today the FDI's primary function is to establish worldwide standards and to promote research on an international level.

Many national organizations came on the scene during the twentieth century. Reflecting a new trend in the profession toward specialization, some of these were devoted to a specific branch of dentistry: in 1918 were formed both the National Society of Denture Prosthetists and the American Society of Oral Surgeons and Exodontists, and two years later the International Association for Dental Research came into being. Since that time, about two hundred more have formed: among them are the Association of Women Dentists, the American Prosthodontic Society, the Society for Clinical Dental Hypnosis, and the Society of Forensic Odontology, to name a few.

The year 1920 also saw the launching of the American College of Dentists (ACD), conceived by four men, John V. Conzett, H. Edmund Friesell, Otto U. King, and Arthur D. Black. On August 22 twenty-five leaders of the profession met and adopted a constitution and bylaws and promulgated the objectives that the ACD still seeks: to elevate the standards of dentistry, to encourage graduate study, and to grant fellowships to those who have done meritorious work. Over the years the organization has served as a catalyst to bring out the best in the profession and to act as a promoter of dentistry to the public. Soon thereafter, in 1928, an International College of Dentists was incorporated.

Afro-Americans Enter the Profession

Until the 1950s the dental schools and dental organizations of the United States were sadly discriminatory. Black dentists were denied admission to most educational institutions and professional societies. With the increase in civil-rights activities after World War II came a flood of demands that discrimination in dentistry be done away with. In 1962 the American Dental Association resolved that its House of Delegates might refuse to seat the delegation of any state

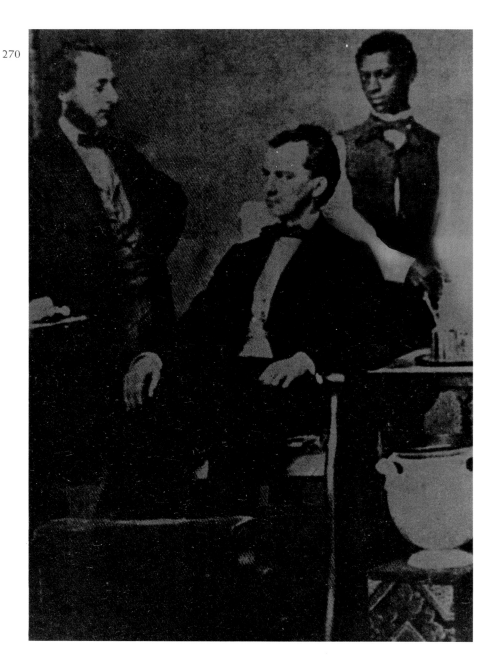

At some time in the mid-1860s, when this photograph was taken, Robert Tanner Freeman, at right, was engaged as an apprentice to a Dr. Noble of Washington, D.C., shown at left. By the decade's end Freeman had become the first black to graduate from an American dental school, Harvard's School of Dental Medicine.

whose bylaws conflicted with those of the ADA prohibiting racial discrimination. This action effectively opened the door for greater participation by blacks in mainstream dental activities.

Yet Afro-Americans have had a long history in American dentistry. At the time the first dental school in the world, the Baltimore College of Dental Surgery, was established, 120 black dentists, products of the apprenticeship system, were practicing in the country. One of them, Robert Tanner Freeman (fig. 270), resigned from his apprenticeship with a white dentist in Washington, D.C., in order to enroll in the first class of Harvard University's School of Dental Medicine, becoming, in 1869, one of the first six students to receive a dental degree from that institution.

In 1867, the United States government, under the aegis of the Freedmen's Bureau, established Howard University in Washington, D.C. Departments of dentistry were organized there in 1881, and in 1886 at Meharry Medical College in Nashville, Tennessee, a private school originally set up to train black physicians. These two institutions educated nearly all the black dentists in the United States until the 1954 United States Supreme Court desegregation decision, which changed the situation significantly.

Blacks slowly made their presence felt in the dental professional community of the nation. In 1910 there were only 478 black dentists, and by 1930 the number had reached a mere 1,773. By the end of the second decade of the century, however, a small cadre of educated black professionals had begun to fill leadership roles and inspire the generation that followed. Prominent among them was Dr. Charles Edwin Bentley, a graduate in 1887 of the Chicago College of Dental Surgery, who became a prolific contributor to dental literature and distinguished himself as clinician, researcher, and administrator, as well as a professor of oral surgery at Harvey Medical College, Chicago. Because of pioneering work in pressing the adoption of dental hygiene measures, Bentley is called the father of preventive dentistry.

Dr. David A. Ferguson, a graduate in 1900 of the Howard University College of Dentistry, was the first dentist to serve as president of the National Medical Association, an organization of black physicians, pharmacists, and dentists. Ferguson was instrumental in establishing a separate organization of black dentists, which ultimately became the National Dental Association (NDA). Dr. Stephen J. Lewis, a graduate of Howard in 1909, played an active role in the Pennsylvania Dental Society, a component of the then predominantly white ADA. In 1924 Dr. Lewis founded the first publication of the NDA and became its first editor.

Americans can pride themselves that discrimination in dental education has largely been done away with and that energetic efforts are being made to attract qualified young black men and women to the dental profession. Today, the many contributions of black dentists in the fields of education, research, and practice are widely appreciated and applauded.

The *Index to Dental Literature*

The twentieth century brought to dentistry, as to the other professions, a proliferation of publications—texts, reference works, and articles. Arthur D. Black (fig. 271), who followed his illustrious father, G. V. Black, as dean of the dental school at Northwestern University, knew how important is professional literature not only to researchers but to general practitioners who wish to maintain their skills. He was also aware of the need for an index to the thousands of periodical articles published each year and decided to tackle the job himself. But first came the problem of classification. In 1898, in association with Frederick B. Noyes, Black devised a workable method based on Melvil Dewey's decimal classification. To test their system over a five-year period, Black and Noyes indexed the articles published in two journals from 1898 to 1903, when they found they had accumulated a stack of more than 25,000 index cards for subjects and authors!

The profession was but slowly attracted to Black's index. In 1908 a group of teachers of dentistry organized a Dental Index Bureau (DIB) but appropriated no funds for it. A committee then solicited the profession at large and by 1910 had collected about a thousand dollars, which was quickly spent on indexing. Undaunted, Black and his committee opened a drive to secure subscriptions to the *Index*, but in the end it took twenty-three years to secure enough money to issue the first compilation! In 1921 the first volume of the *Index to the Dental Periodical Literature in the English Language* was issued for the years 1911 to 1915. Black had originally planned to index only 10 journals, but as the work progressed the number expanded to include 65 periodicals (more than 2,500 journals are indexed today).

The Dental Index Bureau, headquartered in Buffalo, continued to work—forward as well as retrospectively, so that eventually all the dental journals, from the very first issue of the *American Journal of Dental Science* in 1839, were indexed. At the eve of World War II the task had become too formidable for the DIB, and the ADA's Bureau of Library and Indexing Services assumed the charge. In 1965 the work was taken over by the National Library of Medicine (which also produced the *Index Medicus*), but the library director of the ADA remains the editor of the *Index to Dental Literature*.

271

Arthur D. Black was responsible for organizing and launching the indispensable *Index to the Dental Periodical Literature in the English Language*, the first volume of which was published in 1921. This photograph was taken about 1930, when Black was dean of Northwestern University Dental School, in Chicago.

The Dental Hygiene Movement: The Contribution of Alfred C. Fones

The introduction of the paraprofessional into the ranks of healers in dentistry proved a tremendous step forward in countering the ravages of dental disease. To Dr. Alfred Civilion Fones (1869–1938), of Bridgeport, Connecticut, goes the credit for raising the profession of dental hygiene to the important position it now occupies.

While attending a meeting of the Northeastern Dental Society in 1899, Fones heard a lecture by Dr. D. D. Smith of Philadelphia on periodic oral prophylaxis. Impressed, Fones returned home and for five years used Smith's techniques. In 1905 he trained his office assistant to do prophylactic work for the children in his practice, and she thus became the first dental hygienist in the world.

Excited by the implications of his innovation, Fones launched a campaign to make oral prophylactic treatment available to all the children in the Bridgeport city schools and proposed the idea of a training school for dental hygienists—a term he coined. Despite strong opposition from the dental profession, he opened the Fones Clinic for Dental Hygienists in November 1913, in his garage. The faculty, whom he had convinced of the project's value, was impressive: the deans of the dental schools of Pennsylvania and Harvard, seven professors from Yale and two from Columbia, and three New York specialists—all of whom served without pay. Twenty-seven women graduated in the first class, and most entered the Bridgeport school system after Fones had persuaded the Board of Education to provide financial support. The benefits of their work exceeded all expectations: dental caries rates in participating children were reduced about 75 percent!

So successful was the experiment that inquiries soon flowed in from all parts of the United States, and similar projects were started in many areas. With the passage of licensure laws governing hygienists (Connecticut's was the first, in 1917), school after school began training hygienists. By 1972 there were about 30,000 working in the United States alone. Today there are more than 120 schools for dental hygienists, turning out about 2,500 graduates each year.

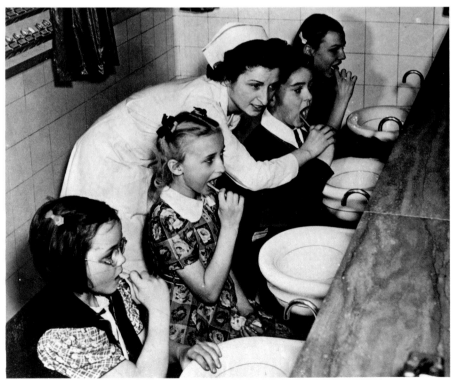

In this photograph of about 1940, a hygienist at the Guggenheim Clinic in New York City teaches young patients correct toothbrushing techniques. Library of Congress, Washington, D.C.

272

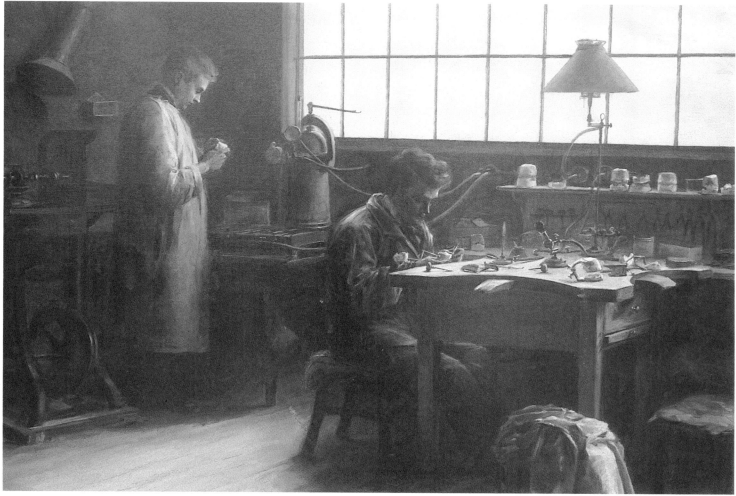

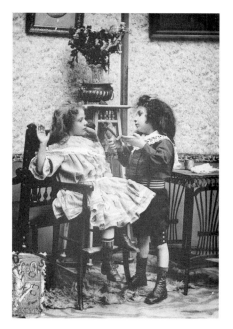

About 1910 an artist named C. Durif-Bedel painted the dental laboratory of her husband, Dr. Durif of Lyons. A peaceful light plays over orderly instruments and containers, and the scene suggests the scientific dentistry of the future rather than the inventive yet artisanlike dentistry of the previous century. Musée de la Chirurgie Dentaire, Lyons.

274

In these French postcards of about 1900, two children play at dentist and patient. Collection Samuel X. Radbill, M.D., Philadelphia.

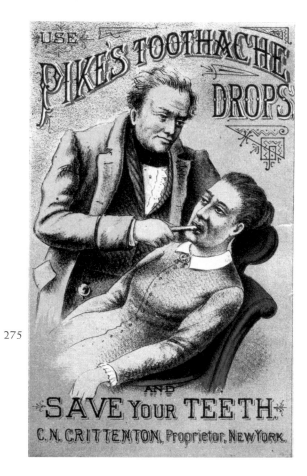

275

The extreme pallor of the patient in the dental chair depicted in this turn-of-the century poster suggests that she may have waited too long to profit from Pike's Toothache Drops. New-York Historical Society, New York City.

Fluoride

Dentists had recognized as early as 1874 that fluorine had a preventive effect on the development of dental caries. In that year a German physician named Erhardt observed changes in the enamel of the teeth of dogs fed the substance. In 1902 a Danish pharmaceutical company promoted the sale of a fluoride compound to strengthen the teeth, but its use was repudiated by the Danish dental profession because scientific studies of its effects had not been carried out.

At about the same time, in May 1908, Dr. Fredrick McKay, who practiced in Colorado Springs, read a paper before the El Paso County Odontological Society concerning the brown mottling, or "Colorado stain," found on the teeth of children of his city, which we now know is caused by excessive consumption of fluorides. McKay suggested the cause was something in the water supply but lacked the sophisticated equipment necessary to determine exactly what it might be. He turned to the great G. V. Black for help, and in 1918 they published their classic report "Mottled Teeth, an Endemic Developmental Imperfection of the Teeth, Heretofore Unknown in the Literature of Dentistry," in which fluorine was suggested as agent. They failed, however, to ascribe a lower incidence of caries to fluorine.

In 1917 McKay moved to New York City and limited his practice to periodontics, but he still maintained his interest in the study of fluorides and the teeth. In 1925 he was consulted by the municipal authorities of Oakley, Idaho, about the mottled teeth of all children of that town, who drank deep-well water. McKay persuaded the local authorities to tap a new source of surface water. Seven years later McKay went back to Oakley to examine the children's teeth and observed no new cases of mottling of tooth enamel. He then suggested that "caries was inhibited by the same water which produced mottled enamel." His announcement paved the way for team investigation of the phenomenon.

The task was undertaken by a Public Health Service team headed by Dr. H. Trendley Dean. Dean realized that in order to determine any relationship between fluoride and caries, he would need a quantitative measuring device, and it was he who developed the DMF Index of decayed, missing, and filled teeth. Dean, who was largely responsible for the development of the new field of dental epidemiology, spent the greater part of his thirty-two-year career studying the relationship between different amounts of fluoride in the water supply and caries susceptibility, and his work paved the way for the large-scale controlled studies of fluoride-containing and fluoride-deficient water carried out during the 1940s in the cities of Grand Rapids and Muskegon, Michigan, and Newburgh and Kingston, New York.

Since that time fluoridation of public water has been adopted in many cities in this country and abroad. As early as 1962, 2,302 communities in the United States had fluoridated public water. By the 1980s, 100 million people drank it. Unfortunately, despite fluoridation's proved safety and effectiveness (caries rates are reduced by 65 percent), the task of introducing the process has not been an easy one, for small groups vociferously opposed to it have thwarted its adoption in many places. The first description of a fluoridation conflict—in Williamstown, Massachusetts—appeared in a report of 1953 by Dr. J. M. Burns. Systematic studies of the issue followed. They pointed out that whereas the basic position of the antifluoridationists was simple, the weaknesses of their arguments were difficult for the layman to grasp; moreover, they appealed to widely held American political doctrines, such as individual rights, and to fear of the unknown and fear of bodily harm. These studies also showed that the higher the socioeconomic and educational level of the voter, the more likely was he or she to support fluoridation. Be that as it may, as a result of the conflict, the universal adoption of this proven health measure is still some years away.

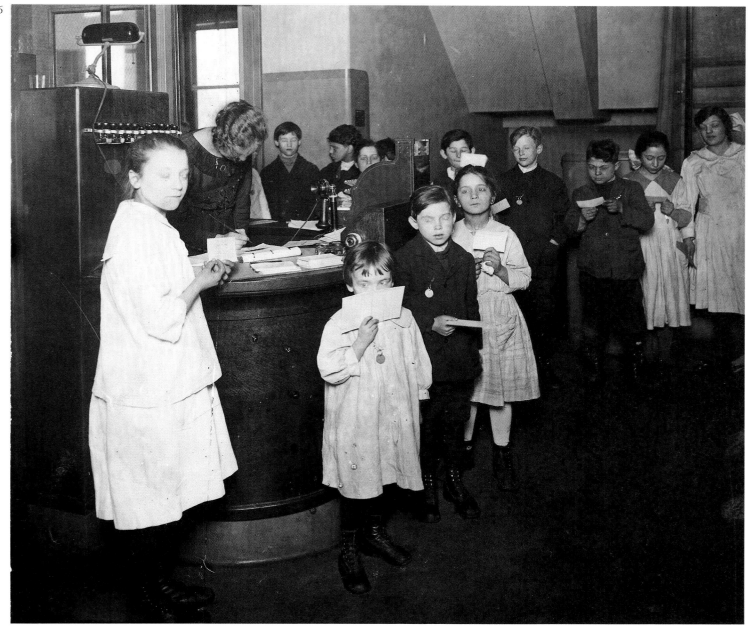

These children have lined up in the reception room of the Eastman Dental Dispensary, newly opened in Rochester, New York, in 1917.

Bringing Dental Care to the People

The first free dental clinic for children in the world was probably the one established about 1902 by Dr. Ernst Jessen of Strassburg, Germany, and eventually taken over by the municipal government. Which was the first in the United States is debatable. There is evidence that a clinic for children was set up in Camden, New Jersey, in 1899, but credit is usually given to a clinic established by the members of the Rochester, New York, Dental Society in 1901 to provide services to needy children. This humanitarian endeavor in time caught the eye and heart of the most powerful man in the city, George Eastman.

The Rochester Dental Society had had a hard struggle to keep its clinic going. It was staffed by local dentists volunteering half a day a month, but this arrangement was unsatisfactory since their attendance was irregular. In 1909 Eastman gave his financial support to a plan to bring the free clinics into the public schools, but funds remained insufficient. Then Eastman offered to shoulder the burden of support if three conditions were met: that treatment be rendered in a central clinic; that the city provide funds for a dental prophylaxis program in the schools; and that ten local citizens contribute $1,000 to the clinic each year for five years. The outcome was that in October 1915, a fledgling corporation

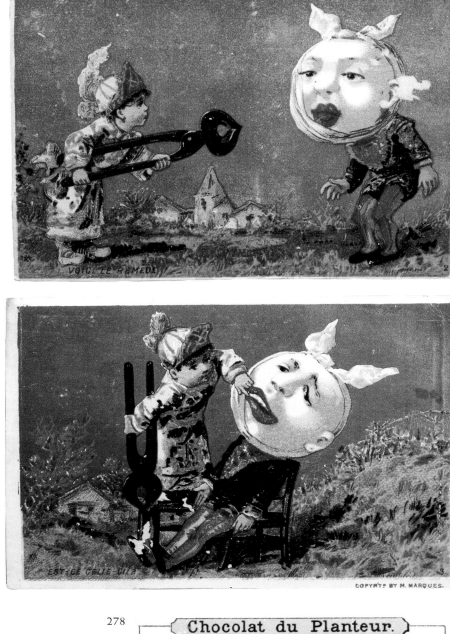

This pair of advertising cards was designed in the early twentieth century by M. Marques for the Great A&P Tea Company. On the back were listed the company's stores—108 in all. Collection William Helfand, New York.

Why the Compagnie Coloniale, importers of tea and chocolate at the turn of the century, should have chosen the image of a street dentist and his patient to advertise their Chocolat du Planteur seems puzzling today. Collection William Helfand, New York.

279

The first lithographed advertising poster was designed about 1867 in France, and French advertising art soon reached a very high aesthetic level. These French, Italian, and Spanish dentifrice advertisements of about 1900 reflect the influence of the posters of Toulouse-Lautrec and Bonnard. Musée de la Chirurgie Dentaire, and (right) Collection William Helfand, New York.

278

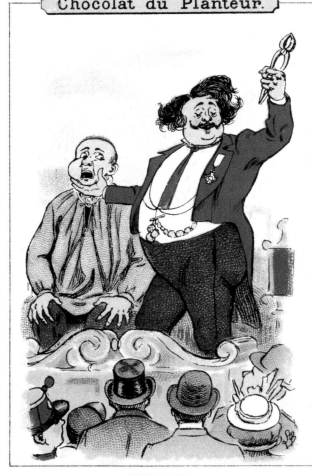

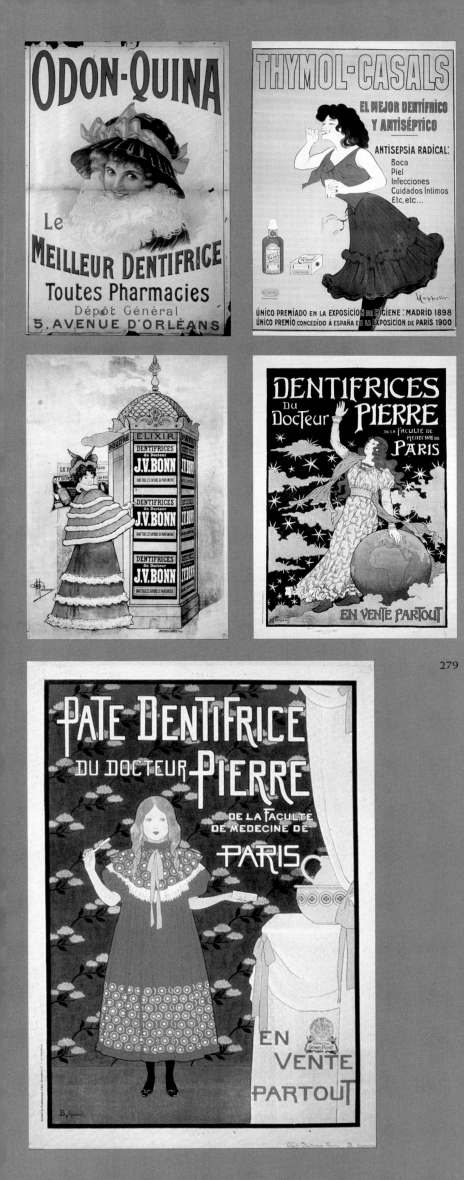

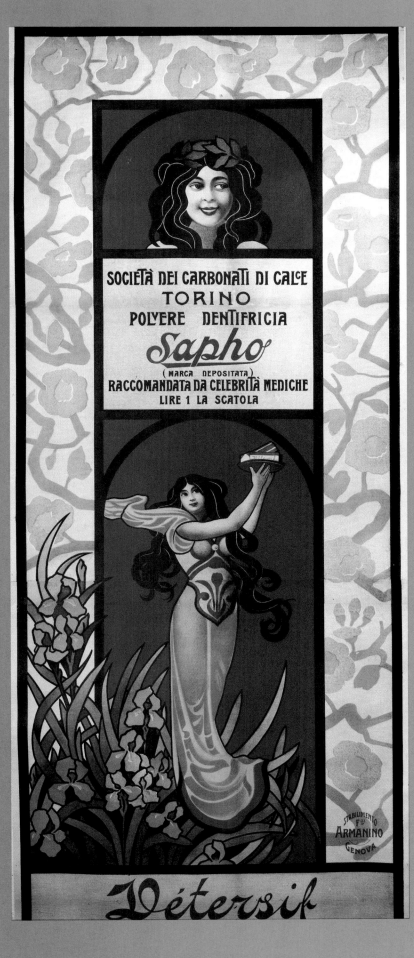

known as the Eastman Dental Dispensary (EDD), with Harvey J. Burkhart as its director, was formed. Eastman put up the money for the building, which cost $400,000—a large sum in those days—and in 1917, amid great fanfare, the building was dedicated before an audience that included numerous dignitaries of the dental profession, among them Truman W. Brophy, president of the Fédération Dentaire Internationale, and Lafayette Barber, president of the National Dental Association.

Envisioned as a clinic to render dental service to needy children, the EDD soon became an advanced training center for young dental graduates, offering a rotating internship program. In October 1916 the EDD program was expanded to include a school for dental hygienists. The first class of thirty-six hygienists graduated in June 1917.

Following Eastman's lead, philanthropists in other cities endowed similar clinics. Among the best known is the Guggenheim Clinic, which opened in New York City in 1929. (The well-known Forsythe Clinic opened earlier still, in 1914 in Boston.) So successful was the Rochester center that Eastman decided to open additional ones in Europe, and by the end of the 1930s Eastman clinics were operating in London, Rome, Brussels, Paris, and Stockholm, with Burkhart acting as international director.

World War II brought about profound changes in Americans' attitude toward dentistry. Citizens were shocked to learn from the office of the Surgeon General that the dental health of the nation's young men was truly deplorable. The Selective Service System had adopted as a minimum dental standard that a potential recruit need have only twelve teeth—three pairs of matching incisors and three pairs of chewing teeth—to be accepted into the armed forces. Among the first two million men summoned for service, one out of five lacked even the minimum number, and dental defects constituted the chief cause for physical rejection for active duty. The Selective Service was obliged to eliminate all dental standards to avoid mass-disqualification of selectees. As a consequence, after the war the United States, and European countries as well, made a vigorous effort to improve the dental health of the world's population.

During the 1950s the new field of public-health dentistry emerged in America. Before World War II, dentists had no established place on the public-health team, and scarcely any dental schools were teaching anything at all on the subject. In 1954 Dr. D. M. Hadjimarkos of the University of Oregon made a nationwide survey and found that though thirty schools at that time included public health in their curriculum, in fact little time was devoted to it: only five schools allocated as much as sixteen hours to the subject.

The first graduate course of study in dental public health was established in the 1940s by the University of Michigan under the direction of Dr. Kenneth A. Easlick, a member of the faculty of the School of Public Health. Easlick trained other dental public-health specialists, and today a number of schools have followed Michigan's lead and established courses leading to advanced degrees in the field.

In 1960 Philip E. Blackerby, then director of the division of dentistry of the W. K. Kellogg Foundation, presented a paper before the American Association of Dental Schools entitled "Why Not a Department of Social Dentistry?" He envisioned a discipline that would relate dentistry to the environment, and since then almost all schools have taken up the idea, although the names they have given their departments are many and various, ranging from environmental dentistry, community dentistry, preventive and public-health dentistry, to ecological dentistry. They all, however, have as their objective the improvement of the dental health of the population by a variety of means, including clinics, examination of schoolchildren, and public-health education.

The establishment in 1950 of the American Board of Dental Public Health has immeasurably aided in promoting dental health throughout the world. This country has been the undisputed leader in the field, and dentists of many other nations have come to American schools to gain knowledge and experience that they then have carried back to their homelands.

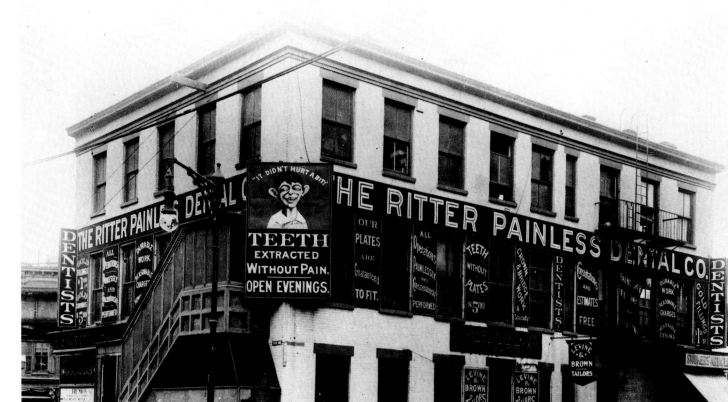

Dental parlors sprang up in major American cities at the end of the nineteenth century. Ritter's, located at Third Avenue and Schermerhorn Street in Brooklyn, advertised its painless procedures, as would "Painless Parker's" famous chain of dental offices during the 1920s and 1930s (see pages 4–5). New-York Historical Society, New York City.

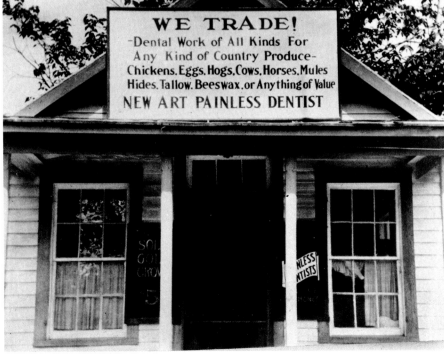

The sign over the door of this dental office in rural Georgia during the depths of the Great Depression indicates that dentists were not spared the economic hardships plaguing the country. Library of Congress, Washington, D.C.

UN HOMME SUR LES DENTS, par Tybalt.

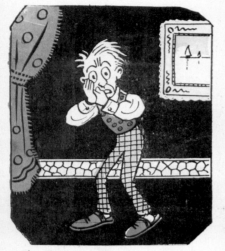

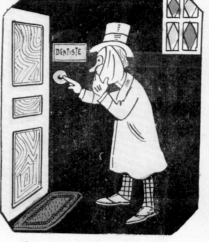

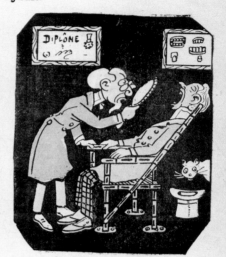

1. — Un jour, souffrant d'une épouvantable rage de dents — Dante a oublié ce supplice dans son Enfer — ...

2. — Je me rendis chez un dentiste pour me faire extirper la dent malade. *Sublata causa tollitur effectus* disaient les anciens.

3. — Excusez-moi, je suis un peu myope, me déclare l'éminent chirurgien... je ne vois pas très bien la dent qui vous gène ; mais cela ne fait rien. Pour plus de sûreté ..

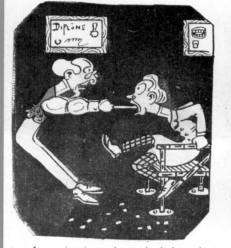

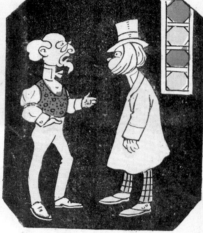

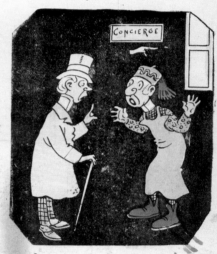

4. — ... je vais vous les arracher toutes... et je vous confectionnerai ensuite un joli petit ratelier, discret, parfumé, dont vous serez satisfait.

5. — M'ayant arraché incisives, canines et molaires sauf deux, il me fit verser la forte somme, et m'engagea à revenir dans quinze jours : tout serait prêt.

6. — Quinze jours plus tard, j'appris par son portier que le dentiste ayant mis la clef sous la porte, mobilier, outils et accessoires, avaient été vendus aux enchères.

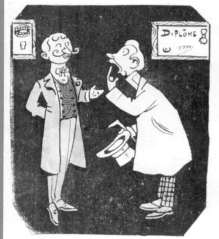

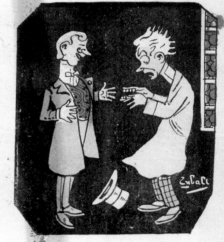

7. — Désolé, j'allai chez un autre dentiste à qui j'exposai mon cas.
— J'ai justement ce qu'il vous faut, me dit-il ; d'ailleurs vous allez en juger.

8. — Et il tira d'une armoire un ratelier superbement monté.

9. — Soudain mes cheveux se dressèrent sur ma tête : je venais de reconnaître dans l'or mes pauvres dents que cette vieille fripouille de premier dentiste m'avait arrachées le mois précédent.

DIE WUNDERBARE ZAHNKUR. — **1.** Da ich eines Tages an heftigen Zahnschmerzen litt-Dante hat diese Qualen in seiner « Hölle » vergessen. — **2.** So begab ich mich zu einem Zahnarzt, um den kranken Zahn ausziehen zu lassen. Sublata causa tollitur effectus sagten die Alten. — **3.** Entschuldigen Sie mich, bitte, ich bin ein bischen kurzsichtig sagte mir der berühmte Chirurg. — Ich kann den Zahn, der Ihnen Schmerzen bereitet zwar nicht gut sehen, aber das ist nichts zur Sache. Um ganz sicher zu sein. — **4.** Werde ich Ihnen sämtliche Zähne ausziehen und Ihnen sodann ein hübsches, nettes Gebisschen herstellen, das sehr diskret und parfümiert sein wird. Sie werden damit zufrieden sein. — **5.** Nachdem er mir sämtliche Schneidezähne, Reisszähne und Backenzähne bis auf 2 ausgezogen hatte, liess er mich eine bedeutende Anzahlung machen und hat mich, in 14 Tagen wieder vorzusprechen. Bis dahin sollte alles bereit sein. — **6.** 14 Tage später vernahm ich durch seinem Portier, dass der Zahnarzt davongegangen sei und sein Mobiliar, seine Werkzeuge usw. versteigertworden seien. — **7.** In meiner Verzweiflung besuchte ich einen andern Arzt, dem ich meinen Fall erzählte. — Ich kann Ihnen just dienen, sagte er, Sie sollen übrigens selbst urteilen. — **8.** Und er zog ein superbes Gebiss aus einem Schrank hervor. — **9.** Plötzlich sträubten sich meine Haare vor Entsetzen : Ich erkannte in der Goldfassung meine armen Zähne, die der obengenannte Halunke von einem Zahnarzt mir im vorigen Monat ausgezogen hatte.

Le Gérant: L. TAUZIAC.

Paris. — Typ. A. DAVY, 52, rue Madame. — *Téléphone.*

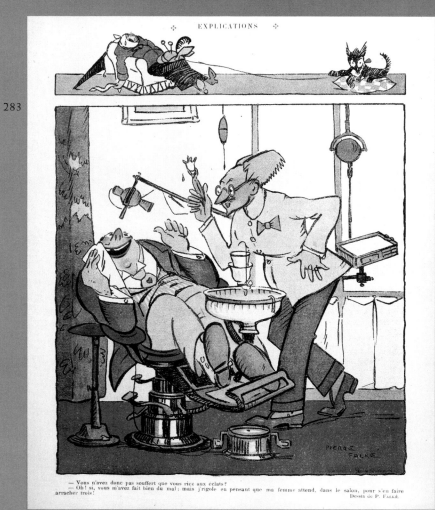

283

—— EXPLICATIONS ——

— Vous n'avez donc pas souffert que vous riez aux éclats?
— Oh! si, vous m'avez fait bien du mal; mais j'rigole en pensant que ma femme attend, dans le salon, pour s'en faire arracher trois!

Dessin de P. FALKÉ.

19e ANNÉE. — No 12.   10 Centimes.   23 Mars 1913.

Le Pêle-Mêle

POUR TOUS – PAR TOUS

L'UTILE ACCOUTREMENT, par Paul d'ESPAGNAT.

Le dentiste du Muséum arrache une dent à un de ses pensionnaires

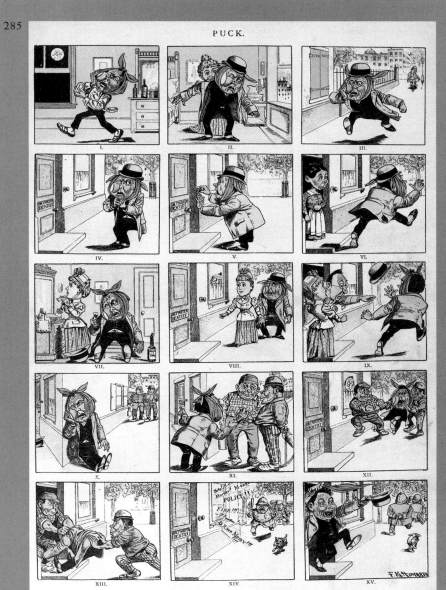

PUCK.

TOOTHACHE AND TERROR;
THE ADVENTURES OF A MAN WITH BOTH.

282

In March 1905, *Chronique Amusante* published this cartoon by Tybalt, which tells an infamous tale of dental malpractice. Collection William Helfand, New York.

283

This cartoon by P. Falké in *Le Rire*, November 22, 1913, shows a postoperative dental patient who is actually laughing. He is happy because his wife is outside waiting to have three of her teeth pulled. Collection William Helfand, New York.

284

The cover illustration of the March 23, 1913, issue of *Le Pêle-Mêle* was this delightfully absurd drawing of a zoo attendant pulling the teeth of one of his more formidable charges. Collection William Helfand, New York.

285

In 1892, the year this cartoon by F. M. Howarth appeared in *Puck*, toothache still held its terrors. Though anesthesia had made extractions painless, dental restorations were still performed with a nerve-rending low-speed drill. Collection William Helfand, New York.

The decades that followed World War II also saw a great change in the means by which dental care is made available to the people of the United States and Europe. In this country there has been a tremendous increase in group practices and clinics. No longer an almost exclusively one-man, one-office profession, dentistry in many areas is organized into groups of practitioners operating under one roof, who pool their skills for the patients' benefit.

Advertising by dentists, a development in the 1970s that followed a Supreme Court ruling permitting advertising by attorneys, has changed the character and image of the profession, as well as the way its skills are being utilized. Studies have shown that most people who respond to advertisements by dentists have had no dental care or only minimal or emergency treatment. Many of the dentists who advertise have set up offices in retail stores and shopping centers, offering working people, who might not otherwise get it, access to care on evenings, weekends, and holidays. Although advertising has encouraged patients to choose their dentist on the basis of who is cheapest or who keeps the longest hours, rather than who is the best qualified, it has at the same time helped to make dental care available to more people than ever before.

Also beneficial has been the increase during the postwar years of "third-party payers." These are essentially insurance group plans that provide payment for basic, routine dental care, plus, in certain instances, more extensive dentistry at an additional premium. During the 1960s and 1970s many unions secured such dental plans in their collective-bargaining agreements, and by 1980 almost 100 million Americans were covered, to some degree, by a dental insurance plan.

The American experience with dental prepayment plans is quite different from that in Europe, where some form of government-sponsored dental insurance has existed in a number of countries for many years. Great Britain took the lead immediately after World War II with its socialized-medicine plan, which included dental care. Other countries, such as Norway and Denmark, provide free dental care to schoolchildren only, offering government insurance plans to adults. In France, dental care is incorporated into the social security system, which reimburses the patient for 75 percent of his costs. Similar government-run insurance plans are operative in West Germany (in which 97 percent of the population is enrolled) and in Denmark and Luxembourg, where patients are reimbursed for up to 80 percent of their costs. Luxembourg has recently pioneered a novel procedure to encourage preventive dentistry: if a person visits the dentist every year for preventive care, the insurance plan pays 100 percent of the charges! Sweden, too, fosters prevention, and its 1973 Law of General Dental Health Insurance also ensures increased payment for preventive dentistry.

One of the Farm Security Administration's mobile dental teams provided dental treatment for migrant farm workers in a camp in Caldwell, Idaho, in 1941. Library of Congress, Washington, D.C.

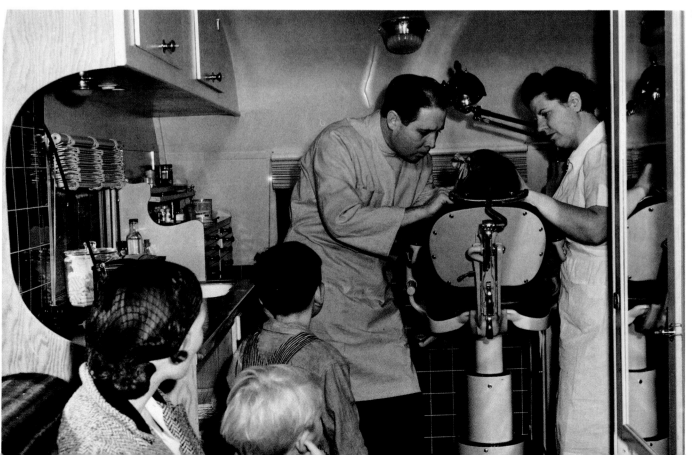

The Development of Professional Specialties

During the twentieth century, eight specialties have developed in dentistry. Today in the United States each has its own official journal (the first of these appeared in 1930, the *Journal of Periodontology*), and each is monitored by its own examining board established in the following order: Orthodontics (1930), Oral Surgery (1946), Oral Pathology (1948), Prosthodontics (1948), Pedodontics (1949), Dental Public Health (1951), and Endodontics (1964).

Orthodontics

During the second half of the nineteenth century, a great deal of attention was paid by the dental profession to irregularities of the teeth, and many articles appeared in the literature. In the early days, their treatment was considered part of prosthetic dentistry and was handled as a purely mechanical procedure. In 1880 Dr. Norman W. Kingsley (1829–1913), widely considered the father of orthodontics, published his *Treatise on Oral Deformities as a Branch of Mechanical Surgery*. Kingsley's contribution was invaluable, for in addition to offering many practical procedures of his own devising—such as occipital anchorage—he made the first attempt at systematizing the treatment of occlusal abnormalities. Eight years later John N. Farrar published the first volume of his useful *Treatise on the Irregulations of the Teeth and Their Correction*, but his work was superseded the following year by Simeon Guilford's *Orthodontia*, which became a standard text in dental colleges.

The emergence of orthodontics as a true specialty is largely the result of the efforts of one man, Edward Hartley Angle (1855–1930). Having graduated from the Pennsylvania College of Dental Surgery in 1878, Angle moved to Minnesota, and his interest in and skill in treating anomalies of the jaw led to his appointment in 1886 to the chair of orthodontics in the dental department of the University of Minnesota. The next year he presented his first paper, "Notes on Orthodontia with a New System of Regulation and Retention," before the Ninth International Medical Congress (at that time, rhinologists felt that the correction of oral irregularities was a part of their medical specialty). Angle's paper served as the basis for his first book, *Malocclusion of the Teeth*, published in 1887. In 1895 Angle moved to St. Louis to teach orthodontics at what was later to become the St. Louis University School of Dentistry. Recognizing the need for a basic scientific foundation to support his teachings, he developed a classification of malocclusion based on the relationship of the first molars, a system that is still used today. Angle believed that orthodontics could best be taught in a school devoted exclusively to that specialty, and in 1900 Angle's School of Orthodontia began to attract students from all parts of the nation.

In 1901 Angle approached the men who were already prominent in the field of orthodontics, as well as some of his students, and together they organized the American Society of Orthodontists, designating Angle as its first president. The first article of the constitution boldly proclaimed their intention "to establish the science of orthodontia" as a specialty of the healing arts—the second one formed, following that of ophthalmology.

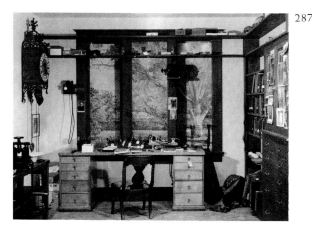

The father of modern orthodontics, Edward Hartley Angle, worked in this study in California until his death in 1930. It is now on display at the National Museum of American History, Smithsonian Institution, Washington, D.C.

Oral Surgery

Oral surgery has its origins as a specialty of dentistry in the work of Simon P. Hullihen (1810–1857), of Wheeling, West Virginia, who established an extensive oral-surgical practice in the 1840s and 1850s. A physician by training, he was awarded an honorary D.D.S. degree by the Baltimore College of Dental Surgery in 1843. He lectured extensively on his methods and established a small hospital in Wheeling devoted exclusively to his oral-surgical patients.

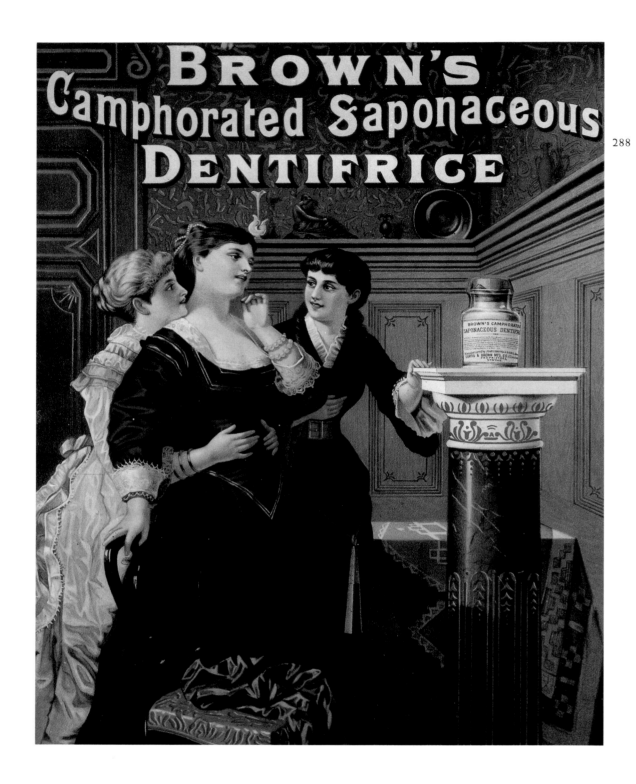

288

Today, advertisements emphasize the hygienic properties of toothpastes, but in earlier times dentifrices were marketed as much for their cosmetic as for their health-giving benefits. In this turn-of-the-century poster, a container of Brown's Camphorated Saponaceous Dentifrice elevated on a Grecian column is contemplated by three ladies in morning and evening dress (suggesting use around the clock). New-York Historical Society, New York City.

289

By comparison with the rather cluttered office of Dr. Lentz (see figure 300), this trim and convenient Danish operating room of about 1900 looks surprisingly modern. Yet the basic equipment is the same: drill, reclining chair, instrument chest, and window as light source. Medicinsk-Historisk Museum, University of Copenhagen.

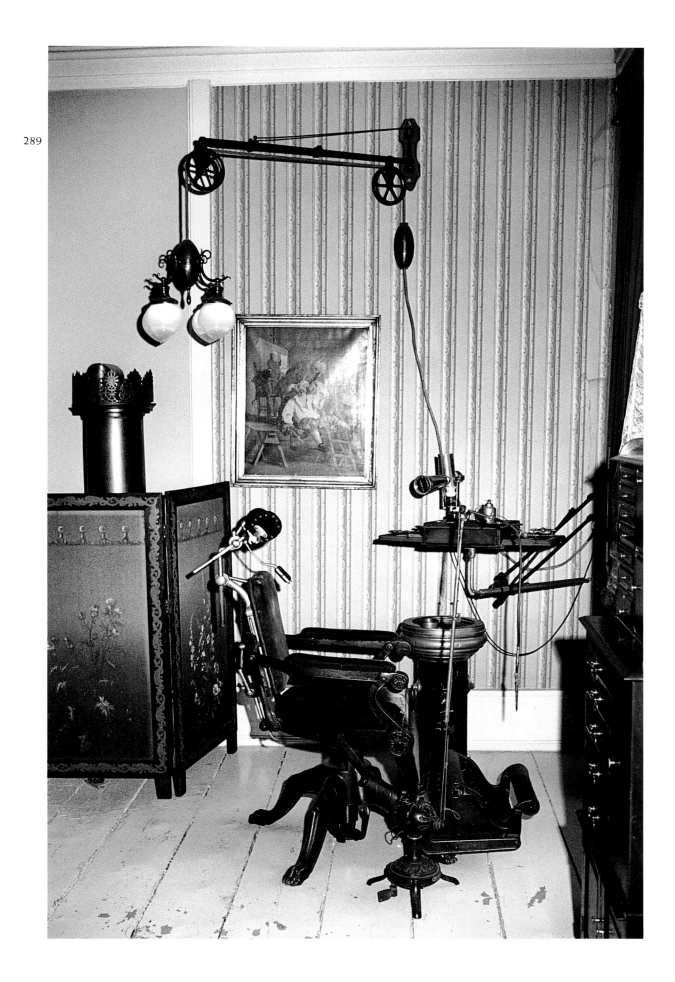

James E. Garretson (1828–1895), often considered the founder of the specialty, received a dental degree in 1856, a year before Hullihen's death, and an M.D. degree in 1859. He began his career as a teacher at the Philadelphia School of Anatomy. In 1869 he was appointed to the hospital of the University of Pennsylvania as "Oral Surgeon"—a title that represents the first official recognition of that field of dentistry. Six years later he was appointed professor of oral surgery at the Philadelphia Dental College, and in 1869 published the first oral-surgery textbook, *A Treatise on the Diseases and Surgery of the Mouth, Jaws and Associated Parts*.

Other dentists soon began limiting their activities to surgery of the oral regions and many made substantial contributions, among them: Truman W. Brophy, who achieved international renown for his special operation for a cleft lip and cleft palate; Matthew W. Cryer, a student of Garretson's and later professor of oral surgery at the dental school of the University of Pennsylvania, who pioneered the technique of removing a portion of the mandible to correct prognathism; and Thomas L. Gilmer of the faculty of the dental school at Northwestern University, who became celebrated for his innovative treatment of maxillary and mandibular fractures.

One of the most outstanding oral surgeons of the twentieth century was Varaztad H. Kazanjian, who in 1915 volunteered with a group of his colleagues at Harvard University to serve in the battle zones of Europe. When the time came for his unit to return, Kazanjian was invited to remain as an honorary major in the British army and to head a unique service. His extraordinary proficiency in constructing splints for facial wounds, and his wonderful results in a highly specialized type of plastic surgery followed by well-planned prosthetic restorations spread his fame rapidly over France. His marvelous achievements brought him the epithet Miracle Man of the Western Front, and he was personally decorated by George V. Returning to America, Kazanjian attended medical school and after earning a degree devoted himself exclusively to the repair of facial defects. Though he is chiefly remembered as the father of modern plastic surgery, it was as a dentist that Kazanjian began his career—a fact that he himself never forgot.

Oral surgery was generally recognized as a dental specialty before any other in America, though the oral surgeons did not formally organize until 1918. Their official organ, the *Journal of Oral Surgery*, was not launched until 1942. In 1978 the name of the examining board was changed from American Board of Oral Surgery to American Board of Oral and Maxillofacial Surgeons.

290

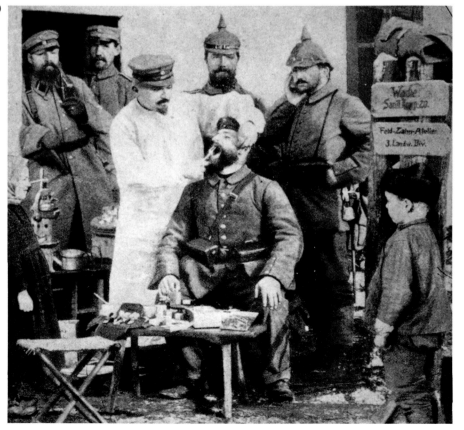

A German dental surgeon is shown operating under rather primitive conditions at a field station during World War I in this magazine illustration of about 1915.

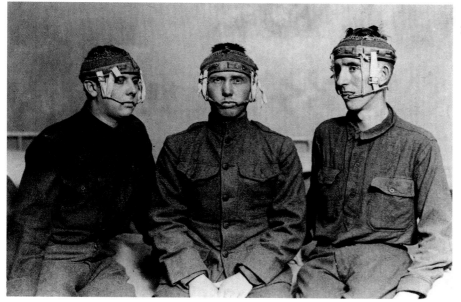

These American soldiers on active duty in France during World War I have been treated for fractures of the jaw with stabilizing dental splints. National Library of Medicine, Bethesda.

Pedodontics

In 1923 fourteen Detroit dentists, led by Dr. Walter McBride, formed the Pedodontic Study Club to improve their skills and knowledge in the field of dentistry for children. Dr. Samuel Harris, who joined in 1925, urged the group to form a national organization, and two years later the American Society for the Promotion of Children's Dentistry was founded, with McBride as president and Harris as secretary. Its aims were twofold: to facilitate the exchange of information among those interested in dentistry for children, and to arouse the public and the profession to an awareness of the need for more and better dentistry for children.

At the group's first annual meeting, in Minneapolis in 1928, the question of an official publication was broached, and out of this eventually came the present *Journal of Dentistry for Children*.

In 1940, the organization changed its name to the American Society of Dentistry for Children, and the first examination of the Board of Pedodontics was held at Northwestern University in February 1949.

Periodontics

Periodontics traces its origins back to the work of John M. Riggs, who, it will be remembered, extracted the first tooth under anesthesia, that of Horace Wells. Riggs introduced his techniques for the treatment of periodontal disease at the 1881 International Medical Congress in London, and thereafter the affliction was called Riggs' Disease.

Surgical treatment of periodontal inflammation was undertaken by numerous dentists in the early part of the twentieth century. Occasionally medical, rather than surgical, treatment was attempted, particularly after C. C. Bass claimed erroneously that *endameba buccalis* was responsible for "pyorrhea" (the now-antiquated term for periodontal disease) and that progress would be made in the development of a suitable vaccine. This approach was effectively countered, however, by Dr. Thomas B. Hartzell in a paper, read before the First District (of New York) Dental Society in 1915, urging instead comprehensive methods of treatment that included deep scaling as well as surgery.

The year 1922 saw the publication of the first authoritative book in the field, *A Textbook of Clinical Periodontia*, by Dr. Paul Stillman and Dr. John Oppie McCall of New York City. In 1914, Stillman and McCall, along with Dr. Grace Rogers Spaulding of Detroit and Dr. Gillette Hayden of Columbus, Ohio, took the initiative and formed the American Academy of Periodontology.

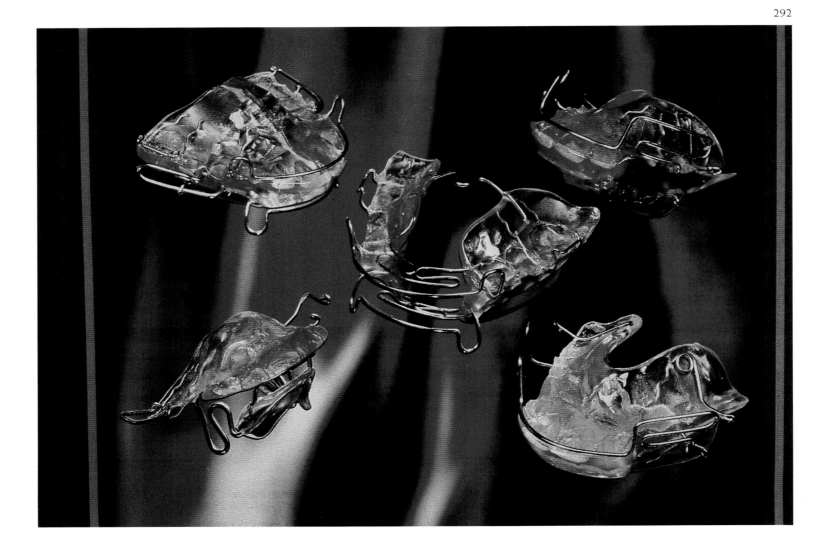

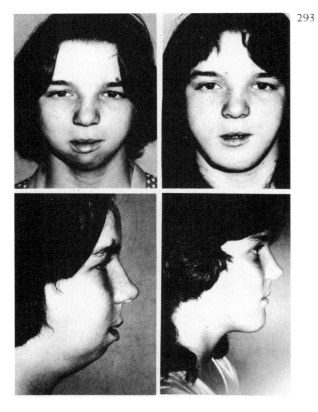

292,293

In the eighteenth and nineteenth centuries, dentists made gross corrections in tooth alignment by means of splints and ligatures (see figure 147). Today fine positioning of teeth can be accomplished by conventional banding and wiring, and sophisticated applicances, such as those shown in figure 292, have been designed to apply force to specific teeth and correct irregularities without banding. Orthognathic surgery represents one of the great accomplishments of modern dentistry, as the before-and-after pictures in figure 293 indicate. An oral surgeon sectioned the patient's mandible and moved the front fragment forward; an orthodontist then realigned the teeth in her jaw.

Advances in Technique, Equipment, and Practice

Restorations

At the beginning of the century, extensive tooth restorations could only be made by using the many types of crowns that had been developed during the preceding thirty years. Inserting most of these crowns into the mouth required devitalization of the damaged tooth and, in addition, they were often ill-fitting and unsightly. Small restorations were made with silver amalgam or else laboriously constructed of gold foil. As we have seen, attempts had long been made to inlay teeth with cemented fillings of one sort or another. One rather ingenious invention of the 1890s called for inserting a tiny factory-made cylinder of glass into a hole prepared in the tooth with a cylindrical drill of the same diameter as the inlay. The technique was never perfected, however, and an excess of cement was needed to hold such inlays in place. Other methods, such as flowing gold solder into a metal matrix, resulted in a poor seal because the gold shrank while cooling and would not fit the cavity tightly.

In the 1880s William H. Taggart (1855–1933), a dentist of Freeport, Illinois, conceived of an alternative to the soldered inlay that could be precisely cast by the ancient disappearing-wax process. An unusually skillful and inventive technician, he experimented with various procedures and by 1907 had perfected a method of casting the first accurately fitting gold inlays. He demonstrated his process, which required the use of a casting machine he had patented (fig. 294), before the New York Odontological Society on the evening of January 15, 1907. The new technique, which the audience received enthusiastically, consisted of carving directly in the mouth a wax model of the cavity to be filled. The model with a small sprue attachment was embedded in a special plaster investment and the plaster heated, "burning out" the wax. Gold melted with a blowpipe was then forced into the plaster mold by means of Taggart's casting machine, which utilized compressed air. The resulting inlay fit the cavity so closely that only a very thin film of cement was needed, serving more as a sealant than a retainer.

Taggart had invested much money and nearly twenty years of work in developing his idea as well as his casting machine and, in order to recoup some of his expenses, he attempted to patent his method as well as his machine. The profession, however, began using his technique almost at once, ignoring his attempts to secure legal rights to it. Taggart tried to interest dentists in buying his expensive machine, but within a few years many practitioners were fashioning their own. Eventually Taggart became involved in extensive litigation over the legality of his patents. He was on the verge of winning his suit when it was discovered that an obscure Iowa dentist had demonstrated a somewhat similar though less sophisticated process before his local dental society in 1896. Embittered and broken, angry at the profession that he felt had betrayed him, Taggart spent his remaining years in retirement. Dentistry has not forgotten Taggart, however, and will forever be in his debt. Because of his ingenious idea and the skill and perseverance that made it work, we are able to manufacture the many intricate castings that have helped to make modern dentistry so successful.

The introduction in the 1960s of crowns consisting of porcelain bonded to metal has enabled dentists to construct extensive, yet esthetic fixed restorations. These crowns have supplanted the once-popular gold crowns with acrylic veneers, for in time the veneers wore away, exposing the gold underneath. But the individual all-porcelain jacket crown still has a place, especially since the invention of aluminized porcelain, a far stronger and less friable material.

A major recent innovation has been the use of composite filling materials and filled resins—the end result of research aimed at reducing caries in the surfaces of children's teeth through the use of sealants. As early as 1910 a dentist had demonstrated a method of sealing the grooves in the biting surfaces of teeth with zinc oxyphosphate cement, which could be replaced periodically as it wore away. A number of investigators experimented with other materials, but the es-

294

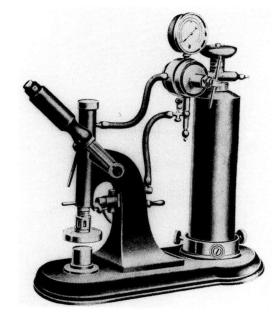

By 1907 William H. Taggart had perfected a new method of casting gold inlays and a machine to do it. The method is still in use today but the machine, seen here in an advertisement of 1908, was expensive and did not sell as well as Taggart had hoped.

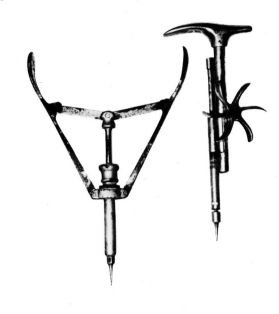

Many innovative and useful dental instruments became available during the early twentieth century. This advertisement of about 1915 by the firm of Wilcox Jewett shows two new pressure syringes used to administer local anesthetics—an invention that has recently been reintroduced.

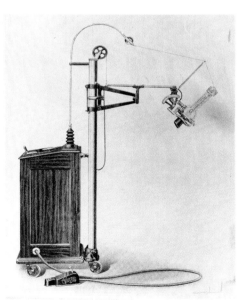

Victor Electric Company manufactured this X-ray machine soon after the turn of the century. The exposed high-tension wire posed a significant shock hazard to the dentists who used it.

sential and critically successful work was done in 1955 by Michael Buonocore while he was employed in research at the Eastman Dental Center in Rochester. He first etched the tooth surface with a mild acid solution and then painted on a thin layer of self-polymerizing acrylic. Acrylic proved too soft to withstand chewing stresses, however, so Buonocore experimented with various other resins and in 1967 introduced the composite, or filled, resins, which depend for their strength on microscopic particles of glass or quartz incorporated into the resin base. This new material made possible "bonding" procedures hitherto undreamed of. The preparation of the enamel surface by acid-etching (which created millions of irregularities to which a liquid plastic could adhere) followed by the application of resins allowed teeth to be built up in many ways. Thin tooth-shaped veneers could be bonded to unsightly teeth, obviating the need for the construction of full crowns. Fractured teeth could be restored without resorting to gold castings. Orthodontic brackets could be fixed to the surfaces of the teeth, eliminating the need for banding the teeth with metal, a procedure both time consuming and unesthetic. Spaces between the teeth could be eliminated and even the shapes of teeth changed. In fact, with the advent in the late 1970s of still more sophisticated plastics and resins and more effective sources of light (almost all bonding materials harden, or cure, when exposed to light), a dentist is limited only by his imagination as to what he can do for his patient.

Profound changes in dental procedures followed the invention in the early postwar period of the high-speed turbine drill, which has made dental restoration easier for the patient to bear and for the dentist to perform; moreover, far more intricate operations can be undertaken because of the increased control possible when drilling at a high speed. During the first half of the century, innovative dentists found that their patients' discomfort decreased as the rate of rotation of the drill bur increased because vibration was reduced, and some early efforts were directed toward increasing drill speeds through complicated pulley arrangements. The Page-Chayes handpiece, introduced in 1958, was the first belt-driven angle-handpiece to operate successfully at speeds over 100,000 rpm. In this instrument all gears were eliminated; instead, a small belt inside the handpiece sheath ran over ball-bearing pulleys. The first true all-turbine (gearless) handpiece was developed in the early 1950s by Dr. Robert J. Nelsen while he was employed in the Dental Research Unit of Washington's National Bureau of Standards. His water-driven machine used a pump driving 1.6 gallons per minute to rotate a small turbine in the head of the handpiece. It was marketed in 1954 under the trade name Turbo-Jet (fig. 297). But Turbo-Jet's top speed was only 60,000 rpm.

Two years earlier Ivor Norlén of Sweden had secured a United States patent on an air-driven turbine handpiece. This instrument could reach a speed of 70,000 rpm. The motive force was transmitted through a series of gears to the handpiece head, which held the bur. In 1957 the big breakthrough came with the introduction by the S. S. White Company of the Borden Airotor, the first clinically successful air-driven handpiece, which developed speeds of 300,000 rpm and used no gears at all. Since then, handpiece design has been only slightly modified, with all new models utilizing a tiny turbine directly driven by compressed air. A small but significant improvement was made in the 1970s, when, through the utilization of fiber-optic components built into the drill handpiece, light could be played on the working area.

This century has also seen the increased use of preformed implants, which are driven into the bones of the upper or lower jaws to act as anchors for fixed prostheses. Although the technique is not new, having first been introduced by Dr. E. J. Greenfield in 1918, it nevertheless is still regarded by many dentists as experimental; however, many practitioners have used these implants with great success to restore partially or totally edentulous mouths. Promising work utilizing nonmetallic implants such as pyrolytic carbon is being carried on in a number of institutions, and eventually a material may be found to which living tissue, such as the gingivae, and cemental fibers will attach themselves.

Denture Construction

Although American dentists were still considered the trendsetters in improving instruments, materials, and techniques, dentists in other lands have also made important contributions during the twentieth century. Alfred Gysi of Switzerland brought out the first truly satisfactory articulator in 1909, and this, together with the face-bow (a device used to measure the spatial relationship of the upper jaw to the lower jaw, both in movement and at rest), which had been invented earlier by Dr. George B. Snow of Buffalo, New York, made it possible to construct better fitting dentures. Dentures were also vastly improved esthetically as a result of the work of James Leon Williams, an expatriate American practicing in London, who in 1914 announced his study of facial form in relation to tooth form. His description of typal forms led to the manufacture of exceedingly natural-looking denture teeth, and when in 1919 pink rubber was introduced, denture bases, too, could be wonderfully lifelike.

Further improvements were made in partial dentures with the introduction of the first chrome-cobalt alloy, Vitallium, in 1930. In 1932 Vinylite, the first of the plastic denture-base materials, was brought out, but it was supplanted by the methyl-methacrylate resins that completely dominated the field by the mid-1930s.

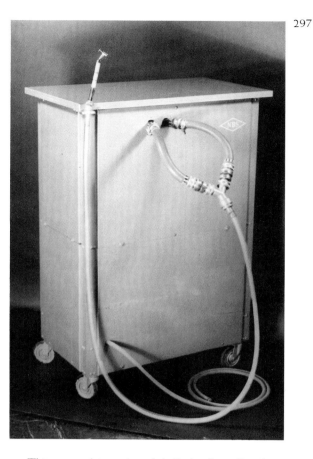

This water-driven dental drill, the first all-turbine model, came on the market in the 1950s. The invention of Dr. Robert J. Nelsen, the Turbo-Jet could achieve speeds of 60,000 rpm. National Museum of American History, Smithsonian Institution, Washington, D.C.

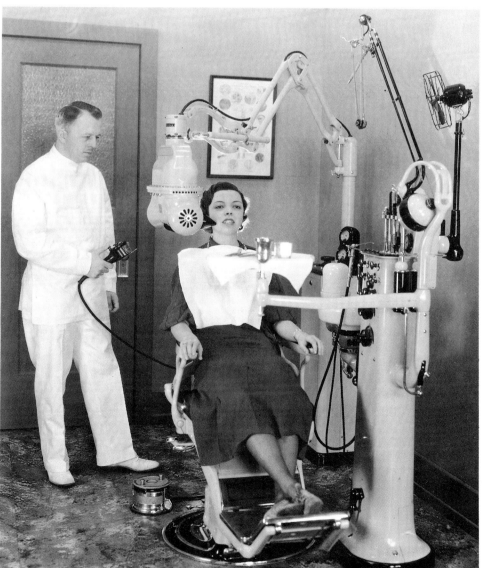

The dental unit, chair, and X-ray machine seen in this well-equipped office of 1940 were made by the Ritter Company of Rochester, New York. The unit combined many elements in a single piece of equipment—drill, air blower, and cuspidor—and marked a great step forward in efficiency. Unfortunately, the profession was not yet fully aware of the dangers of radiation: the dentist stands close to his X-ray machine and the patient wears no protective lead apron.

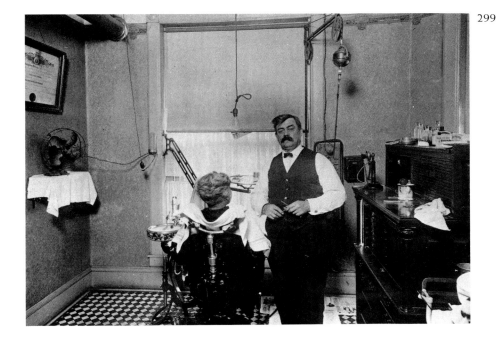

About 1905 a progressive Oklahoma dentist, Dr. R. H. Pendleton, maintained this office. It boasted all the modern conveniences: electric drill, electric fan, and a telephone. Western History Collections, University of Oklahoma, Norman.

Office Equipment and Procedure

Local anesthesia had widely supplanted general anesthesia in the dental office by the end of the first decade of the century. Although cocaine was frequently used after its introduction into medical practice by Karl Koller in 1884, its shortcomings—especially its addictive properties and its tendency to cause tissue-sloughing—were keenly felt. The development of Novocain by the German chemist Alfred Einhorn in 1904 revolutionized dental practice by eliminating pain from most dental procedures.

By the early 1920s most dentists had X-ray machines, and sterilizers were to be found in every dental office. Today, the autoclave has almost universally replaced the old-fashioned sterilizer containing boiling water, and a new panoramic X-ray machine introduced at the end of World War II allows survey radiographs of both entire jaws to be made on one film. Dental chairs have also been redesigned to permit the patient to recline completely, minimizing the discomfort of both patient and operator.

Changes in office procedure during the postwar decades also rendered the routine visit more comfortable and quick. Assistants had become indispensable (the American Dental Assistants Association was organized as early as 1923), and so-called four-handed dentistry, in which the dentist and his or her assistant, both seated, work as a smoothly functioning team in handling instruments, high-volume evacuation equipment, and placement of restorations, has proved an enormous advance.

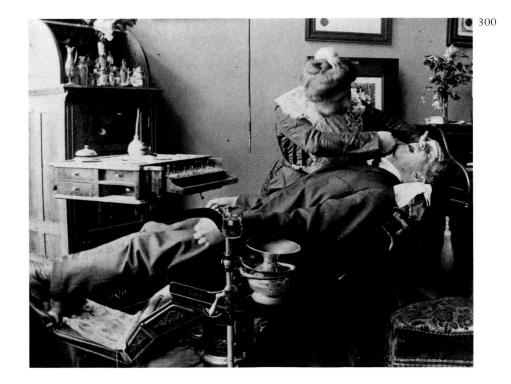

Dr. Olga Lentz, of Minneapolis–St. Paul, one of the very few women who practiced dentistry in her day, is seen extracting a tooth in her office in 1910. Minnesota Historical Society, St. Paul.

299

300

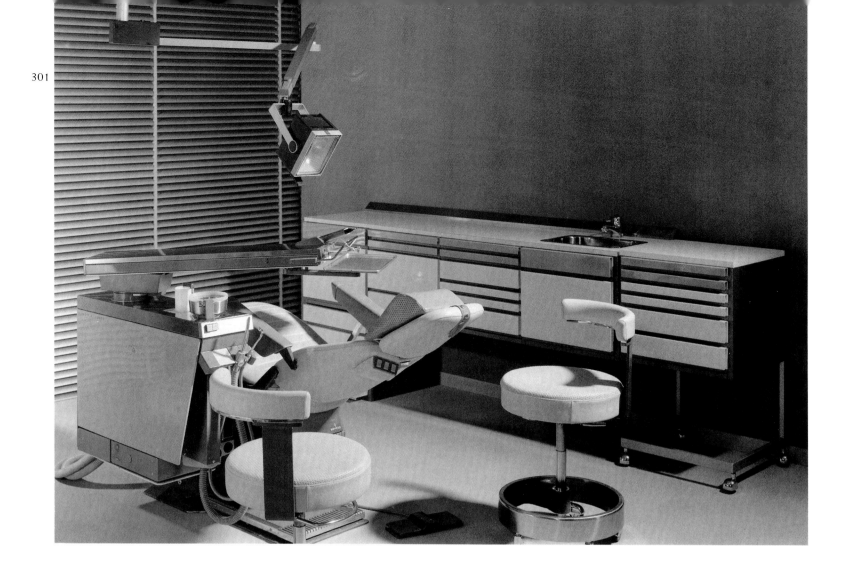

The streamlined office of the 1970s seen in figure 301 was designed to permit a dentist and his assistant to work together with maximum convenience and efficiency. In figure 302, in a classic illustration of "four-handed dentistry," Dr. Robert M. Pick, a periodontist of Chicago, and his assistant treat a patient sedated under nitrous oxide–oxygen analgesia. Both operators wear rubber gloves, and Dr. Pick also wears a mask to reduce the chance of infection.

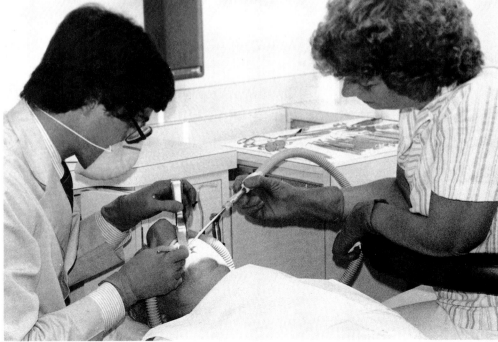

302

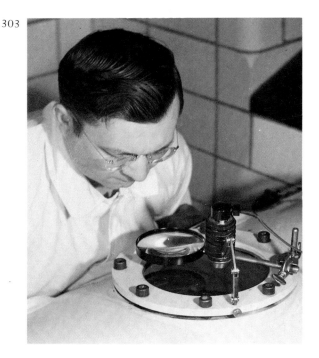

Dr. Frank J. Orland of the University of Chicago peers at rats kept in a germfree unit in his laboratory. Orland's research has proved that the precipitating factor in the development of caries is the presence of *Streptococcus mutans* bacteria in the mouth.

Research

A major step forward was taken in 1948 when the National Institute of Dental Research (NIDR) was established by the United States Public Health Service. Ultimately incorporated into the National Institutes of Health, headquartered in Bethesda, Maryland, just outside Washington, D.C., the NIDR has played a major role in furthering basic and applied research. In addition to conducting original research, it is responsible for approving research grants to other institutions and to individuals. The establishment of NIDR may be considered one of the outstanding developments of recent years in that it represented formal recognition by Congress of the importance of dental health.

One of the principal areas of dental research has been in the field of caries, and some of the most important findings have been made by Dr. Frank J. Orland (fig. 303) of the University of Chicago, who has selectively exposed rats kept in a sterile laboratory environment to various types of bacteria. Orland has determined that caries results principally from the action of *streptococcus mutans* bacteria, giving rise to the hope that someday a suitable anticaries vaccine may become a reality. Orland's research showed that caries is a multifactorial disease that develops in the presence of a susceptible tooth, a diet conducive to caries formation, and the cariogenic microbiota that create the lactic acid that ultimately demineralizes the tooth surface.

Biomedical engineering has played an increasing role in dental research, with amazing results. One of our major areas of ignorance has been the criteria for defining the characteristics of the masticatory apparatus in health and disease. For example: What is a normal bite? What is the normal path of occlusion—that is, the path the mandible takes as it moves during chewing? Modern techniques have allowed us to implant into tooth surfaces miniature transducers that measure pressure. In 1971 Messerman and Gibbs, working at Case Western Reserve University in Cleveland, cemented tiny light-transducers with photoelectric cells to the labial surfaces of both dental arches. These recorded mandibular movement relative to maxillary movement, and the data were stored in a computer. Then the jaw function could be played back and reproduced on a model of the patient's jaws, permitting more intensive study. Other biomechanical engineering marvels allow us to study the demineralization of tooth surfaces with ultrasound or electricity. With the latter we found that the more highly mineralized the tooth surface the higher was its resistance to microelectric currents. In periodontology, improved collection and sampling systems permit the quantitative and qualitative analyses of fluids secured from the gingival crevice by micromethod techniques. In anticaries research, microcapsules that will deliver caries-preventing agents are being incorporated in a polymer that is applied to the tooth surface by aerosol spray. And in the field of radiology, computer-enhanced imaging upgraded the interpretation of radiographs and led to more accurate diagnoses.

In sum, the developments made possible by biomedical engineering will most surely change the face of dental practice, promising an exciting future.

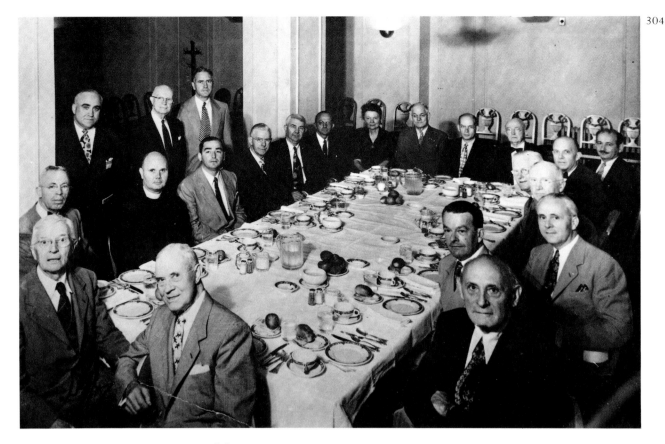

History

The only guide to the future is the study of the past. Excited by this idea, Dr. J. Ben Robinson, then dean of the Baltimore College of Dental Surgery, Dental School, University of Maryland, in 1950 consulted some of his colleagues who were also interested in the practical, theoretical, and moral insights to be derived from a study of dental history. Associated with him in founding the organization born from their deliberations were four dental historians: Dr. Milton B. Asbell, of Camden, New Jersey; Dr. Harold L. Faggart, of Philadelphia; Professor Gardner Foley, of Baltimore; and Dr. William N. Hodgkin, of Warrenton, Virginia. On October 16, 1951, twenty-one enthusiasts convened at the Mayflower Hotel in Washington, D.C., for the charter meeting of the American Academy of the History of Dentistry (AAHD). Robinson presided and outlined the organization's goals: to increase interest among dentists in the history of their profession; to encourage dental schools to develop historical collections and to offer adequate instruction in dental history; to interest the leaders of the profession in dental history so that they might tackle problems in education and practice with the advantage of hindsight; and to create an authoritative body to which important questions relating to dental history could be referred for factual verification.

The AAHD was established on a permanent basis at its first annual meeting, held in St. Louis in 1952 (fig. 304). An official publication, the *Bulletin of the History of Dentistry* (*BHD*), was launched in March 1953, with Dr. George B. Denton as editor. In 1963, Dr. Donald Washburn assumed the editorship, upon Dr. Denton's death. He was followed in 1968 by the author of this book, who has been at the helm of the journal since that time. The *BHD* is the only publication in the English-speaking world devoted to dental history and bibliography. It is recognized worldwide as the authoritative journal on its subject and has attracted subscribers around the globe.

The AAHD has grown since its founding in 1952 to a membership of about 600. It sponsors an annual essay-writing contest among dental students in the United States and Canada and confers an annual Hayden-Harris Award for distinguished contributions to dental history (the first recipient, in 1967, was J. Ben Robinson). The AAHD has also conferred honorary membership upon leading dental historians of other lands in recognition of their outstanding contributions to a vital scholastic field.

The first annual meeting of the American Academy of the History of Dentistry was held in St. Louis on September 6, 1952. Seated in the second row, third and eighth from the left, respectively, are Dr. Milton B. Asbell and Dr. J. Ben Robinson. Standing third from the left in the third row is Professor Gardner Foley.

SELECTED BIBLIOGRAPHY

ADAMS, F. R. *The Genuine Works of Hippocrates.* New York: William Wood, 1891

ADAMSON, JOY. *The Peoples of Kenya.* New York: Harcourt Brace & World, 1965

ALBUCASIS (ABU-AL-QASIM). *La Chirurgie d'Albucasis.* Trans. Lucien Leclerc. Paris: Baillière, 1861

ALLBUTT, T. CLIFFORD. *Greek Medicine in Rome.* New York: Benjamin Blom, 1970

AMERICAN ACADEMY OF DENTAL SCIENCE. *A History of Dental and Oral Science in America.* Philadelphia: S. S. White, 1876

ANDRÉ-BONNET, J. L. *Histoire générale de la chirurgie dentaire.* Paris: Société Auteurs Moderne, 1910

ARISTOTLE. *Works.* Trans. D. W. Thompson. Oxford: Clarendon, 1910

ASBELL, MILTON B. *A Bibliography of Dentistry in America: 1790–1840.* Cherry Hill, N.J.: Sussex House, 1973

————. *A Century of Dentistry: A History of the University of Pennsylvania School of Dental Medicine.* Philadelphia: University of Pennsylvania, 1977

BAKAY, LOUIS. *The Treatment of Head Injuries in the Thirty Years' War (1618–1648): Joannis Scultetus and His Age.* Springfield, Ill.: Charles C. Thomas, 1971

BALTIMORE COLLEGE OF DENTAL SURGERY. *Proceedings of the One Hundred Twenty-Fifth Anniversary Celebration of the Baltimore College of Dental Surgery.* Edited by Gardner P. H. Foley. Baltimore: Baltimore College of Dental Surgery, 1965

BANDINELLI, RANUCCIO B. *Rome: The Center of Power.* New York: Braziller, 1970

BEALL, OTHO T., and SHRYOCK, RICHARD H. *Cotton Mather: First Significant Figure in American Medicine.* Baltimore: Johns Hopkins Press, 1954

BECK, R. THEODORE. *The Cutting Edge: Early History of the Surgeons of London.* London: Lund Humphries, 1974

BENION, ELISABETH. *Antique Medical Instruments.* Berkeley: University of California Press, 1979

BENTLEY, NICHOLAS. *The Victorian Scene: A Picture Book of the Period.* London: Weidenfeld & Nicolson, 1968

BETTMANN, OTTO L. *A Pictorial History of Medicine.* Springfield, Ill.: Charles C. Thomas, 1956

BIDLOO, GOVARD. *Anatomia humani corporis.* Amsterdam: Joannis & Someren, 1685

BLOCK, WERNER. *Der Arzt und der Tod in Bildern aus sechs Jahrhunderten.* Stuttgart: Ferdinand Enke, 1966

BOWERS, J. Z. *When the Twain Meet: The Rise of Western Medicine in Japan.* Baltimore: Johns Hopkins Press, 1980

BRATTON, FRED G. *Maimonides, Medieval Modernist.* Boston: Beacon, 1967

BREASTED, JAMES H. *The Edwin Smith Surgical Papyrus.* Chicago: University of Chicago Press, 1930

BREMNER, M. D. K. *The Story of Dentistry.* Brooklyn, N.Y.: Dental Items of Interest, 1954

BRENDLE, THOMAS R., and UNGER, CLAUDE W. *Folk Medicine of the Pennsylvania Germans.* New York: Augustus M. Kelly, 1970

BRIEGER, GERT H., ed. *Medical America in the Nineteenth Century.* Baltimore: Johns Hopkins Press, 1972

BROWNE, EDWARD G. *Arabian Medicine.* Cambridge: Cambridge University Press, 1921

BRUCK, WALTHER. *Das Martyrium der heiligen Apollonia und seine Darstellung in der bildenden Kunst.* Berlin: Hermann Meusser, 1915

BRUNSCHWIG, HIERONYMUS. *The Book of Cirurgia.* Milan: Lier, 1923

BULLOUGH, VERN L. *The Development of Medicine as a Profession.* Basel: S. Karger, 1966

BURFORD, ALISON. *The Greek Temple Builders at Epidauros.* Toronto, University of Toronto Press, 1969

CAMERON, J. M., and SIMS, B. G. *Forensic Dentistry.* Edinburgh: Churchill Livingstone, 1974

CAMPBELL, J. MENZIES. *Dentistry Then and Now.* Glasgow: privately printed, 1981

CASTIGLIONI, ARTURO. *A History of Medicine.* 2d ed. Trans. E. B. Krumbhaar. New York: Knopf, 1947

CELSUS. *De medicina.* Trans. W. G. Spencer, Cambridge, Mass.: Harvard University Press, 1938

CHARLES, ALLAN D. *History of Dentistry in South Carolina.* Greenville: A Press, Inc., 1982

CIGRAND, B. J. *The Rise, Fall and Revival of Dental Prosthesis.* Chicago: Periodical Pub. Co., 1892

CLENDENING, LOGAN. *A Source Book of Medical History.* New York: Paul B. Hoeber, 1942

COLYER, FRANK. *Old Instruments Used for Extracting Teeth.* London: Staples, 1952

DALE, PHILIP M. *Medical Biographies: The Ailments of Thirty-Three Famous Persons.* Norman: University of Oklahoma Press, 1952

DAMMANN, GORDON. *A Pictorial Encyclopedia of Civil War Medical Instruments and Equipment.* Missoula, Mont.: Pictorial Histories, 1983

DAVY, HUMPHRY. *Researches, Chemical and Philosophical, Chiefly Concerning Nitrous Oxide.* London: J. Johnson: 1800

DAWSON, WARREN R. *The Beginnings: Egypt and Assyria.* New York: Paul B. Hoeber, 1930

DEMAAR, F. E. R., ed. *Van tandmeesters en tandartsen: 100 jaar tandheelkundig onderwits in Nederland.* Amsterdam: 't Koggeschip, 1978

DOBELL, C. *Anthony van Leeuwen Hoek and His "Little Animals."* New York: Harcourt, Brace, 1932

DOBSON, JESSIE. *John Hunter.* Edinburgh: E. & S. Livingstone, 1969

DOBSON, J., and MILNE, R. *Barbers and Barber-Surgeons of London.* Oxford: Blackwell Scientific Publications, 1979

DUKE, MARC. *Acupuncture.* New York: Pyramid House, 1972

DUMESNIL, RENÉ. *Histoire illustrée de la médecine.* Paris: Librairie Plon, 1935

DUMMETT, CLIFTON O., and DUMMETT, LOIS D. *Afro-Americans in Dentistry: Sequence and Consequence of Events.* Los Angeles: privately printed, 1977

EDWARDS, CHILPERIC. *The Hammurabi Code.* London: Watts, 1921

ELLIOTT, JAMES S. *Outlines of Greek and Roman Medicine.* Boston: Milford House, 1971

ENNIS, JOHN. *The Story of the Fédération Dentaire Internationale, 1900–1962.* London: Fédération Dentaire Internationale, 1967

ENTRALGO, PEDRO L., et al. *Historia universal de la medicina.* 7 vols. Barcelona: Salvat Editores, 1974

FARRAR, JOHN N. *A Treatise on the Irregularity of the Teeth and Their Correction.* New York: privately printed, 1888

FASTLICHT, SAMUEL. *Tooth Mutilations and Dentistry in Pre-Columbian Mexico.* Chicago: Quintessence, 1976

FAUCHARD, PIERRE. *Le chirurgien dentiste; ou, traité des dents,* Paris: Jean Mariette, 1728

FEBRES-CORDERO, FOCION. *Origenes de la odontologia.* Caracas: Soc. Venez. Hist. Med., 1966

FITCH, SAMUEL S. *A System of Dental Surgery.* New York: G., C., and H. Carvill, 1829

FOLEY, GARDNER P. H. *Foley's Footnotes: A Treasury of Dentistry.* Wallingford, Pa.: Washington Square East, 1972

FOX, JOSEPH. *The Histology and Treatment of the Diseases of the Teeth.* London: Thomas Cox, 1806

————. *The Natural History of the Human Teeth.* London: Thomas Cox, 1803

GABKA, JOACHIM. *Die erste Zahnung in der Geschichte des Aberglaubens der Volksmedizin und Medizin.* Berlin: Quintessenz, 1970

GALEN. *Hygiene.* Trans. R. M. Green. Springfield, Ill.: Charles C. Thomas, 1951

GARIOT, J. B. *Treatise on the Diseases of the Mouth.* Trans. J. B. Savier. Baltimore: American Society of Dental Surgeons, 1843

GAROSI, ALCIDE. *Inter artium et medicinae doctores.* Florence: Leo S. Olschki, 1958

GARRETSON, JAMES E. *A System of Oral Surgery.* Philadelphia: J. B. Lippincott, 1873

GARRISON, FIELDING H. *An Introduction to the History of Medicine.* 4th ed. Philadelphia: W. B. Saunders, 1929

GEORGE, M. DOROTHY. *Hogarth to Cruikshank: Social Change in Graphic Satire.* New York: Walker, 1967

GHALIOUNGUI, PAUL. *The House of Life: Magic and Medical Science in Ancient Egypt.* Amsterdam: B. M. Israel, 1973

————. *The Physicians of Pharaonic Egypt.* Cairo: Al-Ahram Center for Scientific Translations, 1983

GIES, WILLIAM J. *Dental Education in the United States and Canada: A Report to the Carnegie Foundation for the Advancement of Teaching.* New York: Carnegie Foundation, 1926

GLENNER, RICHARD A. *The Dental Office: A Pictorial History*. Missoula, Mont.: Pictorial Histories, 1984

GORDON, BENJAMIN L. *Medicine throughout Antiquity*. Philadelphia: F. A. Davis, 1949

———. *Medieval and Renaissance Medicine*. New York: Philosophical Library, 1959

GORDON, MAURICE B. *Naval and Maritime Medicine during the American Revolution*. Ventnor, N.J.: Ventnor, 1978

GORDON, RICHARD. *The Sleep of Life*. New York: Dial, 1975

GRANT, MICHAEL, ed. *The Birth of Western Civilization*. New York: McGraw-Hill, 1964

GRAPE-ALBERS, HEIDE. *Spätantike Bilder aus der Welt des Arztes*. Wiesbaden: Guido Pressler, 1977

GUERINI, VINCENZO. *A History of Dentistry from the Most Ancient Times until the End of the Eighteenth Century*. Philadelphia and New York: Lea and Febiger, 1909. (Reprinted Pound Ridge, N.Y.: Milford House, 1969)

GULLETT, D. W. *A History of Dentistry in Canada*. Toronto: University of Toronto Press, 1971

GUTHRIE, DOUGLAS. *A History of Medicine*. Philadelphia: J. B. Lippincott, 1946

HAMARNEH, SAMI K. *The Genius of Arab Civilization, Source of Renaissance*. New York: New York University Press, 1975

HAMBY, WALLACE B. *Ambroise Paré, Surgeon of the Renaissance*. St. Louis: Warren H. Green, 1967

HAND, WAYLAND D., ed. *American Folk Medicine: A Symposium*. Berkeley: University of California Press, 1976

HARGRAVE, JOHN. *The Life and Soul of Paracelsus*. London: Victor Gollancz, 1951

HARRIS, CHAPIN A. *A Dictionary of Medical Terminology, Dental Surgery and the Collateral Sciences*. Philadelphia: Lindsay and Blakiston, 1867

———. *The Principles and Practice of Dental Surgery*. Philadelphia: Lindsay and Blakiston, 1845

HARRIS, JAMES E., and WEEKS, KENT R. *X-Raying the Pharaohs*. New York: Charles Scribner's Sons, 1973

HAY, DENYS, ed. *The Age of the Renaissance*. New York: McGraw-Hill, 1967

HECHTLINGER, ADELAIDE. *The Great Patent Medicine Era; or, without Benefit of Doctor*. New York: Madison Square, 1970

HECKSCHER, WILLIAM S. *Rembrandt's Anatomy of Dr. Nicolas Tulp: An Iconological Study*. New York: New York University Press, 1958

HELFAND, WILLIAM H. *Medicine and Pharmacy in American Political Prints*. Madison, Wis.: American Institute of the History of Pharmacy, 1978

———, and ROCCHIETTA, SERGIO. *Medicina e farmacia nelle caricature politiche Italiane: 1848–1914*. Milan: Edizioni Scientifiche Internazionali, 1982

HENSCHEN, FOLKE. *The History of Diseases*. Trans. John Tate. London: Longmans, 1966

HERRLINGER, ROBERT. *History of Medical Illustration from Antiquity to 1600*. Trans. Graham Fulton-Smith. Munich: Heinz Moos, 1967.

HOFFMANN-AXTHELM, WALTER. *History of Dentistry*. Trans. H. M. Koehler. Chicago: Quintessence, 1981

HOLLÄNDER, EUGEN. *Die Karikatur und Satire in der Medizin*. Stuttgart: Ferdinand Enke, 1921

———. *Die Medizin in der klassischen Malerei*. Stuttgart: Ferdinand Enke, 1923

———. *Plastik und Medizin*. Stuttgart: Ferdinand Enke, 1912

HUNTER, JOHN. *The Natural History of the Human Teeth*. 2d ed. London: J. Johnson, 1778

INGLIS, BRIAN. *A History of Medicine*. Cleveland and New York: World, 1975

JAGGI, O. P. *The Indian System of Medicine*. New Delhi: Atma Ram and Sons, 1973

JONES, RUSSELL M., ed. *The Parisian Education of an American Surgeon: Letters of Jonathan Mason Warren (1832–1835)*. Philadelphia: American Philosophical Society, 1978

KANNER, LEO. *Folklore of the Teeth*. New York: Macmillan, 1934

KEEN, HARRY; JARRETT, JOHN; and LEVY, ARTHUR. *Triumphs of Medicine*. London: Paul Elek, 1976

KEYS, THOMAS E. *The History of Surgical Anesthesia*, Rev. and enl. ed. New York: Dover, 1963

KIDD, FOSTER. *Profile of the Negro in American Dentistry*. Washington, D.C.: Howard University Press, 1979

KIRKPATRICK, T. P. *A Note on the Early History of Dentistry*. Dublin: Gaelic, 1925

KNIPPING, HUGO W., and KENTER, H. *Heilkunst und Kunstwerk: Probleme zwischen Kunst und Medizin aus ärztlicher Sicht*. Stuttgart: F. K. Schattauer, 1966

KOCH, CHARLES R. E. *History of Dental Surgery*. 3 vols. Fort Wayne, Ind.: National Art, 1910

KOMROFF, MANUEL. *The History of Herodotus*. New York: Tudor, 1928

KREMERS, E., and URDANG, G. *A History of Pharmacy*. Philadelphia: J. B. Lippincott, 1976

KUTUMBIAH, P. *Ancient Indian Medicine*. Bombay: Orient Longmans, 1962

LECA, ANGE-PIERRE. *La médecine egyptienne au temps des pharaohs*, Paris: Editions Robert Dacosta, 1971

LEEUWENHOEK, ANTONI VAN. *Collected Letters in Eight Volumes*. Amsterdam: Swets & Zeitlinger, 1941

LeFANU, WILLIAM R. *Notable Medical Books from the Lilly Library, Indiana University*. Indianapolis: Lilly Research Laboratories, 1976

LEGRAND, NOÉ. *Les collections artistiques de la Faculté de Médecine de Paris*. Paris: Masson, 1911

LENNMALM, HERMAN. *World's History and Review of Dentistry*. Chicago: W. B. Conkey, 1894

LINDSAY, LILIAN. *A Short History of Dentistry*. London: Bale and Danielsson, 1933

LUFKIN, ARTHUR W. *A History of Dentistry*. 2d ed. Philadelphia: Lea and Febiger, 1948

McCLUGGAGE, ROBERT W. *A History of the American Dental Association*. Chicago: American Dental Association, 1959

MacLEAN, UNA. *Magical Medicine: A Nigerian Case-Study*. London: Penguin, 1971

MacQUITTY, BETTY. *The Battle for Oblivion: The Discovery of Anesthesia*. London: Geo. Harrap, 1969

MAJNO, GUIDO. *The Healing Hand: Man and Wound in the Ancient World*. Cambridge, Mass.: Harvard University Press, 1975

MAPLE, ERICH. *Magic, Medicine and Quackery*. London: Robert Hale, 1968

MARGOTTA, R. *An Illustrated History of Medicine*. Geltham, Eng.: Paul Hamblyn, 1967

MARRY, LOUIS B. "Pratique odontologique ancienne en Provence." Ph.D. diss., Faculté de Chirurgie Dentaire de Marseilles, 1974

MARTÍ-IBÁÑEZ, FELIX. *The Epic of Medicine*. New York: Bramhall House, 1962

MATHER, COTTON. *The Angel of Bethesda*. Edited by G. W. Jones. Worcester, Mass.: American Antiquarian Society, 1972

MEYER, CLARENCE. *American Folk Medicine*. New York: Thomas Y. Crowell Co., 1973

MEZ-MANGOLD, LYDIA. *A History of Drugs*. Basel: Hoffmann-LaRoche, 1971

MONDOR, HENRI. *Doctors and Medicine in the Work of Daumier*. Boston: Boston Book and Art Shop, 1960

MOSKOW, BERNARD S. *Art and the Dentist*. Tokyo: Shorin, 1982

MUKHOPADHYAYA, GIRINDRANATH. *The Surgical Instruments of the Hindus*. Calcutta: Calcutta University Press, 1914

NABAVI, MIR-HOSSEIN. *Hygiene und Medizin im Koran*. Stuttgart: Ferdinand Enke, 1967

NAKAHARA, KEN; SHINDO, YOSHIHISA; and HOMMA, KUNINORI. *Manners and Customs of Dentistry in Ukiyoe*. Tokyo: Ishiyaku, 1980

NIMS, CHARLES F. *Thebes of the Pharaohs*. New York: Stein and Day, 1965

NITSKE, W. ROBERT. *The Life of Wilhelm Conrad Roentgen, Discoverer of the X-Ray*. Tucson: University of Arizona Press, 1971

NOBLE, IRIS. *Master Surgeon, John Hunter*. New York: Julian Messner, 1971

NOVOTNY, ANN, and SMITH, CARTER, eds. *Images of Healing: A Portfolio of American Medical and Pharmaceutical Practice in the Eighteenth, Nineteenth and Early Twentieth Centuries*. New York: Macmillan, 1980

ORLAND, FRANK J., ed. *The First Fifty-Year History of the International Association for Dental Research*. Chicago: University of Chicago Press, 1973

PAOLI, UGO E. *Rome: Its People, Life and Customs.* New York: David McKay, 1963

PARÉ, AMBROISE. *The Collected Works of Ambroise Paré.* Trans. T. Johnson. Pound Ridge, N.Y.: Milford House, 1948

————. *Ten Books of Surgery with the Magazine of the Instruments Necessary for It.* Athens: University of Georgia Press, 1969

PARROT, ANDRÉ. *Nineveh and Babylon.* London: Thames and Hudson, 1961

PEACHY, GEORGE C. *A Memoir of William and John Hunter.* Plymouth: William Brendon & Son, 1924

PINDBORG, JENS J., and MARVITZ, LEIF. *The Dentist in Art.* London: George Proffer, 1961

PITRE, GIUSEPPE. *Sicilian Folk Medicine.* Lawrence, Kan.: Coronado, 1971

POLO, MARCO. *Travels.* New York: Orion, 1958

PRINZ, HERMANN. *Dental Chronology: A Record of the More Important Historic Events in the Evolution of Dentistry.* Philadelphia: Lea and Febiger, 1945

PROSKAUER, CURT. *Iconographia odontologica.* Berlin: Hermann Meusser, 1915

————. *Kulturgeschichte der Zahnheilkunde,* 4 vols. Berlin: Hermann Meusser, 1913–26

————, and WITT, FRITZ H. *Pictorial History of Dentistry.* Cologne: Du-Mont Schauberg, 1962

PUTSCHER, MARIELENE. *Geschichte der medizinischen Abbildung.* Munich: Heinz Moos, 1972

QVIST, GEORGE. *John Hunter.* London: William Heinemann Medical Books, 1981

RANKE, HERMANN. *Medicine and Surgery in Ancient Egypt.* Philadelphia: University of Pennsylvania Press, 1941

RAPER, HOWARD. R. *Man against Pain: The Epic of Anesthesia.* New York: Prentice-Hall, 1945

RICHARDS, N. DAVID. "The Dental Profession in the 1860's." In *Medicine and Science in the 1860's.* Edited by F.N.L. Poynter. London: Wellcome Institute of the History of Medicine, 1968

RICHER, PAUL. *L'art et la médecine.* Paris: Gaultier, Magnier, 1902

ROBINSON, J. BEN. *The Foundations of Professional Dentistry.* Baltimore: Waverly, 1940

ROGERS, FRED B., and SAYRE, A. REASONER. *The Healing Art: A History of the Medical Society of New Jersey.* Trenton: Medical Society of New Jersey, 1966

ROSNER, FRED. *Julius Preuss' Biblical and Talmudic Medicine.* New York: Sanhedrin, 1978

ROTH, CECIL. *The Jews in the Renaissance.* New York: Harper and Row, 1965

ROTHSTEIN, ROBERT J. *History of Dental Laboratories and Their Contributions to Dentistry.* Philadelphia: J. B. Lippincott, 1958

ROUSSELOT, JEAN, ed. *Medicine in Art: A Cultural History.* New York: McGraw-Hill, 1967

RUBIN, STANLEY. *Medieval English Medicine.* London and Vancouver: David & Charles, 1974

SACHS, HANS. *Der Zahnstocher und seine Geschichte.* Berlin: Hermann Meusser, 1913

SAID, HAKIM M. *Medicine in China.* Karachi: Hamdard Academy, 1965

SCARBOROUGH, JOHN. *Roman Medicine.* Ithaca, N.Y.: Cornell University Press, 1969

SIEGEL, RUDOLF E. *Galen's System of Physiology and Medicine.* Basel and New York: S. Karger, 1968

SINGER, CHARLES, and UNDERWOOD, E. ASHWORTH. *A Short History of Medicine.* Oxford: Oxford University Press, 1962

SISSMAN, ISAAC. *Seventy-Five Years of Dentistry, University of Pittsburgh.* Pittsburgh: University of Pittsburgh, 1970

SKINNER, R. C. *A Treatise on the Human Teeth.* New York: Johnson and Stryker, 1801

SMITH, W. D. A. *Under the Influence: A History of Nitrous Oxide and Oxygen Anesthesia.* Park Ridge, Ill.: Wood Library-Museum of Anesthesiology, 1982

SOULE, ALPHONSE. *Histoire de l'art dentaire dans l'antiquité.* Paris: Jouve, 1913

SPOONER, SHEARJASHUB. *Guide to Sound Teeth.* New York: Wiley & Long, 1836

STODDART, ANNA M. *The Life of Paracelsus, Theophrastus von Hohenheim, 1493–1541.* London: John Murray, 1911

STRÖMGREN, HEDVIG. *Tandläkekonsten hos Romarna.* Copenhagen: H. Koeppel, 1919

————. *Die Zahnheilkunde im achtzehnten Jahrhundert.* Copenhagen: Levin & Munksgaard, 1935

————. *Die Zahnheilkunde im neunzehnten Jahrhundert.* Copenhagen: Levin & Munksgaard, 1945

SUDHOFF, KARL. *Geschichte der Zahnheilkunde.* Leipzig: A. Barth, 1921

TAFT, JONATHAN. *A Practical Treatise on Operative Dentistry.* Philadelphia: Lindsay & Blakiston, 1859

TALBOT, C. H., and HAMMOND, E. A. *The Medical Practitioners in Medieval England.* London: Wellcome Historical Medical Library, 1965

TANTAQUIDGEON, GLADYS. *Folk Medicine of the Delaware and Related Algonkian Indians.* Harrisburg, Pa.: Pennsylvania Historical and Museum Commission, 1972

TAYLOR, JAMES. *History of Dentistry: A Practical Treatise.* London: H. Kimpton, 1922

TERZIOGLU, ARSLAN, and KNEBS, LINDA M. *The History of Old Turkish Dentistry.* Munich: Demeter, 1980

THORNTON, JOHN, and REEVES, CAROL. *Medical Book Illustration.* New York: Oleander, 1983

THORWALD, JÜRGEN. *Histoire de la médecine dans l'antiquité.* Trans. Henri Daussy. Munich: Droemersche Verlageranstalt, 1962

TOMES, JOHN. *A Course of Lectures on Dental Physiology and Surgery.* London: John W. Parker, 1848.

USSERY, HULING E. *Chaucer's Physician: Medicine and Literature in Fourteenth-Century England.* New Orleans: Tulane University Press, 1971

VAKIL, R. J. *Our Glorious Heritage.* Bombay: Times of India, 1966

VENZMER, GERHARD. *Five Thousand Years of Medicine.* New York: Taplinger, 1968

VOGEL, VIRGIL J. *American Indian Medicine.* Norman: University of Oklahoma Press, 1970

VOGT, HELMUT. *Das Bild des Kranken.* Munich: J. F. Lehmann's, 1969

WAIN, HARRY. *A History of Preventive Medicine.* Springfield, Ill.: Charles C. Thomas, 1970

WALLNÖFER, HEINRICH, and ROTTAUSCHER, ANNA VON. *Chinese Folk Medicine.* New York: Crown, 1965

WANGENSTEEN, OWEN, H., and WANGENSTEEN, SARAH D. *The Rise of Surgery from Empiric Craft to Scientific Discipline.* Minneapolis: University of Minnesota Press, 1978.

WATSON, B. *New York—Then and Now.* New York: Dover, 1976

WEBSTER, C. *Health, Medicine and Mortality in the Sixteenth Century, Cambridge, England.* Cambridge: Cambridge University Press, 1979

WEINBERGER, BERNHARD W. *An Introduction to the History of Dentistry.* 2 vols. St. Louis: C. V. Mosby, 1948

————. *Orthodontics: An Historical Review of Its Origins and Evolution.* St. Louis: C. V. Mosby, 1926

WELKER, LOIS E. "A History of Medicine in the Middle Ages." Master's thesis, University of Rochester, 1938

WESLAGER, CLINTON A. *Magic Medicines of the Indians.* Somerset, N.J.: Middle Atlantic, 1973

WILLIAMS, FLOYD E. *A History of Dentistry in New Hampshire.* Milford, N.H.: Cabinet, 1971

WOLF-HEIDEGGER, G., and CETTO, A. M. *Die anatomische Sektion in bildlicher Darstellung.* Basel: S. Karger, 1967

WONG, K. C., and WU, L. T. *History of Chinese Medicine,* 2 vols. New York: Gordon, 1976

WOODFORDE, JOHN. *The Strange Story of False Teeth.* London: Routledge & Kegan Paul, 1983

YOUNG, SIDNEY. *The Annals of the Barber-Surgeons of London.* London: Blades, East & Blades, 1890

ZIGROSSER, CARL. *Medicine and the Artist.* New York: Dover, 1955

Index

Numbers in *italics* refer to pages with illustrations.

Editor: Ellyn Childs Allison

Designer: Carol Robson

Photographic Research: Barbara Lyons

Library of Congress Cataloging-in-Publication Data
Ring, Malvin E.
    Dentistry: an illustrated history / by Malvin E. Ring.
        p.   cm.
    Originally published: New York: Abrams, 1985.
    Includes bibliographical references and index.
    ISBN 0–8109–8116–5
    1. Dentistry—History.   2. Dentistry—History—Pictorial works.
I. Title.
    [DNLM: 1. History of Dentistry.   WU 11.1 R581d 1985a]
RK29.R54   1992
617.6'009—dc20
DNLM/DLC
for Library of Congress   92–10417
                                                                              CIP

Printed and bound in Japan

Photograph Credits

The author and publisher wish to thank the libraries, museums, and private collectors for permitting the reproduction of various objects and works of art in their collections and for supplying the necessary photographs. Photographers and photographs from other sources are gratefully acknowledged below. Unless otherwise indicated, references are to picture numbers.

Aesculape magazine (Paris), 69. Agence C.E.D.R.I., Paris (photo Gerard Sioen), 12. Archiv Funk, Cologne, 194. Dr. Milton Asbell, Cherry Hill, New Jersey, 292. Dr. Zafer Attar, Baghdad, 55. Paul Baker, Northwestern University, 145, 151, 172, 176, 195, 202, 251, 255, 257, 258, 269, 271, 290. A. Tennyson Beals, 264. Bibliothèque Nationale, Paris, 40. Dr. Amadeo Bobbio, São Paulo, Brazil, 53. Steve Borack, 126, 149, 178, 185, 192, 203, 238, 239. Dr. François Brunner, Musée de la Chirurgie Dentaire, Lyons, France, 56, 179, 217, 273, 279 (left). Caisse Nationale, Paris, 15. Joan Lebold Cohen (from Joan Lebold Cohen and Jerome Alan Cohen, *China Today and Her Ancient Treasures*, New York, 1973), 70. Dr. Gordon Dammann, Lena, Illinois, 212. Haluk Doganbey, Istanbul, 48. Dr. Clifton O. Dummett, School of Dentistry, University of Southern California Los Angeles, 270. Egyptian Exploration Society, 26. Dr. Samuel Fastlich, Mexico City, 1–3. Dr. Focion Febres-Cordero, Caracas, 11. Dr. O. C. Francke, Stockholm, 252. © W. O. Funk, Cologne, 17, 36, 130. Giraudon, Paris, 80. Dr. Richard A. Glenner, Chicago, 228, 295, 296, 302. Tony Grylla, Paris, 19. David Gunnar, Boston, 160, 163, 177, 216, 242–47. Dr. James Harris, University of Michigan, Ann Arbor, 24, 25. Hirmer Verlag, Munich, Germany, 21, 33, 34. Dr. W. Hoffmann-Axthelm, Freiburg, Germany, 6, 187. Bill Holland, 191. Dr. Kuninori Homma, Museum of Nippon Dental University, Niigata, Japan, 74 (photo James Ulrich), 77–79 (from Nakahara, Shindo, and Homma, *Manners and Customs of Dentistry in Ukiyoe*, Tokyo, 1980; photo James Ulrich). Dr. Yasuo Ishii, 76. Dr. Ake B. Löfgren, Göteborg, Sweden, 154. Dr. Louis B. Marry, Villeneuve-lès-Avignon, France, 124, 125. Dr. Leif Marvitz, Copenhagen, 259. C. V. Mosby Company, St. Louis (from Epker-Wolford, *Dentofacial Deformities: Surgical Orthodontic Correction*, St. Louis, 1980), 293. Dr. Sataro Motoyama, 73. Dr. L. L. Mulcahy, Jr., Batavia, New York, 260. Albert Munson, 300. National Library of Medicine, Bethesda, 189. Otto Nelson, New York, 221–23, 226, 227, 233, 234, 282–85, 277, 278, 279 (right). Northwestern University Dental School, Chicago (photo Paul Baker), 142. F. P. Orchard, 5. Dr. Frank J. Orland, Chicago, 241. Preussischer Kulturbesitz, Berlin, 66. Dr. Jean-Jacques Quenouille, Orchamps, France, 13, 22, 23, 29, 57. Dr. Malvin Ring, Batavia, New York, 38, 54, 64, 120, 159, 213, 215, 304. Ritter Dental Manufacturing Company, Rochester, 298. Guido Sansoni, 42. George Shelton, Biomedical Communications Department, University of Miami (from Girindranath Mukhopadhyaya, *The Surgical Instruments of the Hindus*, vol. 2, Calcutta, 1914), 58, 59, 61. Siemans Medical of America, 301. Snow, 9. Philip Szczepanski, 150, 186, 193, 241, 266. Dr. Ben Z. Swanson, Jr., London, 49. James Ulrich, State University of New York, Buffalo, 10, 47, 95, 98, 101, 104, 108–12, 122, 132–39, 144, 147, 148, 165, 166, 171, 190, 198, 205, 207, 228, 232, 240, 249, 274, and page 7. Dr. Ralph Voorhees, Montgomery, Texas, 262, 265, 276. World Health Organization, 99. Dr. Mitsuo Yatsu, Matsudo, Japan, 71, 72.